Hidden Hunger

World Review of Nutrition and Dietetics

Vol. 115

Series Editor

Berthold Koletzko Munich

Hidden Hunger

Malnutrition and the First 1,000 Days of Life: Causes, Consequences and Solutions

Volume Editors

Hans K. Biesalski Stuttgart

Robert E. Black Baltimore, MD

24 figures, and 25 tables, 2016

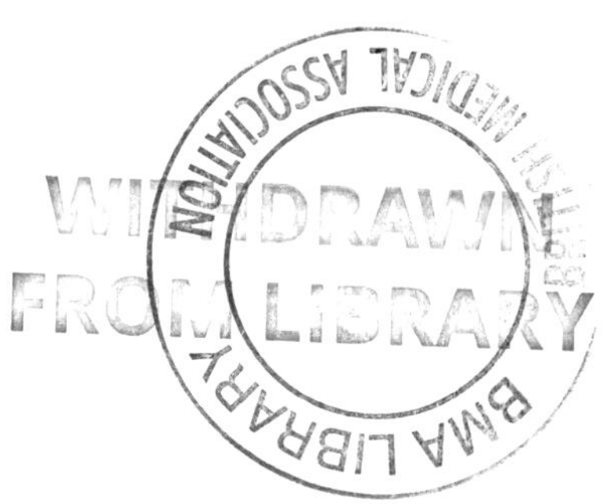

KARGER Basel · Freiburg · Paris · London · New York · Chennai · New Delhi · Bangkok · Beijing · Shanghai · Tokyo · Kuala Lumpur · Singapore · Sydney

Hans K. Biesalski
Institute of Biological Chemistry and
Nutritional Science
University of Hohenheim
Stuttgart
Germany

Robert E. Black
Johns Hopkins Bloomberg
School of Public Health
Baltimore, MD
USA

Library of Congress Cataloging-in-Publication Data

Names: Biesalski, Hans Konrad, editor. | Black, Robert E., editor.
Title: Hidden hunger : malnutrition and the first 1,000 days of life : causes, consequences, and solutions / volume editors, Hans K. Biesalski, Robert E. Black.
Other titles: Hidden hunger (Biesalski) | World review of nutrition and dietetics ; v. 115. 0084-2230
Description: Basel ; New York : Karger, 2016. | Series: World review of nutrition and dietetics, ISSN 0084-2230 ; vol. 115 | Includes bibliographical references and indexes.
Identifiers: LCCN 2016012044| ISBN 9783318056846 (hard cover : alk. paper) | ISBN 9783318056853 (electronic version)
Subjects: | MESH: Fetal Nutrition Disorders | Infant Nutrition Disorders | Developed Countries | Developing Countries | Socioeconomic Factors
Classification: LCC RJ216 | NLM WQ 211 | DDC 362.1963/9--dc23 LC record available at http://lccn.loc.gov/2016012044

Bibliographic Indices. This publication is listed in bibliographic services, including Current Contents® and Index Medicus.

www.karger.com
Printed in Germany on acid-free and non-aging paper (ISO 9706) by Kraft Druck GmbH, Ettlingen
ISSN 0084–2230
eISSN 1662–3975
ISBN 978–3–318–05684–6
e-ISBN 978–3–318–05685–3

Contents

Preface

Hidden Hunger describes a state of deficiency in humans of essential vitamins and minerals (referred to collectively as micronutrients) that occurs largely without signs and symptoms of micronutrient deficiency diseases. There is a long history of discovery of essential vitamins and minerals, and considerable success has been made in the prevention and treatment of related classic deficiency disorders (e.g. rickets, scurvy, and anemia). Only more recently has it been appreciated that an inadequate intake of micronutrients may have health consequences even without overt signs of disease. The 1,000-day window, from conception till the end of the second year of life, is a very critical period for growth and development requiring an adequate supply of micronutrients. Hidden hunger during this period is a problem not only in low-income countries but also in middle- and high-income countries. Poverty and poor knowledge of the importance of dietary diversity are the basic conditions leading to food insecurity and a poor-quality diet. Hidden hunger during pregnancy results in intrauterine growth restriction with consequences for the development of the child. Babies who are too small for their gestational age, as well as premature births, are the visible consequences of maternal malnutrition. Growth restriction of several organs may have an impact on the development of diseases in a child's later life. Poor-quality complementary feeding limited in calories and micronutrients, suboptimal breastfeeding, and an inadequate diet of the preschool child will adversely impact physical and cognitive development with consequences for adult health and productivity. The articles in the book describe the causes and consequences of hidden hunger during the 1,000-day window, as well as possible interventions and program-based responses. Knowledge about hidden hunger may help to detect, prevent, and treat these avoidable conditions and improve the health and prosperity of the next generation.

Hans K. Biesalski, Stuttgart
Robert E. Black, Baltimore, MD

We thank the Food Security Center, University Hohenheim, the German Academic Exchange Service (DAAD) and the German Ministry of Cooperation and Development for their generous support for the 2nd International Congress Hidden Hunger.

Biesalski HK, Black RE (eds): Hidden Hunger. Malnutrition and the First 1,000 Days of Life: Causes, Consequences and Solutions. World Rev Nutr Diet. Basel, Karger, 2016, vol 115, pp 1–15
DOI: 10.1159/000442377

The 1,000-Day Window and Cognitive Development

Hans Konrad Biesalski

Institut für Biologische Chemie und Ernährungswissenschaft, Institut Hohenheim, BIO I, Stuttgart, Germany

During the first 1,000 days of a human life, lasting from conception until the second year of life, the most important developmental steps occur. The nutritional status of a mother at the time of conception is a critical condition with respect to embryonic development.

Intrauterine growth retardation results in low birth weight of the newborn. Major determinants of low birth weight, particularly in developing countries, are poor nutritional status of the mother and subsequent low nutrient flow to the developing child. Newborns with low birth weights (<2,500 g) are four times more likely to die during their first 28 days of life than those weighing between 2,500 and 2,999 g and 10 times more likely to die than those weighing between 3,000 and 3,499 g [1]. Low birth weight is often a phenotype resulting from intrauterine stunting and consequently also a visible marker of potentially impaired brain development. Indeed, it has been documented that the effect of stunting on short-term memory is equivalent to the differences in short-term memory observed between children in US families that had experienced poverty for 13 years and children in families with incomes of at least three times the poverty level [2]. Malnutrition is a frequent companion of poverty in both developing and developed countries, and it has a strong impact on brain development.

Brain Development and Poverty: A Fateful Relationship

The human brain develops in different steps during embryogenesis. Interneuron connections develop within the so-called cortical plate during weeks 8–16 and are replaced by cortical neurons from week 24 until the perinatal period. A brain growth spurt begins in the last trimester of pregnancy and continues through the first 2 years of life. During this time, the majority of dendritic growth, synaptogenesis and glial cell proliferation occurs [3, 4]. During the first 2 years of life (by the age of 2, a child's brain has reached 80–90% of the weight of an adult brain), a child is highly sensitive to deficiencies in micronutrients [5, 6].

The structure of the brain at any given time is a product of interactions between genetic, epigenetic and environmental factors [7]. These environmental factors include both outside events and the internal physiological milieu. Consequently, poor nutrition or stress will have an impact on both brain structure and function. One connection between stress and poor nutrition is poverty. Developmental cognitive neuroscience dealing with poverty and social gradients is a new field of research that has recently emerged. It has recently been shown that being pregnant with and growing up under a low socio-economic status (SES) will have neural and cognitive consequences [8, 9].

Children living in poverty have poorer cognitive outcomes and school performance. Poor SES is related to reductions in attention, literacy and numeracy function, which, in addition to other factors, may explain the poor educational levels of children living in poverty [10]. Language and memory functions are related to brain regions that are sensitive to environmental and nutritional influences. Research in both animals and humans suggests that the experience of stress has important negative effects on the hippocampus and the amygdala, both of which are highly susceptible during the late fetal and early neonatal periods.

The amygdala and the hippocampus subserve emotion, language, and memory, functions that change markedly between the ages of 4 and 18 years [11]. Amygdala and hippocampal volumes increase with age. Both structures are involved in stress regulation and emotion processing, and both are sensitive to environmental stimuli, including nutrition. Different studies have reported lower hippocampal volumes in children and adolescents (aged between 5 and 17 years) from lower income backgrounds compared to those in the same age group but with higher SES [12–14].

Poor nutrition resulting from poor income is not the only reason for developmental changes in the brain. Poverty is strongly associated with other factors that impact brain development; such factors include unsupportive parenting, poor education, lack of caregiver education and high levels of stressful events. In particular, the income-to-need ratio necessary to ensure daily nutrition might become a source of stress that influences brain development [11]. Indeed, income-to-need ratio, but not parental education, has been positively associated with hippocampal size [15, 16]. Stressors more directly related to income, such as limited access to material resources (e.g. a variety of food), may have greater influence on hippocampal size than parental education with respect to cognitive stimulation and parenting style.

A study of healthy children in France showed a positive correlation between SES, reading and verbal abilities, and literacy [17]. The neural correlate was a significant correlation between SES and local gray matter volumes of the bilateral hippocampi.

Similar results were obtained from a study of US households. This study documented a significant positive relationship between income and hippocampal-gray-matter volume. The authors suggested that differences in the hippocampus, perhaps due to the stress associated with growing up in poverty, might partially explain differences in long-term memory, learning, neuroendocrine function control, and emotional behavior modulation. Lower family income may cause limited access to material resources, including food, which may be more important for predicting hippocampal size [18].

Two independent studies that potentially assessed the same group of children in Germany (Brandenburg) documented that SES impacts physical and cognitive outcomes. The first study [19] investigated children at admission into primary school (aged 6 years in the year 2000) and documented impairments in literacy in 18.2% of children of low SES compared to 8.2% of children of average SES and 4.3% of children of high SES, as well as impairments in cognitive development of 13.2 versus 2.8 versus 0.9%, respectively.

In another study, anthropometric data collected from children living in Brandenburg was used to investigate the effect of unemployment on childhood development [20]. Data from 253,050 preschool-aged children collected from 1994 to 2006 were used, and the authors stated:

> After an initial substantial height increase of school starters in the Eastern German Land of Brandenburg between the re-unification of 1990 and 1995, the upward trend stopped suddenly and even developed into a downturn in children's heights between 1997 and 2000. Since 2000, heights have been stagnating at a low level. This is all the more remarkable, as heights have never declined over longer time spans in Eastern German Laender since 1880 – except for the most recent period 1997–2006.

They further concluded:

> The interaction terms of unemployment and additional children are remarkably large. Above, it was already shown that households with four and more children fall behind smaller households with regard to children's height, the former's children being significantly shorter (–1.8 cm). The unemployment variable subtracts another height coefficient of –0.3 cm, in addition to the 'normal' sibling effect! In addition, if the parents are unemployed, the detriment is even larger.

The height difference was around 1 standard deviation from the 95th percentile of the children within that area, so it cannot be defined as stunting, although it must be taken seriously. Together with data from another Brandenburg study showing a massive impact of SES on cognitive development in one of the richest countries in the world, the trends are alarming because they have consequences for the later successes of children in terms of education, income, and escape from poverty. Accordingly, it was very recently reported in an analysis of ten European countries that economic conditions at the time of birth significantly influence cognitive function in later life [15]. The authors argued that children born during a time of recession may experience low quality and/or quantities of food, which impact development during that time and have consequences for later life.

Poor nutrition has been documented not only in low-income countries but also in families living in poverty in high-income countries [16]. Diet quality is not only affected by age, traditions or personal preferences but also by education, living conditions and income, all of which are important indices of SES and social class. If the income-to-need ratio is not sufficient to ensure an adequate food pattern, then other needs (e.g. education and medicine) are reduced or the diet becomes more and more poor with respect to quality. If food costs rise, food selection narrows to those items that provide the most energy at the lowest cost. When these conditions persist, essential nutrients disappear from the diet and malnutrition develops [17, 21]. Indeed, a recent study on the effects of poverty on children's living conditions showed that, in addition to a lack of cognitive stimulation, food insecurity has a strong association with income [22]. There is clear evidence that SES has a strong impact on dietary quality because diet costs are positively related to foods that are of higher quality [23].

The individual driving force for food selection is to reduce hunger with an appropriate quantity of food; food quality is a secondary motivation. Indeed, when indicators of well-being in children living in poverty were compared in the USA [24], the most obvious difference was related to those who had 'experienced hunger (food insecurity) at least once in past year'. Indeed, 15.9% of poor children had experienced hunger in the past year compared to 1.6% of children who were not poor, which is a nearly 10-fold difference. Considering other indicators of well-being, there was a 6.8-fold difference in child abuse and neglect between poor and nonpoor children, a 3.5-fold difference in lead poisoning, and 2-fold differences in victimization via violent crime, length of hospital stay, stunting, grade repetition and high school drop-out frequency.

Poverty and low income are often associated with poor dietary quality and, consequently, malnutrition. Although many other factors (e.g. parental care and education) are involved, the impact of an inadequate supply of essential nutrients on physical and, in particular, brain development should not be underestimated.

Micronutrients and Brain Development

There is scientific evidence that several micronutrients are critically involved in both prenatal and postnatal brain development, particularly, iron, iodine, zinc, folate, vitamin A and vitamin D. Micronutrients, whether alone or in combination, are a major missing source in the diets of one third of the world's population. In addition to micronutrients, protein, energy intake and n-3 fatty acids may also impact brain development.

Table 1 summarizes specific brain-related micronutrients and their impacts on brain development during the late fetal and neonatal periods. The magnitudes of impairments in brain development and brain function depend on the severity of a micronutrient deficiency. In many cases, deficiencies do not exist in an isolated form.

Table 1. Impact of selected nutrients on brain development

Nutrient	Requirement	Brain area
Iron	Myelin formation Monoamine synthesis Neuronal and glial energy metabolism	White matter Striatal frontal Hippocampal-frontal
Iodine	Myelination, neuronal proliferation	Cortex, striatum, hippocampus
Zinc	DNA synthesis Neurotransmitter	Autonomic nervous system Hippocampus, cerebellum
Copper	Neurotransmitter synthesis, energy metabolism	Cerebellum
Vitamin A	Neurogenesis Neurotrophic factors	Hippocampus
Vitamin D	Neurogenesis Neurotrophic factors	Hippocampus White matter
LC-PUFA	Synaptogenesis Myelin	Eye Cortex

LC-PUFA = Long-chain polyunsaturated fatty acids.

Other micronutrients may also be involved, depending on food intake pattern, and malnutrition resulting from protein and energy intake might also be present. The latter also has a negative impact on brain development [25], but this relationship will not be discussed any further in this article.

Furthermore, vitamins are suggested to play a role in brain development, although studies investigating this effect within the first 1,000 days of life are not available. n-3 fatty acids are mainly derived from fatty fish. Studies (n = 6) investigating the effects of fish consumption during pregnancy on cognitive outcome have shown that a higher intake of fish by pregnant women is linked to higher scores on tests of cognitive function in their children between 18 months and 14 years of age [26]. However, n-3 fatty acid consumption is not further discussed in this review because it cannot really be attributed to hidden hunger.

Iron

Anemia due to inadequate iron supply from food is the most common single-nutrient deficiency in the world. Two billion people are affected, including approximately 50% of pregnant women and children. Iron accumulates during the last trimester in a significant quantity, creating approximately 80% of a newborn's iron store. Inadequate supply during this time places the newborn at risk for iron deficiency anemia. In particular, infants born prematurely are at high risk for iron inadequacy due to the shortened period of accumulation. Even mild iron deficiency in the mother reduces the accumulation of iron in the fetus, resulting in neonatal iron deficiency. The majority of iron is used for erythropoiesis (red blood cell production) in the newborn. As a consequence, the developing brain of a newborn is at particular risk under a state of iron deficiency. The most affected part of the brain seems to be the hippocampus. The human hippocampus is highly susceptible to iron deficiency during the late fetal and early neonatal periods. In addition, poorer myelination has been described. Poorer myelination means that the speed of neural transmission is reduced, resulting in decreased responses to stimuli in the auditory and visual brain areas [27]. Children (aged 9–15 months) born to iron-deficient mothers or experiencing iron deficiency during the first years of life show delayed electrophysiological responses to recognition memory stimuli associated with delayed hippocampal function (established as impaired attention and recognition memory) compared to children with sufficient iron supplies [28]. Indeed, it has been shown that iron deficiency results in long-term alterations in the expression of genes that are critical for hippocampal differentiation and plasticity [29]. This might lead one to question whether a complete recovery is possible under iron supplementation.

A review of 14 different studies found associations between iron deficiency anemia, poor cognitive and motor development, and behavioral problems in all 14 studies. Longitudinal studies consistently indicate that children who were anemic in infancy continue to have poorer cognition and school achievement, as well as more behavioral problems, into middle childhood [30]. Despite the relationship between low iron intake and cognition, intervention studies and meta-analyses have not found an improvement in global cognitive scores [31]. What might be the reason for this discrepancy? The reason may be that iron deficiency is usually not isolated to only iron; rather, it is associated with a diet of low diversity and, consequently, with poor sources of easy-to-absorb heme iron (e.g. meat, meat-derived products, and liver). Such sources are also excellent reservoirs of additional important nutrients, such as proteins, minerals, and vitamins.

Zinc

Severe zinc deficiency is rare, but moderate deficiency or inadequate supply affects up to 40% of the world's population [32]. Diets low in animal-derived foods (the best source of zinc) or high in starchy foods (which have low bioavailability of zinc) promote deficiency. Indeed, zinc deficiency during pregnancy as a consequence of a diet high in starchy food with high phytate content (which lowers the bioavailability of zinc and iron) has been reported to be associated with lower scores on the psychomotor index in infants [33]. Diarrhea, which frequently occurs in response to zinc deficiency and is a major disease in children in developing countries, impairs zinc uptake and subsequently accelerates both zinc deficiency and additional micronutrient deficiencies. Children with zinc deficiencies often suffer from uncontrollable diarrhea and pneumonia as well as increased susceptibility to malaria. Even a moderate zinc deficiency is enough to promote infection, especially in the intestines. Diarrhea inhibits the proper absorption of micronutrients, which further exacerbates the situations faced by these children.

Zinc is one of the major micronutrients that are important during rapid growth, which places infants at risk for zinc deficiency during their first years of life. The impact of zinc deficiency on brain structure coincides with the period of rapid brain development that occurs mainly during the first 2 years of life. Zinc is indeed a vital nutrient for the brain, with important functional and structural roles. Indeed, more than 200 enzymes involved in protein, DNA and RNA synthesis need zinc as a cofactor. In synaptic vesicles (important for signal transmission) in hippocampal neurons, zinc is found in high concentrations [34].

Different studies evaluating zinc supplementation during pregnancy have revealed controversial results regarding cognitive development. Zinc supplementation alone may cause imbalances in the availability of other nutrients; thus, zinc deficiency may not occur alone. Indeed, it has been documented that supplementation with a combination of zinc and iron leads to an improvement in cognition [35]. In this double-blind trial, 221 infants were randomly assigned to 1 of 5 treatment conditions, which were administered weekly from 6 to 12 months in age. These conditions included supplementation with iron (20 mg), zinc (20 mg), iron + zinc, a multivitamin/mineral supplement (16 vitamins and minerals, including iron and zinc), or riboflavin. Iron and zinc, whether administered together or with other micronutrients, had a beneficial effect on infant motor development. Iron and zinc, administered individually and in combination, also had a beneficial effect on orientation-engagement. From animal experiments, there is good evidence that zinc deficiency affects cognitive development (via increased emotional reactions and impaired memory and learning capacity). Experiments comparing zinc-deficient rats to zinc-sufficient rats showed changes in hippocampal neuronal morphology and, as a consequence, impairments in memory and learning behavior [36]. Similar observations regarding memory have been made in newborns and infants at 6 months of age born to zinc-deficient mothers [37].

Another important facet of zinc can be noted during early childhood development. Stunting is an early sign of zinc deficiency in a child's first 2 years of life. For this reason, zinc deficiency alone is believed to be a cause for developmental disorders that occur during early childhood [38]. A meta-analysis of 36 studies that examined the effects of zinc supplementation on stunting among children under the age of 5 years showed that zinc did indeed have a positive effect in promoting growth [39].

Iodine

The World Health Organization considers iodine deficiency to be 'the single most important preventable cause of brain damage' worldwide. Approximately one third of the world's population is estimated to have insufficient iodine intake, in particular in Southeast Asia and Europe [40]. Adequate maternal iodine stores within the thyroid are important for normal fetal and infant neurodevelopment. Adequate thyroid iodine stores (in iodine-sufficient regions) fulfill the increased demand for iodine during pregnancy if optimal intake is maintained. In iodine-deficient regions, however, potentially inadequate iodine stores are rapidly depleted during pregnancy, leading the fetus to be at risk for developmental impairment, especially in the brain.

Severe iodine deficiency during pregnancy may cause 'cretinism', which may include mental retardation as well as speech and hearing impairments. In particular, impaired cochlear (inner ear) development results in congenital deafness, which is a severe burden particularly in developing countries, which have inadequate clinical care and special education resources to help a child develop the ability to communicate. Children with both deafness and vitamin A deficiency (VAD), which has resulted in blindness, are the most pitiful results of hidden hunger.

Iodine deficiency causes hypothyroxinemia (low levels of the hormone thyroxin) in the fetal brain. Within the brain, thyroid hormones regulate metabolic rate and myelination, and they play a special role in glucose transport to astrocytes. Astrocytes are important for energy and nutrient supply to neuronal cells. The fetal brain may become irreversibly damaged due to intrauterine iodine deficiency. Very recently, it was documented that mild maternal iodine deficiency in rats causes a delay in the development of hippocampal nerve fibers (i.e. axons) [41].

The effect of mild-to-moderate iodine deficiency on fetal brain development, however, is less clear. Observational studies from different countries in Europe and the USA have documented a significant association between mild maternal iodine deficiency and cognitive impairment in children. The severity and onset of iodine deficiency during pregnancy will affect how the clinical signs are expressed. In particular, the severity of cognitive impairment seems to be associated with the degree of iodine deficiency [42]. In early childhood, iodine deficiency impairs cognition; however, in contrast to fetal iodine deficiency, there is evidence that improvement can be achieved with iodine treatment. Children from iodine-deficient areas have greater cognitive impairment compared with children from areas with sufficient iodine [43]. Several European studies have shown that isolated iodine deficiency during pregnancy is associated with impaired cognitive development in children [reviewed in 44].

In a recent observational trial in the UK, the effect of inadequate iodine status on cognitive outcome was evaluated in 14,551 pregnant women and their children (13,988). The data support the hypothesis that inadequate iodine status during early pregnancy is adversely associated with child cognitive development. Low maternal iodine status was associated with an increased risk of suboptimal scores for verbal IQ at an age of 8 years, as well as suboptimal reading accuracy, comprehension, and reading score at an age of 9 years. The authors showed that the risk of suboptimal cognitive scores in children is not confined to those who were born to mothers with very low iodine status (i.e. <50 μg/g), but rather that iodine-to-creatinine ratios between 50 and 150 μg/g (which would suggest a more mild-to-moderate deficiency) are also associated with heightened risk [45].

Based on different intervention studies on children of different ages, it is argued that the developmental effects of iodine deficiency during early gestation are irreversible with later iodine repletion [39]. Supplementation in pregnant women, however, showed a clear benefit in the cognitive outcomes of their children. In iodine-insufficient areas of Spain, the effect of supplementation during pregnancy on the cognitive development of offspring (aged between 3 months and 3 years) could be clearly documented in three out of four studies [46].

In contrast, supplementation after birth has no clear impact on cognitive development [reviewed in 47]. This underlines the importance of adequate nutrition for females, in particular at the onset of and during pregnancy [48, 49]. In addition, it must be considered that a newborn depends on the iodine found in breast milk. In areas with inadequate iodine supplies, breast-milk iodine concentration is not sufficient to meet the needs of the infant, even when mothers are supplemented with 150 μg daily iodine during the first 6 postpartum months [50].

Vitamin A

Inadequate vitamin A intake increases the risk for infectious diseases, particularly of the respiratory tract. As a consequence, deficiencies in additional micronutrients arise due to higher turnover, disturbances in tissue distribution or impaired absorption. In addition, VAD is often accompanied by anemia. Vitamin A and iron are found in the same sources. Consequently, it is not easy to discriminate between their effects. However, based on recent data, vitamin A seems to have an isolated effect on brain development. In the brain, levels of retinoic acid (RA), the active metabolite of vitamin A, are relatively high, being highest in the hippocampus [51]. RA is critically involved in the induction of neurogenesis (i.e. the formation of neurons) and controls neuronal patterning (i.e. interactions and networking between neurons) in the brain. This effect can be explained by the strict control exerted over the formation of RA concentration gradients. VAD may have a negative impact on the plasticity of the hippocampus. Plasticity is required for neural networks to adapt to changes in the environment. This is important for the learning brain, and in cases of VAD problems in learning and memory may occur [44]. The hippocampus is a region of the brain whose function is critically dependent on plasticity. Reduced hippocampal sizes and reduced learning abilities have been described in rats with VAD [52]. According to Barth and co-workers [45], it might be assumed that VAD seldom occurs in the Western world but recent results have pointed to high levels of RA signaling in hippocampus and it has been shown that human supplementation with RA results in improved learning and memory [53]. This suggests that normal human brain may have suboptimal levels of RA, perhaps of its high demand for the vitamin A.

VAD during pregnancy and early childhood may influence hippocampal plasticity and, consequently, learning and memory. However, supplementation with vitamin A during pregnancy or even later might help improve hippocampal function in case of poor vitamin A status.

Vitamin D

Vitamin D (VDD) deficiency is a worldwide problem with several health consequences in children and adults. VDD is observed in 60% of Caucasian women; in women with dark skin, the rate is estimated to be even higher [54].

It has been frequently described that maternal VDD during pregnancy is associated with adverse health outcomes in offspring, including intrauterine growth restriction and impaired bone mass. VDD is also related to different cognitive and behavioral dysfunctions, such as schizophrenia [55]. VDD is more pronounced during wintertime, especially in northern regions, because sunlight is a major trigger for vitamin D synthesis in the skin. Indeed, schizophrenia is more frequent at high latitudes and in children who were born during the winter [56].

The fetus depends on the plasma vitamin D levels [i.e. $25(OH)D_3$] of the mother because vitamin D passes through the placenta and is metabolized to form the active metabolite $1,25(OH)_2D_3$ in the fetal kidney. If plasma levels of vitamin D are low in the mother, the fetus develops in a state of hypovitaminosis D, which may have consequences such as low bone mineral density and increased risk for osteoporosis in later life [57]. Infants born to mothers with VDD have significantly lower birth weights and an increased risk of being small for their gestational age compared with infants born to mothers with adequate plasma levels of vitamin D [58]. In cases with sufficient medical care, this may not lead to notable consequences, but in developing countries with missing or poor medical care the lives of these children are in great danger.

In a study of 743 Caucasian women in Australia, low maternal serum vitamin D levels during pregnancy were significantly associated with language impairments in their offspring at 5 and 10 years of age [59]. In addition to its well-known effects on bone development and immune system functioning, vitamin D seems to have an important role in the developing brain by controlling the expression of genes encoding so-called neurotrophins, which are important for neurogenesis [60].

The developing fetus depends on the vitamin D status of the mother. If the mother's status is not sufficient, the supply to the fetus might be inadequate. Because the only natural sources of vitamin D are fatty ocean fish and sun-dried mushrooms (which are present in some traditional diets), the dietary supply of vitamin D for women living in poverty is rather poor. The most important source for vitamin D is solar irradiation, which allows the skin to synthesize the vitamin. In cases of high pigmentation and poor sun exposure, for either seasonal reasons or because of clothing traditions, the formation of vitamin D becomes critical. The high prevalence of VDD in northern Europe [61], particularly in migrants from the south (up to 70%), should be further investigated with respect to its impact on pregnancy and fetal development.

Conclusion

Nutrition plays an important role in fetal and newborn brain development. If malnutrition reduces optimal metabolic functioning during sensitive periods of cognitive development, it may have lasting negative consequences by affecting a child's development and reducing the chances that a child will escape from poverty. Reduced physical strength and poor brain development are a fateful combination that leaves a child in a hopeless situation with no chance of escape. Malnutrition during the first 1,000 days of life is a basically irreversible, yet preventable, burden for a child. Nearly 170 million children are stunted, and it can be suggested that stunting is accompanied by impaired brain development.

In developed countries, hidden hunger may appear as a single event related to either iron or iodine. Supplementation or the provision of advice on how to compose an adequate diet might be helpful. However, in less developed countries or for people living in poverty and with food insecurity, deficiency of a single micronutrient is a rare case, as overall diet composition is poor in such cases, resulting in hidden hunger for several micronutrients. With respect to development, missing micronutrients might act synergistically to harm development. Supplementation with one or more micronutrients might serve as an emergency intervention, but it is not a sustainable approach.

It should not be overlooked that a selective deficiency in one micronutrient is a rare case, especially in developing countries. If the supply of a single micronutrient is inadequate and creates clinical symptoms, it might not be sufficient to offer only a single supplement, as the deficiency is usually a consequence of overall inadequate dietary intake of micronutrients. For example, the most important sources of vitamin A are liver products followed by egg yolk. Liver is also an excellent source of iron in bioavailable form and of zinc. Other foods, such as meat and milk, are rather poor sources of vitamin A. Vitamin A also exists as provitamin A in yellow fruits and vegetables. However, the conversion of the provitamin into the vitamin is not very efficient, and iron and zinc are only present in small amounts in fruits and vegetables. Therefore, dietary patterns determine whether symptoms of VAD or zinc and iron deficiency develop. The clinical signs of VAD or iron deficiency can reflect poor supplies of either one or both of these nutrients. Depending on dietary intake, the signs of VAD or of iron deficiency might alternate in prominence. Thus, supplementing only one of these nutrients may overlook the importance of the other.

The tragedy of such hidden malnutrition is the fact that missing assessments and clinical symptoms result in a lack of intervention implementation. In particular, in developed countries, it seems hard to believe that there might be a problem. However, different studies have shown that food insecurity is related to both poverty and a risk of malnutrition. A recent study assessed the relationship between growth failure at 24 months and adult outcomes [60] using data from 1,338 Guatemalan adults (25–42 years of age) who were studied as children (1969–1977). Individuals who were stunted scored worse on tests of reading and intelligence. Stunted individuals were also more likely to have lower wages (men) and to live in poor households as adults.

The magnitude of the impact of malnutrition on developmental impairment in children from poor settings is not known and difficult to estimate. However, in contrast to problems arising from missing parental care and environmental factors, adequate nutrition for pregnant women and children might be easier to achieve. However, this requires political will and public awareness. The basic approach is to ensure adequate nutrition for females of childbearing age to avoid deficiencies during the early phases of pregnancy. This approach involves providing education and knowledge about the importance of food quality. In cases of selected deficiencies, supplementation might be an alternative. However, several studies that have investigated the effect of supplementation with iron during the first 1,000 days of life have failed to show a real benefit in cognitive function [62].

Improving nutrition during the first 2 years of life by using a micronutrient-enriched protein supplement showed a positive impact on cognition (i.e. reading comprehension and schooling) in adulthood, even after accounting for the effect of education [63]. Intake of the supplement improved growth rates and reduced the prevalence of stunting at 3 years of age compared to nonsupplemented children, documenting the impact of adequate food quality on development.

Maturation of the brain regions responsible for higher cognitive functioning continues throughout childhood and adolescence [64]. Neuroimaging research suggests that even relatively brief interventions can lead to measurable differences in brain structure in children and that this change is directly related to improvement in cognitive skill [65]. Nevertheless, the earlier adequate nutrition can be ensured, the better the supply to the brain and the better the development.

Malnutrition must be a top priority for national governments and international organizations. It is not acceptable that in a globalized world with rapidly growing markets and per capita incomes millions of children are born into poverty and will remain there. These children are the human capital of the countries in which they are born and will contribute to the economic and intellectual development of these countries. However, if these children remain glued to the hunger carousel they will be a starting point for the next generation, leading them to suffer the same fate. To stop this carousel, we need to address the problem of hidden hunger and intervene as early as possible at the levels of the governments, civil and private sectors, and religious communities of the affected countries, with all of their available power. The costs of applying interventions to protect children from malnutrition are far below those of other life-saving health interventions for children. We must not only feed the world but also nourish the world.

References

1 Podja J, Kelley L: Nutrition Policy Paper 18. Geneva, United Nations Subcommittee on Nutrition, 2000.
2 Korenman S, Miller JE, Sjaastad JE: Long-term poverty and child development in the United States: results from the National Longitudinal Survey of Youth. Child Youth Serv Rev 1995;17:127–151.
3 Gogtay N, Nugent TF, Herman DH, et al: Dynamic mapping of normal human hippocampal development. Hippocampus 2006;16:664–672.
4 Levitt P: Structural and functional maturation of the developing primate brain. J Pediatr 2003;143:35–45.
5 Lenroot RK, Giedd JN: Brain development in children and adolescents: insight from anatomical magnetic resonance imaging. Neurosci Behav Rev 2006; 30:718–729.
6 Georgieff MK: Nutrition and the developing brain: nutrient priorities and measurement. Am J Clin Nutr 2007;85:614–620.
7 Lenroot R, Giedd JN: Brain development in children and adolescents: insights from anatomical magnetic resonance imaging. Neurosci Behav Sci 2006;30: 718–729.
8 Raizada R, Kishiyama M: Effects of socioeconomic status on brain development, and how cognitive neuroscience may contribute to levelling the playing field. Front Hum Neurosci 2010;4:1–11.
9 D'Angiulli A, Lipina JS, Olesinska A: Explicit and implicit issues in the developmental cognitive neuroscience of social inequality. Front Hum Neurosci 2012;6:1–17.
10 Lipina SJ, Posner MI: The impact of poverty on the development of brain networks. Front Hum Neurosci 2012;6:1–12.
11 Luby J, Belden A, Botteron K, et al: The effects of poverty on childhood brain development: the mediating effects of caregiving and stressful life events. JAMA Pediatr 2013;167:1135–1142.
12 Noble KG, Houston SM, Kan E, et al: Neural correlates of socio-economic status in the developing human brain. Dev Sci 2012;15:516–527.
13 Houston JL, Chandra A, Wolfe B, et al: Association between income and the hippocampus. PLoS One 2011;6:19712.
14 Jednorog K, Altarelli I, Monzalvo K, et al: The influence of socio-economic status on childrens brain structure. PLoS One 2012;7:42486.
15 Doblhammer G, van den Berg GJ, Fritze T: Economic conditions at the time of birth and cognitive abilities in late life: evidence from ten European countries. PLoS One 2013;8:e74915.
16 Mabli J, Castner L, Ohls J: Food expenditure and diet quality among low income-households and individuals. Mathematica Policy Research, 2010, ref. No. 06408.600.
17 Karp RJ: Malnutrition among children in the United States. The impact of poverty; in Shils ME, Shike M, Ross AC, et al (eds): Modern Nutrition in Health and Disease, ed 10. Baltimore, Williams Willkins Lippincott, 2005, pp 860–874.
18 Hanson JL, Chandra A, Wolfe BL, et al: Association between income and the hippocampus. PLoS One 2011;6:e18712.
19 Böhm A, Ellsäßer G, Kuhn J, et al: Soziale Lage und Gesundheit von jungen Menschen im Land Brandenburg. Das Gesundheitswesen 2003;65:219–225.
20 Baten J, Böhm A: Trends of children's height and parental unemployment: a large-scale anthropometric study on Eastern Germany, 1994–2006. German Economic Review 2010;11:1–24.
21 Darmon N, Drewnowski A: Does social class predict diet quality? Am J Clin Nutr 2008;87:1107–1117.
22 Berger LM, Paxson C, Waldfogel J: Income and Child Development. Working Paper No. 05-16-FF. Princeton, Center for Research on Child Wellbeing, 2005.
23 Aggarwal A, Monsivais P, Cook AJ, et al: Does diet cost mediate the relation between socioeconomic position and diet quality? Eur J Clin Nutr 2011;65: 1059–1066.
24 Brooks-Gunn J, Duncan GJ: The effects of poverty on children. Future Child 1997;7:55–71.
25 Laus MF, Vales LD, Costa TM, et al: Early postnatal protein-calorie malnutrition and cognition: a review of human and animal studies. Int J Env Res Pub Health 2011;8:590–612.
26 Ryan AS, Astwood JD, Gautier S, et al: Effects of long chain polyunsaturated fatty acids supplementation on neurodevelopment in childhood: a review of human studies. Prostaglandins Leukot Essent Fatty Acids 2010;82:305–314.
27 Algarin C: Iron deficiency anemia in infancy: long lasting effects on auditory- and visual system functioning. Pediatr Res 2003;53:217–221.

28 Burden MJ, Westerlund BA, Armony-Sivan R, et al: An event related potential study of attention and recognition memory in infants with iron-deficient anemia. Pediatrics 2007;120:336–342.
29 Carlson ES, Stead JD, Neal CR, et al: Perinatal iron deficiency results in altered developmental expression of genes mediating energy metabolism and neuronal morphogenesis in hippocampus. Hippocampus 2007;17:679–691.
30 Grantham-McGregor S, Ani C: A review of studies on the effect of iron deficiency on cognitive development in children. J Nutr 2001;131:649–668.
31 Guo X, Liu H, Qian J: Daily iron supplementation on cognitive performance in primary-school-aged children with and without anemia: a meta-analysis. Int J Clin Exp Med 2015;8:16107–16111.
32 Ahmed T, Hossain M, Sanin K: Global burden of maternal and child undernutrition and micronutrient deficiencies. Ann Nutr Metab 2012;61:8–17.
33 Fuglestad A, Ramel SE, Georgieff MK: Micronutrient needs of the developing brain: priorities and assessment; in Packer L (ed): Micronutrients and Brain Health. Abingdon Oxford, Taylor and Francis, 2010.
34 Bathnagar S, Tanejy S: Zinc and cognitive development. Br J Nutr 2001;85:139–145.
35 Black MM, Baqui AH, Zaman K, et al: Iron and zinc supplementation promote motor development and exploratory behavior among Bangladeshi infants. Am J Clin Nutr 2004;80:903–910.
36 Yu X, Jin L, Zhang X, et al: Effects of maternal mild zinc deficiency and zinc supplementation in offspring on spatial memory and hippocampal neuronal ultrastructural changes. Nutrition 2013;29:457–461.
37 Kirksey A, Rahmanifar A, Wachs TD, et al: Relation of maternal zinc nutriture to pregnancy outcome and infant development in an Egyptian village. Am J Clin Nutr 1991;60:782–792.
38 Cole CR, Lifshitz F: Zinc nutrition and growth retardation. Ped Endocrinol 2008;5:88–96.
39 Imdad A, Bhutta Z: Effect of preventive zinc supplementation on linear growth in children under 5 years of age in developing countries: a meta-analysis of studies for input to the lives saved tool. BMC Public Health 2011;11(suppl 3):S22.
40 WHO, UNICEF, ICCIDD: Assessment of iodine deficiency disorders and monitoring their elimination, ed 3. Geneva, World Health Organization, 2007.
41 Wi W, Wang Y, Dong J, et al: Developmental hypothyroxinemia induced by maternal mild iodine deficiency delays hippocampal axonal growth in the rat offspring. J Neuroendocrinol 2013;25:852–862.
42 Azizi F, Sarshar A, Nafarabadi M, et al: Impairment of neuromotor and cognitive development in iodine-deficient schoolchildren with normal physical growth. Acta Endocrinol 1993;129:497.
43 Vermiglio F, Sidoti M, Finocchiaro MD, et al: Defective neuromotor and cognitive ability in iodine-deficient schoolchildren of an endemic goiter region in Sicily. J Clin Endocrinol Metab 1990;70:379.
44 Olson C, Mello CV: Significance of vitamin A to brain function, behavior and learning. Mol Nutr Food Res 2010;54:489–495.
45 Barth S, Steer C, Golding J, et al: Effect of inadequate iodine status in UK pregnant women on cognitive outcomes in their children: results from the Avon Longitudinal Study of Parents and Children (ALSPAC). Lancet 2013;382:331–337.
46 Trumpff C, Schepper JD, Tafforeau J, et al: Mild iodine deficiency in pregnancy in Europe and its consequences for cognitive and psychomotor development of children: a review. J Trace Elem Biol Med 2013;27:174–183.
47 Melse-Boonstra A, Jaiswal N: Iodine deficiency in pregnancy, infancy and childhood and its consequences for brain development. Best Pract and Res Clin Endocrinol Metab 2010;24:29–38.
48 Cao X-Y, Xin-Min J, Zhi-Hong D, et al: Timing of vulnerability of the brain to iodine deficiency in endemic cretinism. N Engl J Med 1994;331:1739–1744.
49 O'Donnell K, Rakeman M, Xue-Yi C, et al: Effects of iodine supplementation during pregnancy on child growth and development at school age. Dev Med Child Neurol 2002;44:76.
50 Mulrine HM, Skeaff SA, Ferguson EL, et al: Breast milk iodine concentration declines over the first 6 mo post-partum in iodine deficient women. Am J Clin Nutr 2010;92:849–856.
51 Werner EA, DeLuca HF: Retinoic acid is detected at relatively high levels in the CNS of adult rats. Am J Physiol Endocrin Metab 2002;282:672–678.
52 Shearer KD, Stoney PM, Morgan P, et al: A vitamin for the brain. Trends Neurosci 2012;35:733–741.
53 Ormerod AD, Thind A, Rice S, et al: Influence of isotretinoin on hippocampal-based learning in human subjects. Psychopharmacology 2011;221:667–674.
54 Bodnar LM, Simhan HN, Powers RW, et al: High prevalence of vitamin D insufficiency in black and white pregnant women residing in the northern United States and their neonates. J Nutr 2007;137:447–452.
55 McCann J, Ames BN: Is there convincing biological and behavioral evidence linking vitamin D to brain function. FASEB J 2008;22:982–1001.
56 McGrath JJ, Burne TH, Féron F: Developmental vitamin D deficiency and risk of schizophrenia: a 10-year update. Schizophr Bull 2010;36:1073–1078.
57 Javaid MK, Crozier SR, Harvey NC, et al: Maternal vitamin D status during pregnancy and childhood bone mass at age 9 years: a longitudinal study. Lancet 2006;367:36–43.

58 Leffelaar ER, Vrijkotte TG, van Eijsden M: Maternal early pregnancy vitamin D status in relation to fetal and neonatal growth: results of the multi-ethnic Amsterdam Born Children and Their Development cohort. Br J Nutr 2010;104:108–117.
59 Whitehouse A, Holt B, Serralha M, et al: Maternal serum vitamin D levels during pregnancy and offspring neurocognitive development. Pediatrics 2012; 129:485–493.
60 Hoddinott J, Behrman J, Maluccio J, et al: Adult consequences of growth failure in early adulthood. Am J Clin Nutr 2013;98:1170–1178.
61 van der Meer I, Karamali N, Boeke A, et al: High prevalence of vitamin D deficiency in pregnant non-Western women in The Hague, Netherlands. Am J Clin Nutr 2006;84:350–353.
62 Grantham-McGregor S, Ani C: A review of studies on the effect of iron deficiency on cognitive development of children. J Nutr 2001;131:649–668.
63 Stein AD, Wang M, DiGirolamo A, et al: Nutritional supplementation in early childhood, schooling, and intellectual functioning in adulthood: a prospective study in Guatemala. Arch Pediatr Adolesc Med 2008; 162:612–618.
64 Toga AW, Thompson PM, Sowell ER: Mapping brain maturation. Trends Neurosci 2006;29:148–159.
65 Keller TA, Just MA: Altering cortical connectivity: remediation-induced changes in the white matter of poor readers. Neuron 2009;64:624–631.

Prof. Dr. Hans Konrad Biesalski
Institut für Biologische Chemie und Ernährungswissenschaft
Institut Hohenheim
Garbenstrasse 30, DE–70599 Stuttgart (Germany)
E-Mail biesal@uni-hohenheim.de

Biesalski HK, Black RE (eds): Hidden Hunger. Malnutrition and the First 1,000 Days of Life: Causes, Consequences and Solutions. World Rev Nutr Diet. Basel, Karger, 2016, vol 115, pp 16–23
DOI: 10.1159/000441882

Hidden and Neglected: Food Poverty in the Global North – The Case of Germany

Sabine Pfeiffer[a] · Elke Oestreicher[a] · Tobias Ritter[b]

[a]Chair of Sociology (550D), University of Hohenheim, Stuttgart, and [b]Institute for Social Science Research (ISF Munich), Munich, Germany

Abstract

Although still a powerful economy, Germany faces rising income inequality and food insecurity. Quantitative data show that nutritional poverty in Germany has become a fact, especially for social welfare recipients. This contribution gives an overview and discusses the limits of results from different data sources, such as German food surveys, and addresses how affected population groups are systematically underrepresented. To give a more thorough impression of food insecurity in Germany, the article compares nutritional consumption data from the Statistics on Income and Living Conditions/Eurostat survey for Germany, the members of the European Union 27 (EU27), and Greece. The figures for Germans with incomes below 60% of the median equivalised income who cannot afford one proper meal every second day are worse than those in the remaining EU27 member nations, and the figures for their children are not so far from the figures for crisis-stricken Greece. As eating is not only about nutrition but also a means of social activity, we consider the ability to eat and drink with friends an issue of alimentary participation. The percentages of Germans who cannot afford a drink or meal with others at least once a month is very high compared to the rates of the remaining EU27 member nations and Greece. The provided quantitative figures prove that we see serious signs of food poverty in portions of Germany, despite its comparatively strong economy. Data from hundreds of qualitative interviews describing how people stricken by food insecurity try to cope with the situation complement these results. Such data are very important, as governments widely underestimate the problem and leave it to be dealt with by food banks as the only institutional solution.

Food Insecurity in Germany

Although Germany is considered the most powerful economy in the European Union, income inequality has risen sharply since 2000 [1]. With rising inequality, food insecurity, meaning the 'inability to acquire or eat an adequate quality or sufficient quantity of food in socially acceptable ways (or the uncertainty of being able to do so)' [2], has become an increasingly serious problem in the Global North and is also becoming a problem in Germany. As the German government widely ignores this issue, leaving it to be dealt with by charities [3], individual coping strategies at the household level are key to understanding the problem.

Based on a variety of evidence drawn from different sources of quantitative data, in 2011, we tried to prove that there is nutritional poverty in Germany and in particular that social welfare recipients are widely excluded from eating out [4]. Since then, the situation has intensified. Physiological hunger and hunger for social inclusion by eating out are realities in contemporary German society. Even so, the predominant responses of the German political and social welfare systems can be characterised by delegation and denial of the problem and by a tendency to stigmatise the poor. We now provide some basic information on the state of food-related research in Germany.

The scientific and public debate on eating patterns in Germany is dominated by the topic of obesity instead of food poverty. According to the German food survey Nationale Verzehrstudie (NVS), one in five people are classified as obese, and excess weight is unequally distributed along the social scale [5]. However, this study was only carried out twice, first in the 1980s (NVS I) and second between 2005 and 2007 (NVS II), and population groups at a higher risk of nutritional poverty (e.g., migrants and homeless or elderly people) are underrepresented. The referenced German food surveys distort food insecurity because of these missing but particularly affected population groups and therefore implicitly indicate that unsatisfactory nutrition in Germany is merely a self-inflicted problem caused by unhealthy eating patterns, such as the consumption of too much alcohol, fat, sugar and nicotine. German food surveys are as lacking in nutritional details as they are biased according to social stratification effects.

Despite the lack of thorough food-related research in Germany, there are some indicators that point to the rising problem of food insecurity in Germany. One indicator to decide whether we face food insecurity in Germany is the lack of items related to nutrition included in the surveys regularly conducted by the Federal Statistical Office. Based on the German Socio-Economic Panel (www.diw.de/soep), we estimated that 1% of the population, or 800,000 people, in Germany spend less than EUR 99 per month of their household expenditures on food and are likely to live in nutritional poverty and experience hunger at least from time to time. This may also hold true for an estimated 300,000 homeless people. As we also noted, food insecurity could be an intermittent reality for some of the 7% of the population – more than 5 million

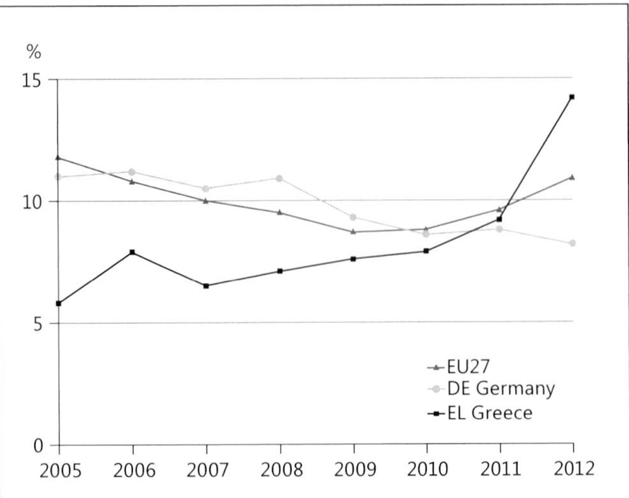

Fig. 1. Data from the Statistics on Income and Living Conditions/Eurostat survey conducted in 2013. Percentage of the total population who cannot afford one meal with meat, chicken or fish (or a vegetarian equivalent) every second day.

people – who have a monthly grocery budget of between EUR 100 and 199. Again, based on the German Socio-Economic Panel dataset, spending on food clearly differs according to employment status: in 2011, employed households in Germany spent EUR 362 a month on food, beverages and tobacco (13.7% of monthly private consumption expenditures), while unemployed households were only able to spend EUR 205, or 19.2% of their consumption expenses. The differences are much more evident if one compares expenditures for hotels and restaurants: employed households in Germany spent EUR 147 per month (5.6% of consumption spending), while unemployed households' equivalent expenses total EUR 21 a month, or 2% of their overall expenditure [6].

As nutrition and food security are considered essentials of life, we will now look into some data related to both nutritional and social aspects by comparing consumption data from the Statistics on Income and Living Conditions/Eurostat survey for Germany, the European Union 27 (EU27), and Greece. We choose to compare Germany and Greece because they are at opposite ends of the European scale for almost all social and economic indicators. For example, the 2012 unemployment rate in Greece was the worst in Europe at 24.5%, while Germany's was the best at 5.5% [7]. This is also true for the number of 'yes' responses to the question 'Have there been times in the past 12 months when you did not have enough money to buy food that you or your family needed?' For Greece, the number jumped from under 10% in 2006/2007 to approximately 18% in 2012, while there was a considerable decline in Germany from approximately 7 to under 5%.

The data only shed light on nutritional behaviour in terms of the ability to afford one meal with meat, chicken or fish (or the vegetarian equivalent) every second day (or at least once a day for children). Comparing the data (fig. 1) for the EU27, Ger-

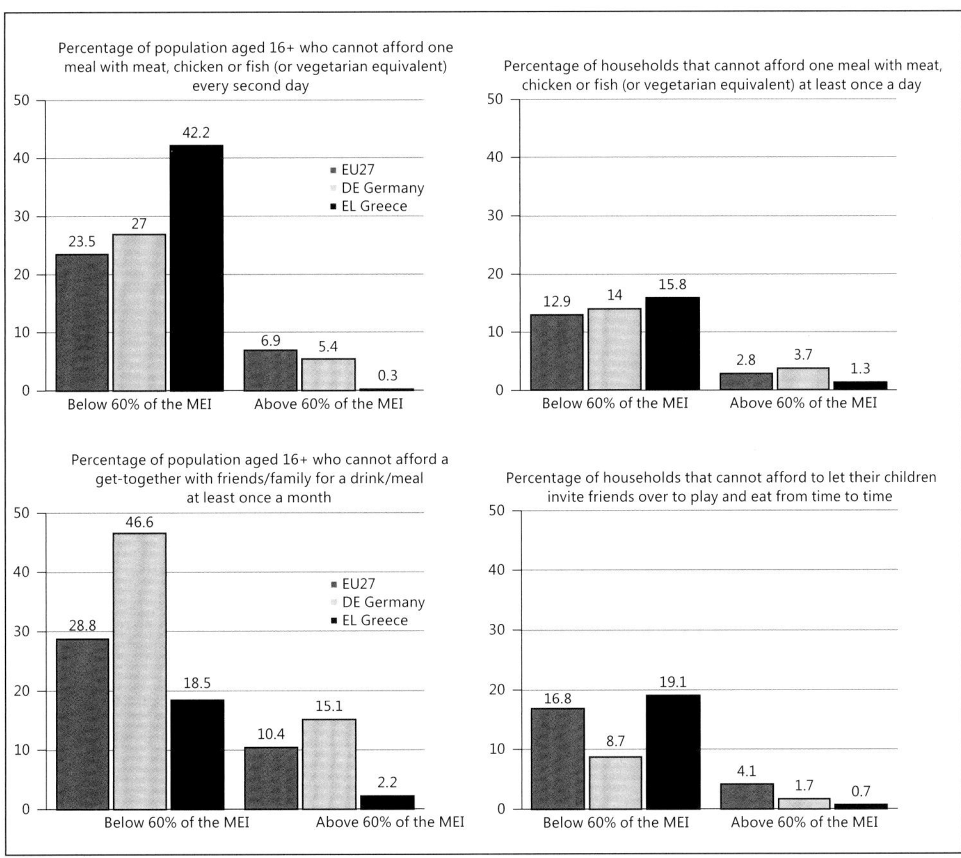

Fig. 2. Data from the Statistics on Income and Living Conditions/Eurostat survey conducted in 2011. The percentage below/above the MEI graphics were created by the authors.

many and Greece shows a moderate decline in the percentage of the total population for Germany: the amount who could not afford the stated meal every second day sank from 11% in 2005 down to 8.2% in 2012. At first sight, nutritional poverty does not seem to be an increasing problem – that is, if German public and political opinion take 8.2% as an acceptable figure – especially as the EU27 shows far higher percentages, and Greece faced a skyrocketing increase from 2011 to 2012 alone.

However, an in-depth look at the data points to a more problematic pattern for Germany. The upper charts in figure 2 show that 27% of Germans with an income below 60% of the median equivalised income (MEI) cannot afford one proper meal every second day, a figure that is without question considerably better than Greece's 42.2%, but higher than the European average of 23.5%. For individuals with incomes above 60% of the MEI in Germany, 5.4% cannot afford a proper meal – this value is not as high as in the EU27, but it is way higher than one would expect from the leading economy in Europe. It is also higher than in other better-performing economies, such as the UK, where 3.6% of non-poor individuals cannot afford a square meal every second day. Even if they cannot afford square meals for the adults every now and then, poor households clearly try hard to provide a substantial meal at least once a day for their children, as indicated by the overall lower percentages on the upper right side of figure 2 for the answer 'cannot afford'. Although Germany, with rates of 14% below 60% of the MEI and 3.7% above 60% of the MEI, shows higher rates than those in the EU27 (12.9%), it almost catches up with the rate (15.8%) of crisis-stricken Greece.

As we previously highlighted, being able to afford meals at home is just one side of nutritional poverty. What we have coined as 'alimentary participation' [8], defined as experiencing the social function of food in public and together with others, has become crucial in a modern and individualised consumer society. We do not learn anything about occasions of eating out in the Statistics on Income and Living Conditions/Eurostat dataset. However, there are some hints, as there is one question aimed at determining how many individuals can afford a get-together with friends or family for a drink/meal at least once a month (for children, this is measured as invitations to play and eat with friends from time to time).

The lower charts in figure 2 show alarmingly high percentages for Germany, especially for those with an income that falls below 60% of the MEI: 46.6% of these individuals cannot afford a drink or meal with others at least once a month, which is a very high percentage compared to the rates for the EU27 (28.8%) and even Greece (18.5%). Even for the population with an income above 60% of the MEI, Germany shows higher percentages of people who cannot afford drinking and/or eating in company. Despite the cultural differences surrounding the social importance of shared meals or drinking with company all over Europe, and despite the fact that Germany might be less social in this respect, the explicit distance between the German and the EU27 averages within the portion of the population earning below 60% of the MEI hints at substantial inequality problems in Germany and not mere cultural distinctions. Again, the figures indicate that parents try hard to avoid letting their children feel the economic squeeze. The percentage of individuals who cannot afford to accept their children's social invitations is considerably lower than that for adult social invitations, and in Germany it is lower than both the EU27 average (16.8%) and the average in Greece (19.1%). For comparison, 8.7% of individuals earning below 60% of the MEI and 1.7% of individuals earning above 60% of the MEI in Germany are affected, which are higher percentages than those found in the UK (5.8 and 0.7%, respectively).

These actual figures, superficial as they are compared to the social complexities of nutritional patterns, poverty consumption and alimentary participation, and despite the relative success of Germany's economy in coping with the crisis, indicate that there are people in the midst of Germany's thriving economy who are experiencing occasional hunger and who are stricken by food insecurity. Denial and stigmatisation of hunger and nutritional poverty in Germany are predominant ways of dealing with food poverty and poverty in general in German society and government. The third and quite unique concept in the domain of social policy is delegating the problem to food banks. These food banks are mostly organised by the German federal association of food banks known as Bundesverband Deutsche Tafeln (www.tafel.de), which was founded 1993 and has since exploded throughout Germany. The rise in food bank consumption has accelerated from 480 food banks in 2005 to 916 food banks in 2013. Currently, 60,000 volunteers serve food to 1.5 million so-called regular customers. These numbers alone could be interpreted as evidence for food insecurity in Germany, although the regional distribution of food banks does not always match the socio-economic distribution of demand (www.tafel.de). Without acknowledging food poverty as an actual and real problem in Germany and by just delegating the problem from the realm of social policy to 'sweet charity' [9], with all its contradictions and immanent problems, there is currently no governmental concept to address food poverty in Germany. As delegation, denial, and stigmatisation are still the predominant societal strategies for tackling food insecurity in Germany, the affected individuals are required to find their own solutions in their daily lives. The next chapter will provide a qualitative insight into this side of the problem.

Coping with Nutritional Scarcity at the Individual Level

In an underlying qualitative longitudinal study, a socio-economically well-balanced initial sample of 106 welfare recipients, as defined by Social Code II, were repeatedly interviewed over a period of 5 years using in-depth biographical interviews [10]. The transcribed material consists of 453 qualitative interviews, of which 81 cases were interviewed over all four waves. The analysis followed the methodology of qualitative content analyses [11], identifying a variety of interacting conditions that shape the ways in which the interviewees were coping with restricted nutritional situations. These conditions included *objective factors*, like accessibility to food banks and other infrastructural features of food supply, as well as facilities for food storing and cooking; *subjective factors*, such as overall attitude to food and eating (e.g., lifestyle, indulgence vs. modest eating, eating culture and health awareness, and shopping patterns and use of food banks), household capabilities (including cooking skills), and money management; *medical factors*, such as illnesses that require special diets, and finally *factors of sociality*, such as caring for others or being cared for, the range and intensity of family and social networks in general, and the corresponding time structure for eating. The way these conditions are entwined with each other was further elaborated. In a dialectical and dynamic form of on-going biographical transformation and sedimentation, these factors are both the reason for and the result of individual representations of coping types, which can be described along three analytical dimensions: nutrition and alimentary experiences, biographical acquisition of eating habits, and overall food-related capabilities. By following the introduced analytical steps, we identified a broad range of eight individual coping types:

- *Against the odds.* People coping actively with the situation, feeling pragmatic and not shameful for using food banks, making the best of it.
- *Children first.* People with subjective feelings of severe restriction of food supply, but who are trying hard to provide their children with good and healthy food.
- *Abandonment of quantity or quality.* People coping with financial restrictions for food by lowering the quality and/or quantity of food they consume, even if this is accompanied by a fatalistic anticipation of serious risks caused by chronic diseases (e.g., diabetes).
- *Surfing the ups and downs.* Due to different financial situations during the month, these people undergo changes in nutrition and food supply strategies, simulating normality in the beginning of the month and then spiralling downward over the course of the month.
- *Embracing nutrition for sense and structure.* For these people, activities like cooking, eating, and managing of food supplies provide not only practical solutions for the restricted nutritional situation but also offer a sense of time structure.
- *Enforcing networks.* In order to maintain their food supplies, these people depend on social networks. Parents, children and friends are visited to improve the nutritional situation.
- *Risky food financing.* These people enhance their food supplies in potentially risky ways, such as by exploiting their bodies (e.g., blood donations) or engaging in illegal work.

The evidence provided here sheds a first light on food consumption patterns and food management practices in unemployed German households. According to lifestyle, accustomed food practices, and family structures, people faced with food poverty are creative in developing coping strategies. This cannot absolve German society from finding structural answers to combat food insecurity, and this endeavour should be started before the on-going positive economic situation changes for the worse.

Discussion

We have provided some current quantitative data on food insecurity in Germany and compared it with qualitative results on nutritional coping strategies. In conclusion, for all coping types, one thing seems to hold true: as long as people have to rely on social benefits, they are very likely to suffer from rigid constraints concerning alimentary participation, even amounting to exclusion. Alimentary participation in modern consumer societies is a complex problem for the poor and a daily experience of exclusions for which no individual coping strategy will satisfactorily compensate. The provided results shed a first light on nutritional consumption patterns in unemployed German households. Understanding individual day-to-day coping strategies will help develop social policy strategies to minimise food insecurity not only in Germany but also throughout Europe, provided that careful policy decisions are made. As an objected problem in Germany, the denial, stigmatisation and delegation of food poverty are closely interrelated and mutually reinforce each other. If they continue to prevail, they might contribute to increases in nutritional poverty and hunger. Here, social sciences have a contribution to make towards challenging the orthodoxy. The best way to do so is to orient its methods and concepts to the realisation that alimentary deprivation can also become an existential problem for many people in German society. As social transfers are more often part of consolidation plans when reacting to the last crisis compared to other areas of public spending, spending cuts are more likely to hurt the poor and therefore food insecurity will remain a problem.

Acknowledgement

This article was made possible by the research framework of the third 'Reporting on Socioeconomic Development in Germany – soeb' (www.soeb.de/en/), funded by the German Federal Ministry of Education and Research.

References

1 OECD: Divided we stand: why inequality keeps rising. Country Note Germany, 2011. http://www.oecd.org/germany/49177659.pdf (accessed April 30, 2015).
2 Dowler E, O'Connor D: Rights based approaches to addressing food poverty and food insecurity in Ireland and UK. Soc Sci Med 2012;74:44–51.
3 Caraher M, Dowler E: Food for poorer people: conventional and 'alternative' transgressions; in Goodman M, Sage C (eds): Food Transgressions: Making Sense of Contemporary Food Politics. Farnham, Ashgate, 2015, pp 227–246.
4 Pfeiffer S, Ritter T, Hirseland A: Hunger and nutritional poverty in Germany: quantitative and qualitative empirical insights. Crit Public Health 2011;21: 417–428.
5 Max Rubner-Institut: Nationale Verzehrstudie II – Ergebnisbericht, Teil 2. Karlsruhe, Bundesforschungsinstitut für Ernährung und Lebensmittel, 2008.
6 Statistisches Bundesamt: Datenreport 2013: Ein Sozialbericht für die Bundesrepublik Deutschland. Wiesbaden, Destatis, 2013.
7 OECD: Society at a glance. OECD social indicators. OECD Publishing, 2014. http://dx.doi.org/10.1787/soc_glance-2014-en (accessed April 30, 2015).
8 Pfeiffer S, Ritter T, Oestreicher E: Food Insecurity in German households: qualitative and quantitative data on coping, poverty consumerism and alimentary participation. Social Policy and Society DOI: 10.1017/S147474641500010X.
9 Poppendieck J: Sweet Charity? Emergency Food and the End of Entitlement. New York, Penguin, 1999.
10 Rosenthal G: Biographical research; in Seale C, Giampieto G, Gubrium GF, Silverman D (eds): Qualitative Research Practice. London, Sage, 2004, pp 48–64.
11 Mayring P: Qualitative Content Analysis. Forum: Qualitative Social Research 2000;1:Art. 20.

Prof. Dr. Sabine Pfeiffer
Chair of Sociology (550D), University of Hohenheim
Wollgrasweg 23
DE–70599 Stuttgart (Germany)
E-Mail soziologie@uni-hohenheim.de

Biesalski HK, Black RE (eds): Hidden Hunger. Malnutrition and the First 1,000 Days of Life: Causes, Consequences and Solutions. World Rev Nutr Diet. Basel, Karger, 2016, vol 115, pp 24–35
DOI: 10.1159/000441885

Critical Dietary Habits in Early Childhood: Principles and Practice

Mathilde Kersting[a] · Ute Alexy[b] · Susanne Schürmann[a]

[a]Research Institute of Child Nutrition Dortmund, University of Bonn, [b]DONALD Study, Nutritional Epidemiology, Institute of Nutrition and Food Science, University of Bonn, Germany

Abstract

The adequacy of a diet is usually evaluated based on nutrient intake. As people eat foods but not nutrients, food-based dietary guidelines (FBDG) are needed. To evaluate dietary habits in infants and young children, the following stepwise approach is suggested: (1) develop country-specific FBDG to identify the potential of common nonfortified foods to ensure adequate nutrient intake and (2) examine potential 'critical' dietary patterns if main food groups are excluded, such as in vegetarian diets or if a family's precarious social status leads to food constraints. The German FBDG for infant and child nutrition demonstrate that a well-designed mixture of common foods results in an adequate supply of nutrients, except for vitamin D, iodine and iron. The following solutions are feasible to address deficiencies in these critical nutrients: routine supplementation (vitamin D), fortified complementary food consumption or supplementation for infants as well as inclusion of table salt in the family diet for children (iodine), and individual pediatric care for infants at risk (iron). In the exclusion of food groups of animal origin from vegetarian diets, several nutrients are at risk of becoming deficient if not substituted. Existing studies characterizing vegetarian children are rare. These were mainly published in the 1980s and 1990s and were biased towards a high social status. Thus, firm conclusions on today's dietary practices and health statuses of European vegetarian children cannot be drawn. A social gradient exists for food patterns and dietary quality in children, but energy intake need not necessarily be affected. Scenarios in Germany suggest that families on unemployment assistance can afford to eat a diet compliant with German FBDG only if they restrict food selection to basic food. Yet, the question of how families cope with financial constraints in everyday life remains. In conclusion, well-designed FBDG provide various opportunities to identify critical nutrients and critical food habits in early childhood and beyond.

Introduction

The adequacy of a diet is traditionally evaluated by comparing the usual nutrient intake of a population or population subgroup with reference values for nutrient intake. Recently, the European Food Safety Authority (EFSA) reviewed the existing data on nutrient requirements and dietary intake for infants and young children in European countries [1]. Subsequently, the EFSA used those reference values judged as most appropriate to evaluate the risk of inadequate nutrient intake as reported from nutrition surveys. Complementary evidence from studies reporting status markers of nutrient adequacy was considered, but this was seldom available. As a result, iron, iodine and vitamin D were identified as 'critical' nutrients in infants and children in Europe, with mean intakes often below the EFSA reference values and low biomarker status in the case of vitamin D and iron.

In day-to-day living, people eat foods rather than nutrients. Therefore, it is mandatory to assess the food habits of at-risk population groups to identify underlying causes for deficiencies in 'critical' nutrients. Subsequently, sound food choices with the potential to prevent or alleviate nutrient inadequacies can be recommended. As almost all foods act as sources of multiple nutrients and because consumers do not eat single foods but rather consume combinations of foods, the dietary food pattern has gained considerable attention in recent decades. Within this concept, potential 'critical' dietary habits that may affect multiple nutrients can be identified in cases of intentional exclusion of basic food groups or when there are constraints in general food availability.

To evaluate critical dietary habits in infant and young child nutrition, we suggest the following stepwise approach:

1. Develop country-specific food-based dietary guidelines (FBDG) and identify the potential of the available food supply to ensure adequate nutrient intake at the population level
2. Examine potential 'critical' dietary patterns deviating from FBDG in cases in which families exclude main food groups from their children's diets, such as in families with vegetarian diets, or if a family's precarious social and financial status leads to food constraints and food insecurity

Step 1: Food-Based Dietary Guidelines

Modular Systems for Infant and Child Nutrition in Germany

Along with the epidemic increase in the prevalence of diet-related chronic diseases in wealthy Western countries, public health nutrition research has opened a new window for dietary recommendations, turning the focus from nutrients to foods. The main objective is to translate classical nutrient-based recommendations into FBDG that should be summarized into short and understandable messages for the public.

These guidelines should consider existing health problems and dietary habits and should address the total diet as opposed to single food groups. Due to population-specific dietary habits, FBDG must be developed for each country [2] and for specific age groups, such as infants or children.

With regard to child nutrition, the EFSA introduced the existing FBDG for infant and child nutrition in Germany as examples of food patterns that ensure an adequate energy and nutrient supply of these age groups. Both of these modular concepts, named 'Dietary schedule for the first year of life' and 'Optimized mixed diet for children and adolescents 1–18 years of age' are based on common, nonfortified food and a traditional meal pattern [3]. Food selection and food amounts were cautiously optimized to meet the German nutrient-based recommendations that are set to cover the requirements of almost all individuals (mean + 2 standard deviations) with various age groups.

Nutrient Adequacy and 'Critical' Nutrients

Evaluation of these FBDG shows that an adequate, and for some nutrients even ample, supply of nutrients for infants and children can be achieved by a well-designed mixture of common foods (fig. 1). However, obvious exceptions to this are vitamin D, iodine and iron, with intakes well below the national reference values. The same nutrients were evaluated as critical to the dietary patterns of European infants and young children by the EFSA as well. Particularly, deficiencies of iodine and iron in early developmental periods may have lasting consequences that lead to impaired cognitive and functional capacities later in life [4, 5]. Thus, fortification and/or supplementation are needed. The German example can demonstrate how the critical nutrient supply inherent in an optimized food pattern can be evaluated and overcome.

Vitamin D

Fortunately, representative biomarker data on vitamin D status in children are available in Germany [6]. They demonstrate an adequate vitamin D status [serum 25(OH) D] as long as infants receive routine vitamin D supplementation. Thereafter, the typical low vitamin D intake in combination with insufficient endogenous vitamin D production via sunlight exposure leads to a sharp decrease in vitamin D levels and high proportions of vitamin D deficiency depending on the cut-offs used. A simple and safe solution recommended by the German Pediatric Society is the continuation of routine vitamin D supplementation from infancy into childhood, at least in high-risk groups if sunlight exposure is insufficient [7].

Iodine

Although the iodine content in cow's milk has increased due to changes in cow-feeding practices in Germany in recent years, iodine intake from food is not sufficient to meet requirements either in dietary practice or in the German FBDG. Therefore, the use of iodized table salt in the household as well as in the food industry is recom-

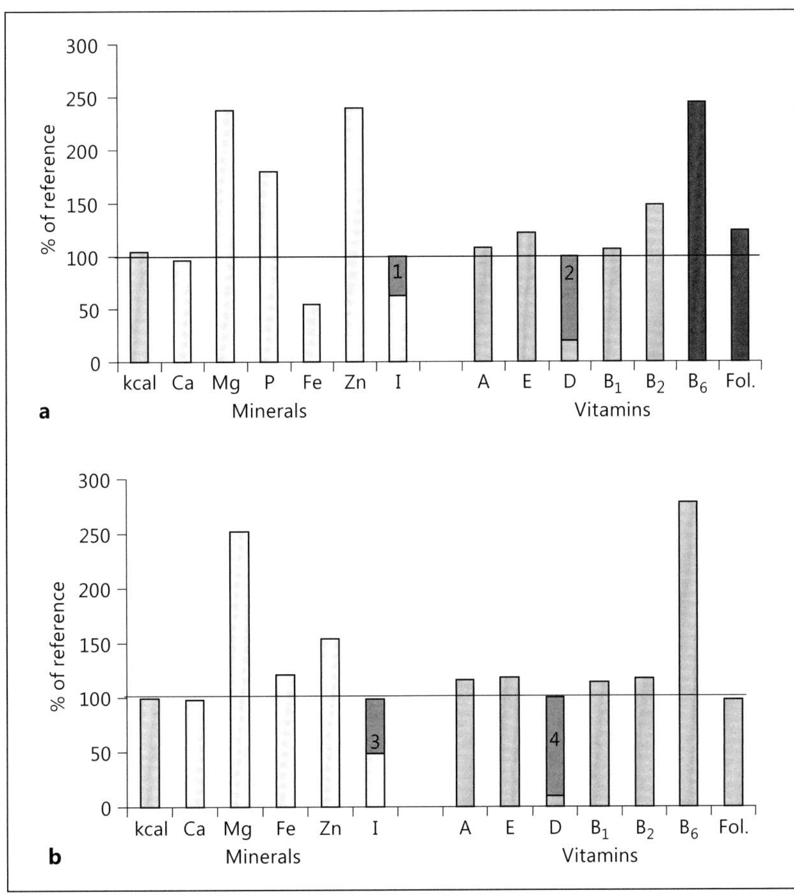

Fig. 1. Nutrient supply according to FBDG for infant and child nutrition in Germany, shown as percentages of German reference values. Solutions to achieve an adequate intake of critical nutrients by supplementation or fortification are marked. **a** Dietary schedule for the 1st year of life. **b** Optimized mixed diet for children and adolescents. 1: Iodine supplementation or fortified commercial complementary food. 2: Vitamin D supplementation. 3: Iodine-fortified salt in household and food industry. 4: Vitamin D supplementation.

mended in Germany. Since iodine status biomarkers are not available for infants and young children, little is known about iodine status in these age groups. In older children, from preschool age onwards, analysis of 24-hour urine samples has shown a decreasing trend in recent years, probably due to decreased use of iodized salt by the food industry [8].

However, infants should not yet receive salted food, since early exposure to the taste of salt may lastingly increase salt preference and blood pressure [9]. Therefore, this age group does not profit from the German population-based iodine fortification strategy [10]. Nevertheless, two alternate solutions are feasible to overcome a deficient iodine supply when homemade complementary food is preferred; these include the supplementation of iodine (50 μg/day) or the use of iodine-fortified commercial complementary food (e.g. cereal-milk gruel, which can be easily integrated as one of the 3 recommended complementary meals in the infant FBDG).

Iron

Data from a double-blind randomized controlled intervention trial examined high and low meat content in complementary food as part of the German FBFG. Overall, the trial showed fully sufficient iron status biomarkers (e.g. serum ferritin, hemoglobin) in the second 6 months of life, despite a mean iron intake far below the German reference values (6 vs. 8 mg/day), which are well in accordance with the latest EFSA reference values [11]. This finding suggests that the current reference values for iron intake in European infants and young children may overestimate iron requirements in infants, at least if they are fed according to the German FBDG for infant nutrition.

However, in the subgroup of infants who are fully breastfed during the first 4–6 months of life as recommended, up to 20% of infants were found to have iron deficiency (ferritin <12 μg/l) and 6% had iron deficiency anemia (ferritin <12 μg/l, hemoglobin <105 g/l) [12]. A similar iron status prevalence was reported from study samples in other European countries [1].

As iron overload should be avoided and a decrease in iron body stores may be physiological during the second half of infancy, pediatric check-ups for infants and young children at risk of iron deficiency could be a feasible and safe approach to assure adequate iron intake instead of routine iron supplementation. In addition, the applicability of the existing reference values for iron intake in infants in Germany should be critically reviewed.

Step 2: Critical Dietary Habits

Food Exclusion in Vegetarian Diets

Principles

In principle, vegetarian diets can be categorized by the exclusion of food groups of animal origin (table 1). Nutrition experts can estimate the potential impact on nutrient supply if the excluded food is not sufficiently substituted.

In general, vegetarian diets are supposed to be healthy and superior to the standard omnivorous Western diet, which is energy dense and high in saturated fatty acids, refined carbohydrates, and salt, but low in dietary fiber, antioxidants and other bioactive plant food components. Although the American Dietetic Association and the American Academy of Pediatrics [15, 16] have stated that well-planned vegetarian diets are appropriate for individuals during all stages of the life cycle, including infancy, childhood, and adolescence, the German Nutrition Society and the Research Institute of

Table 1. Categories of vegetarian diet types and related nutrients [13, 14]

Vegetarian diet type	Excluded food	Reduced nutrients
Semi-vegetarian	Mainly meat and meat products (small amounts of fish and/or meat are consumed)	–
Lacto-ovo-vegetarian	Meat, fish and products made from these	Iron, zinc (highly bioavailable), iodine, n-3 fatty acids
Lacto-vegetarian	Meat, fish, eggs and products made from these	Iron, zinc (highly bioavailable), iodine, n-3 fatty acids + vitamins A, D
Ovo-vegetarian	Meat, fish, milk and products made from these	Iron, zinc (highly bioavailable), iodine, n-3 fatty acids + calcium, vitamins B_2, B_{12}
Vegan	All food of animal origin	Iron, zinc (highly bioavailable), iodine, n-3 fatty acids, calcium, vitamins A, D, B_2, B_{12} + protein, energy
Macrobiotic	Mainly food of animal origin (sometimes small amounts of fish are consumed), specific focus by choosing food of plant origin	Iron, zinc (highly bioavailable), iodine, n-3 fatty acids, calcium, vitamins A, D, B_2, B_{12} + protein, energy

Child Nutrition question whether the specific dietary requirements in childhood can be safely met, particularly with vegan diets.

Remarkably, in the course of restricting food groups of animal origin, only those nutrients that are already critical in an optimized omnivorous food pattern are thought to become insufficient, namely, iron, iodine and vitamin D.

Practice

The prevalence of children consuming vegetarian diets in Germany is assumed to be on the rise, but valid data are missing. Because manifestations of vegetarian diets are blurred in practice, dietary assessment is difficult, and results may depend on survey methodology. In nationwide surveys in Germany, the prevalence of vegetarian children and adolescents was reported to be between 5 and 6% based on parental or self-evaluation and from dietary records [17].

In a recent systematic review, we evaluated studies on dietary intake and health status in infants, children and adolescents on vegetarian diets [unpubl.]. The inclusion criteria were (1) appropriate characterization of the vegetarian diet and (2) evaluation of nutritional and health status. Case reports (e.g. on vitamin B_{12} deficiency in vegan diets) as well as studies from nonindustrialized countries were excluded.

A total of 28 publications [18–45] from 16 studies (13 from Europe, 3 from the USA) were identified, with mostly small samples (<50 participants). These studies were mainly undertaken in the 1980s and 1990s. Most often, the participants came from families of high social status. Nutrient supplementation was common. Nine publications originated from a Dutch study reported in the 1980s that evaluated children and adolescents eating a macrobiotic diet. In around half of the studies, the authors allocated the examined diets to a vegetarian diet category (table 2).

Overall, growth and body weight in these studies was within the lower reference ranges (table 2). Dietary intake and nutrient status were inconsistent between the studies and in comparison to omnivorous control groups. Some potential health benefits, such as beneficial blood lipid levels and high intake of dietary fiber and vitamin C, were observed. Multiple low clinical or biochemical indicators of vitamin status, such as for vitamin B_{12}, vitamin D, and iron, were reported, as well as signs of impaired bone health. Whereas young children on macrobiotic diets suffered from multiple nutrient deficiencies and showed signs of growth retardation, indications for a poor nutritional status were rarely reported within lacto-ovo-vegetarian groups. A poor vitamin B_{12} status was reported in vegan groups if not supplemented.

The existing database is not sufficient, however, to soundly evaluate present-day dietary practices of vegetarian children. Today, the food industry offers more and more specialized vegetarian products, and vegetarian families might be increasingly aware of the need to consume fortified food or to supplement critical nutrients.

Food Constraints in Precarious Socio-Economic Situations

Principles

There is a well-known social gradient for nutritional status characteristics in childhood in Europe with regard to excess weight and obesity [46]. A social gradient is also apparent for food consumption habits in children, but on a weaker basis. Strong evidence exists, however, for breastfeeding, where low maternal educational status is a consistent risk factor for low breastfeeding [47]. Regarding the mixed childhood diet, associations with social status seem to be broadly similar to those reported in adults: low social class populations consume less from the ‘healthy' side of the food palette, in particular fruit and vegetables, and more from the ‘unhealthy' side, in particular confectionary and soft drinks. In contrast, food habits regarding basic food like milk are more similar between the different social classes [48–50]. The differences in dietary quality between social classes have been suggested to impact nutrient status, but biomarker data are rare [51].

While the consequences of specific food group exclusion on the supply of specific nutrients, such as in nonsubstituted vegetarian diets, are predictable, it is more difficult to estimate the consequences of a generally lower quality diet. This could be the case if food consumption is constrained but an omnivorous diet remains, where all food groups contribute their specific nutrient profiles to supply a whole range of

Table 2. Overview of results from a systematic review of studies on children eating vegetarian diets compared to omnivorous groups or reference and normal values (unpublished)

Diet type [Ref.]	Nutrient supply	Nutritional status	Health status
General vegetarian (n = 8) [27, 28, 31–33, 35–37, 41, 43–45]	– Macronutrients = Ref – Vit B_{12} ≤ Ref – Vit D < Ref – Fe ≤ Ref – Folic acid, Vit C > Ref Nutrient supplementation n = 2	– Height = Ref – Weight = Ref	– Vit D* < Norm – Vit B_{12}* = Norm – Fe status* ≤ Norm – Fatty acid pattern* = Ref
Lacto-ovo-vegetarian (n = 3) [20, 21, 34]	– Energy ≤ Ref – *Infants:* Fe ≤ Ref, Zn = Ref No nutrient supplementation	– Height ≤ Ref – Weight ≤ Ref – *Infants:* height and weight = Ref	– Fitness = OM – *Infants:* Fe status* = Norm
Vegan (n = 3) [22, 26, 42]	– Energy ≤ Ref – Fiber > Ref – Vit D < Ref – Ca < Ref – Vit B_{12} with supplementation > Ref, without < Ref Nutrient supplementation n = 2 (Vit B_{12}, Vit D, Vit A)	– Height = Ref – Weight = Ref	– Vit D* < Norm – BMC, BMD < Norm
Macrobiotic (n = 2) [18, 19, 23–25, 29, 30, 38–40]	– Fiber > Ref – Folic acid > Ref – Vit B_{12} < Ref – Ca < Ref – *Infants:* energy, fat and protein < OM, Vit B_{12}, Vit C and Ca < Ref Nutrient supplementation n = 1	– Height ≤ Ref – Weight ≤ Ref – *Infants:* height and weight < Ref	– Vit B_{12}* < Norm – BMC, BMD < OM – Psychomotor and cognitive abilities < Norm – *Infants:* Vit B_{12}*, Ca*, Fe* and Vit D* < Norm; physical and motor development < Norm

BMC = Bone mineral content; BMD = bone mineral density; n = number of studies; Norm = normal value; OM = omnivore; Ref = reference value; Vit = vitamin. * Blood measurements.

nutrients. Yet, the drivers of differences in children's dietary intake related to socioeconomic status have not been well defined to date.

Practice

Reasonable assessment of nutrient supply or nutritional risks due to low social status is difficult in practice. Prospective epidemiological methods, such as dietary records or repeated 24 -hour recalls, are laborious for study participants, decrease compliance and increase selection bias.

Food cost scenarios in Germany suggest that families on unemployment assistance could afford a diet compliant with the German FBDG for children and adolescents only if they restrict their food selection to basic foods and do without the convenience and branded products that are popular in today's family diet [52] (fig. 2). No data are available to show how families cope with such financial constraints in everyday life.

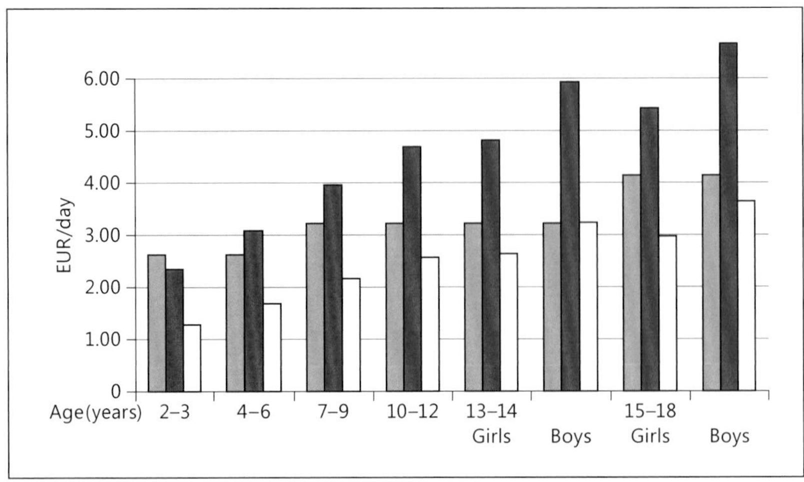

Fig. 2. Food costs (EUR/day) for children and adolescents. Light gray: based on amount provided for nutrition in unemployment assistance. Dark gray: food costs based on the German FBDG, including convenience and brand name foods used in the dietary practice of families. White: food costs based on the German FBDG, excluding convenience and brand foods [52].

Studies in extreme food deprivation suggest that diet quality as well as child growth and health deteriorate with increasing grades of food insecurity. Energy intake need not necessarily be affected, but the energy provided by healthy food is thought to decrease and that provided less healthy food is thought to increase [48–50]. It remains open whether a less healthy diet is primarily caused by lack of money to spend on food or by unwise budget management [50, 53].

A social gradient in dietary quality may be associated with a family's cultural or immigration background, but the proportional contributions of these two factors are difficult to untangle. Differences in dietary habits between immigrant and native populations as well as differences between subgroups of immigrants within a country are most often specific to ethnic group and grade of inculturation [54, 55]. Therefore, findings from observational studies with regard to socio-cultural influences on dietary habits cannot be easily transferred from one country to another.

Conclusion and Perspectives

The German example shows that even well-designed FBDG for infant and young child nutrition that rely on common nonfortified foods present with 'critical' nutrient deficiencies in vitamin D, iodine and iron. Feasible solutions are, however, available, either by routine supplementation (vitamin D), use of fortified commercial complementary food or supplementation for infants and use of table salt for children (iodine), and pediatric check-ups for infants at risk (iron).

The existing database that is available to evaluate present-day food habits that deviate from FBDG, such as in vegetarian children in Europe, is insufficient. Future research should be devoted to the valid assessment of the prevalence and manifestation of vegetarian diets and their effects on nutrient intake and nutrient status in today's food environments. Based on such an assessment, a European science-based position on and up-to-date guidance for vegetarian diets in children could be elaborated.

Although a social gradient has been repeatedly demonstrated for compliance with dietary recommendations in children and in adults, valid markers for socio-economic constellations with detrimental effects on child nutrient status are not yet available. Future research could be devoted to the identification of socio-cultural indicators that have relevance for food patterns and resulting nutrient and health statuses in children, in particular in extreme constellations of food insecurity combined with immigration status.

In summary, the development of well-designed, country-specific FBDG could provide various opportunities to identify critical nutrients and critical food habits in early childhood and beyond.

References

1 EFSA NDA Panel (EFSA Panel on Dietetic Products, Nutrition and Allergies): Scientific opinion on nutrient requirements and dietary intakes of infants and young children in the European Union. EFSA J 2013; 11:3408.

2 EFSA Panel on Dietetic Products, Nutrition, and Allergies (NDA): Scientific opinion on establishing food-based dietary guidelines. EFSA J 2010;8:1460.

3 Hilbig A, Lentze MJ, Kersting M: Introduction and composition of complementary feeding. Scientific evidence and practical guidelines in Germany (in German). Monatsschr Kinderheilkd 2012;160:1089–1095.

4 Remer T, Johner SA, Gärtner R, Thamm M, Kriener M: Iodine deficiency in infancy – a risk for cognitive development (in German). Dtsch Med Wochenschr 2010;135:1551–1556.

5 Pala E, Erguven M, Guven S, Erdogan M, Balta T: Psychomotor development in children with iron deficiency and iron-deficiency anemia. Food Nutr Bull 2010;31:431–435.

6 Hintzpeter B, Scheidt-Nave C, Müller MJ, Schenk L, Mensink GB: Higher prevalence of vitamin D deficiency is associated with immigrant background among children and adolescents in Germany. J Nutr 2008;138:1482–1490.

7 Böhles HJ, Fusch C, Genzel-Boroviczény O, Jochum F, Kauth T, Kersting M, et al: Vitamin D supply in infants, children and adolescents (in German). German Society of Child and Youth Medicine, 2011. http://www.dgkj.de/wissenschaft/stellungnahmen/meldung/meldungsdetail/vitamin_d_versorgung_im_saeuglings_kindes_und_jugendalter/ (accessed October 1, 2015).

8 Johner SA, Thamm M, Nöthlings U, Remer T: Iodine status in preschool children and evaluation of major dietary iodine sources: a German experience. Eur J Nutr 2013;52:1711–1719.

9 Geleijnse JM, Hofman A, Witteman JC, Hazebroek AA, Valkenburg HA, Grobbee DE: Long-term effects of neonatal sodium restriction on blood pressure. Hypertension 1997;29:913–917.

10 Alexy U, Drossard C, Kersting M, Remer T: Iodine intake in the youngest: impact of commercial complementary food. Eur J Clin Nutr 2009;63:1368–1370.

11 Dube K, Schwartz J, Mueller MJ, Kalhoff H, Kersting M: Complementary food with low (8%) or high (12%) meat content as source of dietary iron: a double-blinded randomized controlled trial. Eur J Nutr 2010;49:11–18.

12 Dube K, Schwartz J, Mueller MJ, Kalhoff H, Kersting M: Iron intake and iron status in breastfed infants during the first year of life. Clin Nutr 2010;29:773–778.

13 Kushi M: The Book of Macrobiotics: The Universal Way of Health, Happiness, and Peace. Tokyo, Japan Publications, 1987.

14 Leitzmann C, Keller M: Vegetarian Diets. 74 Tables. Terms and Definitions (in German). Stuttgart, Ulmer, 2010.

15 Craig WJ, Mangels AR: Position of the American Dietetic Association: vegetarian diets. J Am Diet Assoc 2009;109:1266–1282.

16 American Academy of Pediatrics (ed): Pediatric Nutrition Handbook: Nutritional Aspects of Vegetarian Diets. Elk Grove Village, American Academy of Pediatrics, 2009, pp 201–224.

17 Mensink GBM, Kleiser C, Richter A: Food consumption of children and adolescents in Germany. Results of the German Health Interview and Examination Survey for Children and Adolescents (KiGGS) (in German). Bundesgesundheitsblatt Gesundheitsforschung Gesundheitsschutz 2007;50:609–623.

18 van Dusseldorp M, Schneede J, Refsum H, Ueland PM, Thomas CM, de Boer E, et al: Risk of persistent cobalamin deficiency in adolescents fed a macrobiotic diet in early life. Am J Clin Nutr 1999;69:664–671.

19 van Dusseldorp M, Arts IC, Bergsma JS, de Jong N, Dagnelie PC, Van Staveren WA, et al: Catch-up growth in children fed a macrobiotic diet in early childhood. J Nutr 1996;126:2977–2983.

20 Taylor A, Redworth EW, Morgan JB: Influence of diet on iron, copper, and zinc status in children under 24 months of age. Biol Trace Elem Res 2004;97:197–214.

21 Sievers E, Dörner K, Hamm E, Janisch C, Schaub J: Comparative studies on the iron supply of lacto-ovo-vegetarian infants. Ärztezeitschr Naturheilverf 1991;32:106–112.

22 Sanders TA: Growth and development of British vegan children. Am J Clin Nutr 1988;48:822–825.

23 Dhonukshe-Rutten RA, van Dusseldorp M, Schneede J, de Groot LC, van Staveren WA: Low bone mineral density and bone mineral content are associated with low cobalamin status in adolescents. Eur J Nutr 2005;44:341–347.

24 Parsons TJ, van Dusseldorp M, Seibel MJ, van Staveren WA: Are levels of bone turnover related to lower bone mass of adolescents previously fed a macrobiotic diet? Exp Clin Endocrinol Diabetes 2001;109:288–293.

25 Parsons TJ, van Dusseldorp M, van der Vliet M, van de Werken K, Schaafsma G, van Staveren WA: Reduced bone mass in Dutch adolescents fed a macrobiotic diet in early life. J Bone Miner Res 1997;12:1486–1494.

26 O'Connell JM, Dibley MJ, Sierra J, Wallace B, Marks JS, Yip R: Growth of vegetarian children: the Farm Study. Pediatrics 1989;84:475–481.

27 Nathan I, Hackett AF, Kirby S: A longitudinal study of the growth of matched pairs of vegetarian and omnivorous children, aged 7–11 years, in the northwest of England. Eur J Clin Nutr 1997;51:20–25.

28 Nathan I, Hackett AF, Kirby S: The dietary intake of a group of vegetarian children aged 7–11 years compared with matched omnivores. Br J Nutr 1996;75:533–544.

29 Miller DR, Specker BL, Ho ML, Norman EJ: Vitamin B-12 status in a macrobiotic community. Am J Clin Nutr 1991;53:524–529.

30 Louwman MW, van Dusseldorp M, van de Vijver FJ, Thomas CM, Schneede J, Ueland PM, et al: Signs of impaired cognitive function in adolescents with marginal cobalamin status. Am J Clin Nutr 2000;72:762–769.

31 Laskowska-Klita T, Chelchowska M, Ambroszkiewicz J, Gajewska J, Klemarczyk W: The effect of vegetarian diet on selected essential nutrients in children. Med Wieku Rozwoj 2011;15:318–325.

32 Krajcovicová-Kudlácková M, Simoncic R, Béderová A, Grancicová E, Magálová T: Influence of vegetarian and mixed nutrition on selected haematological and biochemical parameters in children. Nahrung 1997;41:311–314.

33 Krajcovicová-Kudlácková M, Simoncic R, Béderová A, Klvanová J: Plasma fatty acid profile and alternative nutrition. Ann Nutr Metab 1997;41:365–370.

34 Hebbelinck M, Clarys P, de Malsche A: Growth, development, and physical fitness of Flemish vegetarian children, adolescents, and young adults. Am J Clin Nutr 1999;70:579S–585S.

35 Gorczyca D, Prescha A, Szeremeta K, Jankowski A: Iron status and dietary iron intake of vegetarian children from Poland. Ann Nutr Metab 2013;62:291–297.

36 Gorczyca D, Pasciak M, Szponar B, Gamian A, Jankowski A: An impact of the diet on serum fatty acid and lipid profiles in Polish vegetarian children and children with allergy. Eur J Clin Nutr 2011;65:191–195.

37 Dwyer JT, Dietz WH Jr, Andrews EM, Suskind RM: Nutritional status of vegetarian children. Am J Clin Nutr 1982;35:204–216.

38 Dagnelie PC, van Staveren WA: Macrobiotic nutrition and child health: results of a population-based, mixed-longitudinal cohort study in The Netherlands. Am J Clin Nutr 1994;59:1187–1196.

39 Dagnelie PC, Vergote FJ, van Staveren WA, van den Berg H, Dingjan PG, Hautvast JG, et al: High prevalence of rickets in infants on macrobiotic diets. Am J Clin Nutr 1990;51:202–208.

40 Dagnelie PC, van Staveren WA, Vergote FJ, Dingjan PG, van den Berg H, Hautvast JG, et al: Increased risk of vitamin B-12 and iron deficiency in infants on macrobiotic diets. Am J Clin Nutr 1989;50:818–824.
41 Ambroszkiewicz J, Klemarczyk W, Gajewska J, Chelchowska M, Rowicka G, Oltarzewski M, et al: Serum concentration of adipocytokines in prepubertal vegetarian and omnivorous children. Med Wieku Rozwoj 2011;15:326–334.
42 Ambroszkiewicz J, Klemarczyk W, Gajewska J, Chelchowska M, Franek E, Laskowska-Klita T: The influence of vegan diet on bone mineral density and biochemical bone turnover markers. Pediatr Endocrinol Diabetes Metab 2010;16:201–204.
43 Ambroszkiewicz J, Klemarczyk W, Gajewska J, Chelchowska M, Laskowska-Klita T: Serum concentration of biochemical bone turnover markers in vegetarian children. Adv Med Sci 2007;52:279–282.
44 Ambroszkiewicz J, Klemarczyk W, Chelchowska M, Gajewska J, Laskowska-Klita T: Serum homocysteine, folate, vitamin B12 and total antioxidant status in vegetarian children. Adv Med Sci 2006;51:265–268.
45 Ambroszkiewicz J, Laskowska-Klita T, Klemarczyk W: Low levels of osteocalcin and leptin in serum of vegetarian prepubertal children. Med Wieku Rozwoj 2003;7:587–591.
46 Kurth BM, Schaffrath Rosario A: Overweight and obesity in children and adolescents in Germany (in German). Bundesgesundheitsblatt Gesundheitsforschung Gesundheitsschutz 2010;53:643–652.
47 von der Lippe E, Brettschneider AK, Gutsche J, Poethko-Müller C: Factors influencing the prevalence and duration of breastfeeding in Germany: results of the KiGGS study: first follow up (KiGGS Wave 1) (in German). Bundesgesundheitsblatt Gesundheitsforschung Gesundheitsschutz 2014;57:849–859.
48 Leung CW, Blumenthal SJ, Hoffnagle EE, Jensen HH, Foerster SB, Nestle M, et al: Associations of food stamp participation with dietary quality and obesity in children. Pediatrics 2013;131:463–472.
49 Zarnowiecki DM, Dollman J, Parletta N: Associations between predictors of children's dietary intake and socioeconomic position: a systematic review of the literature. Obes Rev 2014;15:375–391.
50 Nelson M: Childhood nutrition and poverty. Proc Nutr Soc 2000;59:307–315.
51 Kant AK, Graubard BI: Race-ethnic, family income, and education differentials in nutritional and lipid biomarkers in US children and adolescents: NHANES 2003–2006. Am J Clin Nutr 2012;96:601–612.
52 Alexy U, Kersting M: Food costs and Hartz IV. What is feasible with the present unemployment assistance (in German). Prävention 2012;7:71–74.
53 Pilgrim A, Barker M, Jackson A, Ntani G, Crozier S, Inskip H, et al: Does living in a food insecure household impact on the diets and body composition of young children? Findings from the Southampton Women's Survey. J Epidemiol Community Health 2012;66:e6.
54 Falconer CL, Park MH, Croker H, Kessel AS, Saxena S, Viner RM, et al: Can the relationship between ethnicity and obesity-related behaviours among school-aged children be explained by deprivation? A cross-sectional study. BMJ Open 2014;4:e003949.
55 Kleiser C, Mensink GB, Neuhauser H, Schenk L, Kurth BM: Food intake of young people with a migration background living in Germany. Public Health Nutr 2010;13:324–330.

Prof. Dr. Mathilde Kersting
Forschungsinstitut für Kinderernährung
Heinstück 11
DE–44225 Dortmund (Germany)
E-Mail kersting@fke-do.de

Biesalski HK, Black RE (eds): Hidden Hunger. Malnutrition and the First 1,000 Days of Life: Causes, Consequences and Solutions. World Rev Nutr Diet. Basel, Karger, 2016, vol 115, pp 36–45
DOI: 10.1159/000442069

Food Price Policies May Improve Diet but Increase Socioeconomic Inequalities in Nutrition

Nicole Darmon[a] · Anne Lacroix[b] · Laurent Muller[b] · Bernard Ruffieux[b]

[a]INRA UMR1260, INSERM UMR1062, Aix-Marseille Université, Marseille, and [b]INRA UMR, 1215 GAEL, Grenoble Alpes Université, Grenoble, France

Abstract

Unhealthy eating is more prevalent among women and people with a low socioeconomic status. Policies that affect the price of food have been proposed to improve diet quality. The study's objective was to compare the impact of food price policies on the nutritional quality of food baskets chosen by low-income and medium-income women. Experimental economics was used to simulate a fruit and vegetable subsidy and a mixed policy subsidizing healthy products and taxing unhealthy ones. Food classification was based on the Score of Nutritional Adequacy of Individual Foods, Score of Nutrients to Be Limited nutrient profiling system. Low-income (n = 95) and medium-income (n = 33) women selected a daily food basket first at current prices and then at policy prices. Energy density (ED) and the mean adequacy ratio (MAR) were used as nutritional quality indicators. At baseline, low-income women selected less healthy baskets than medium-income women (less fruit and vegetables, more unhealthy products, higher ED, lower MAR). Both policies improved nutritional quality (fruit and vegetable quantities increased, ED decreased, the MAR increased), but the magnitude of the improvement was often lower among low-income women. For instance, ED decreased by 5.3% with the fruit and vegetable subsidy and by 7.3% with the mixed subsidy, whereas decreases of 13.2 and 12.6%, respectively, were recorded for the medium-income group. Finally, both policies improved dietary quality, but they increased socioeconomic inequalities in nutrition.

Introduction

A large intake of energy-dense foods that are high in fat, salt and sugar but low in vitamins, minerals and other micronutrients is considered to be among the most convincing causes of obesity and overweight [1]. Price is a determining factor in food choices, and unhealthy eating is more prevalent among people with a low socioeconomic status [2]. Low-income (LI) individuals consume less fruit and vegetables and more refined cereals. These socioeconomic differences in food choices have been partly attributed to the low cost of energy-dense, nutrient-poor foods, generally high in fat and sugar, compared with the high cost of energy-diluted, nutrient-rich foods, such as fruit and vegetables [3].

Policies that affect the price of food have been proposed to improve diet quality [4]: foods high in calories, fat, or sugar may be subjected to specific taxes, whereas healthy foods, such as fruit and vegetables, may be subsidized. A vast literature covers this issue [5–10]. An extensive review has concluded that studies estimating price effects on substitutions from unhealthy to healthy food and price responsiveness among LI populations are crucially needed [11]. Simulation-modeling studies have suggested that taxes based on a single nutrient or a single food tend to generate undesired effects on the demand for other nutrients or foods due to substitutions between taxed and non-taxed foods as well as heterogeneous consumer responses depending on income level [5, 6, 12].

The objective of this study was to evaluate the impact of food price policies on the food content and the nutritional quality of daily food baskets selected by LI and medium-income (MI) women. It consisted of an experiment conducted within the framework of experimental economics. Experimental economics estimates the preference that an individual attributes to a choice by placing him or her under experimental conditions that reproduce the real conditions for the choice [13–15]. It allowed us to measure the actual impact on diet of two price policies by comparing the food baskets selected at baseline and under each policy.

Materials and Methods

Participant Selection

We recruited a convenience sample of 160 women, mainly selected according to their household income. Apart from the income criterion, three other eligibility criteria for the participants were used: (i) being in the 20–54 age group; (ii) being in charge of grocery shopping for themselves or their household, and (iii) purchasing from a French food repertoire. Each woman received EUR 25 for participation. The experiment took place between May 20 and July 26, 2008, in six southeastern French suburbs in Grenoble and Lyon.

After eliminating incomplete responses, we had a sample of 128 women. This sample was divided into two groups: (i) the LI group consisted of 95 women below the poverty line (equivalent to 60% of the French median disposable income); (ii) the MI group consisted of 33 women whose disposable incomes per month per consumption unit were around the French median income.

Table 1. The different steps of the experiment

	Learning	Baseline	FV policy	NP policy
Task	Yesterday daily food basket	Tomorrow daily food basket	Tomorrow daily food basket	Tomorrow daily food basket
Prices	No posted price	Observed prices	–30% fruit and vegetables	–30% healthy foods (including fruit and vegetables) +30% unhealthy foods
Data collection		Dietary indexes (baseline) Budget (baseline)	Dietary indexes (distance) Budget (distance)	Dietary indexes (distance) Budget (distance)

Software

The compositions of 180 food items commonly purchased by French adults were used for this experiment (excluding alcoholic beverages). For each selected food item, actual retail prices were collected in May 2008 in the largest French food cyber market (Ooshop). We will call these retail prices 'observed prices'. The participants were informed of this source before the experiment. The software package (Medical Expert Systems), originally developed for food consumption surveys, was adapted for the present purpose. Using it, a participant could compose an individual food basket by 'picking' products on a screen from a tree-structured database. Once a product was chosen, the portion was selected according to pictures.

Score of Nutritional Adequacy of Individual Foods, Score of Nutrients to Be Limited Nutrient Profiling

All fruits and vegetables (n = 43) were aggregated into one food category. This category included soup and canned or frozen vegetables but excluded potatoes, nuts and processed fruits containing added sugars. Other foods were classified using the French Score of Nutritional Adequacy of Individual Foods (SAIN), Score of Nutrients to Be Limited (LIM) nutrient profiling system [16]. This system assigns two independent sub-scores to each food. The positive SAIN sub-score is the mean nutrient adequacy percentage for 5 basic nutrients (proteins, fiber, vitamin C, iron and calcium) and a variable number of optional nutrients and is calculated per 100 kcal. The negative LIM sub-score is the mean percentage of maximal recommended values for 3 nutrients whose intake should be limited, including saturated fatty acids (SFA), added sugar and sodium, and is calculated per 100 g. Using the SAIN and LIM thresholds [16], in the present study, foods other than fruits and vegetables were allocated to 3 classes: high SAIN and low LIM (healthy products, n = 24), low SAIN and low LIM or high SAIN and high LIM (neutral products, n = 51), and low SAIN and high LIM (unhealthy products, n = 62).

Price Policies

Two different policies were tested: (i) the 'Fruit & Vegetables (FV) policy' consisted of a 30% decrease in the observed prices of fruits and vegetables; (ii) the 'Nutrient Profile (NP) policy' consisted of a 30% decrease in the observed prices of fruit and vegetables and of other healthy products and a 30% increase in the observed prices of unhealthy products.

Experiment Implementation and Data Collection
Prior to the experiment, the participants filled out a questionnaire to obtain sociodemographic data, including occupation, income, household size, etc. Table 1 describes the different steps of the experiment. First, in order to familiarize participants with the software, each participant was asked to describe her previous day's daily food intake by selecting a 'yesterday food basket' using the food-purchasing software. Then, the participants were asked to design a 'tomorrow food basket' by selecting all the food that they intended to consume over the next 24 h. Three alternatives were successively designed: (i) the 'baseline', where foods were posted at their observed prices (i.e. no policy implementation), and (ii) the 'FV policy' and (iii) the 'NP policy', where the observed prices were modified according to price policies tested. The rationale of the price manipulations was not explained to the participants. Before ending the experiment, the participants had to fill out another questionnaire on their height, weight, and potential chronic health disorders.

This experiment involved incentives specific to experimental economics: the participants were informed that their food choices would generate real sales. A subset of the 180 products, which was hidden to them, was placed in the room adjacent to the experimentation room. For all of a subject's choices corresponding to the available products and to a food basket that was selected randomly, the actual portions chosen were bought at the end of the session. Each participant paid for her purchases and went back home with her products.

Data Analyses
The impacts of price policies were measured for the LI and MI groups through the distances of the daily food intakes from the baseline. These impacts were analyzed in terms of (i) quantities of each food-category, including fruit and vegetables, other healthy foods, neutral products and unhealthy products, and (ii) dietary quality indexes.

Different dietary indexes were used. (i) Energy density (ED, in kcal/100 g) was used as an indicator of bad nutritional quality [17]. The food weights and energy contents (beverages excluded) were calculated for each basket by summing the edible weight and the energy content of selected foods. (ii) The Mean Adequacy Ratio (MAR) was used as an indicator of good nutritional quality, as it is a truncated index of the percentage of recommended intakes for several key nutrients [18]. Sixteen positive nutrients were included, notably fibers, proteins, vitamins, minerals, and essential fatty acids [19]. (iii) Particular attention was paid to three nutrients whose intake must be limited in a healthy diet: SFA, sodium and free sugars. Three indicators measuring the percentage of the maximum daily recommended values were calculated for these nutrients.

Results

Sample

Table 2 shows the demographic characteristics of the two participant groups. It highlights significant differences in levels of education, household size and employment. The prevalence of overweight and chronic health disorders was as expected (i.e. more overweight and more disorders for LI women), but neither of them was significant. Only the percentage of women who never practiced any sport was significantly different between the two groups, as the likelihood of practicing sport was significantly higher among MI women. The energy contents of the food baskets presented no significant differences between the income groups.

Table 2. Demographic and health characteristics of participants; energy content of daily food baskets purchased at baseline and under each price policy by each group of women; food content of the baseline baskets of each group (mean ± standard deviation or %)

	LI group (n = 95)	MI group (n = 33)	p value[1]
Demographic characteristics			
Age, years	35.3±7.0	34.8±6.9	0.3509
Education, years	4.6±2.1	6.5±2.2	0.0001
Employed, %	17	70	<0.0001
Income, EUR per consumption unit	572±140	1,500±444	<0.0001
Household size, n	3.8±1.6	2.8±1.4	0.0011
Health characteristics			
Body mass index[2]	25.3±5.8	23.9±4.3	0.1921
Overweight, %	44	33	0.2744
At least one chronic health disorder[3], %	20	12	0.3098
No sport, %	58	24	0.0149
Energy content, kcal			
Learning	1,487±584	1,458±679	0.4957
Baseline	1,555±949	1,456±643	0.4546
FV policy	1,471±575	1,409±698	0.2926
NP policy	1,400±570	1,364±550	0.3085

[1] Against the null hypothesis of no differences between income groups (Wilcoxon rank-sum test or χ^2 test). [2] Calculated from height and weight as stated by participants. [3] As stated by participants. Three questions were asked: 'Are you suffering from high blood pressure? Cholesterol? Diabetes?'

Price Policies' Impacts on Quantities

The food baskets selected by LI women, compared with those selected by the MI group, contained fewer fruits and vegetables, fewer 'other healthy products', and more unhealthy products (table 3). Fruit and vegetables were increased with both policies and in both income groups. Other healthy products were increased only for the MI group, and the magnitude of this increase was greater with the NP policy than with the FV policy. Neutral products significantly decreased with both policies, although none of the policies modified the prices of these products. Unhealthy products decreased only under the NP policy, and the reduction was significant only for the MI group. Ultimately, the volumes purchased by the LI group were double those purchased by the MI group.

Price Policies' Impacts on Diet Quality

At baseline, the food baskets selected by the LI women appeared less healthy than those selected by the MI women: they had significantly higher ED and lower MAR (table 4). The three negative nutrients (SFA, sodium and free sugars) exhibited no significant differences. Both policies significantly improved the ED and the MAR for both income groups. However, the magnitude of the improvement was often lower

Table 3. Food content of the daily food baskets purchased at baseline and under each price policy by each group of women (mean ± standard deviation)

	LI (n = 95)	MI (n = 33)	Difference LI-MI
Fruit and vegetables, g			
Baseline	410.3±22.9	514.7±15.5	−104.3[a]
FV policy	511.5±61.3***	712.0±74.4***	−200.5[a]
NP policy	532.6±89.0***	642.9±85.9***	−110.2[a]
Other products, g			
Baseline	518.7±34.0	703.6±23.0	−184.9[a]
FV policy	513.7±9.5, n.s.	737.0±11.5***	−223.3[a]
NP policy	508.9±52.3**	836.4±50.5***	−327.5[a]
Neutral products, g			
Baseline	727.5±93.9	902.9±63.7	−175.5[a]
FV policy	670.0±45.7***	830.7±55.4***	−160.7[a]
NP policy	674.8±90.0***	810.1±86.9***	−135.2[a]
Unhealthy products, g			
Baseline	322.9±309.1	196.0±209.4	+126.9[a]
FV policy	309.3±187.4, n.s.	191.0±227.4, n.s.	+118.4[a]
NP policy	253.5±134.1, n.s.	126.8±130.0***	+126.7[a]

, * Critical probability ($p < 0.05$, $p < 0.01$ Wilcoxon signed-rank test) for difference from baseline values. [a] Critical probability ($p < 0.01$ Wilcoxon rank-sum test) for difference between groups. Values are the mean and the standard deviation of the quantities adjusted for the total energy content of the selected daily basket. Except for fruit and vegetables, foods are classified as other healthy, neutral and unhealthy products according to a nutrient profiling described in the Materials and Methods section.

among LI women. Thus, the two indices remained less favorable for LI women than MI women. The NP policy induced differences in SFA and sodium levels between the income groups that were not present at baseline and that were unfavorable to the LI women. None of the price policies had a significant impact on free sugar quantities, but the FV policy induced a difference that was not present at baseline and that was unfavorable to the LI women.

Discussion

The present results confirmed that the food choices of LI groups are less healthy than those of MI groups. In addition, they showed that the two food price policies tested, i.e. the FV policy and the NP policy subsidizing healthy products and taxing unhealthy ones, were able to improve the nutritional quality of food choices in both income groups. However, the differences observed at baseline were still present or even greater, which suggests that it will be difficult to narrow this gap with food price policies. Other problems associated with the policies need to be mentioned. (i) Both policies

Table 4. Nutritional characteristics of the daily food baskets at baseline and under each price policy (mean ± standard deviation)

	LI (n = 95)	MI (n = 33)	Difference LI-MI
ED, kcal per 100 g			
Baseline	141.8±32.5	122.6±22.0	19.2[a]
FV policy	134.3±22.2**	106.4±27.0***	27.9[a]
NP policy	131.5±17.9***	107.2±17.3***	24.3[a]
MAR, % adequacy per day			
Baseline	55.2±14.2	61.1±9.7	–5.89[a]
FV policy	58.4±11.0***	63.4±13.4**	–4.97[b]
NP policy	56.5±12.1**	63.3±11.7**	–6.81[a]
SFA, % of the maximum recommended daily value			
Baseline	116.2±76.2	101.2±51.6	15.0, n.s.
FV policy	107.1±48.4, n.s.	100.9±58.8, n.s.	6.2, n.s.
NP policy	107.9±47.6, n.s.	88.4±46***	19.4[b]
Sodium, % of the maximum recommended daily value			
Baseline	93.2±36.1	92.9±24.5	0.3, n.s.
FV policy	85.6±26.9**	91.8±32.7, n.s.	–6.2, n.s.
NP policy	93.4±24.2, n.s.	85.8±23.4***	7.6[b]
Free sugars, % of the maximum recommended daily value			
Baseline	92.9±88.5	74.4±60.0	18.5, n.s.
FV policy	83.3±42.0, n.s.	65.6±51.0, n.s.	17.6[a]
NP policy	76.7±40.7, n.s.	71.9±39.2, n.s.	4.8, n.s.

, * Critical probability ($p < 0.05$, $p < 0.01$ Wilcoxon signed-rank test) for difference from baseline values. [a, b] Critical probability ($p < 0.01$, $p < 0.05$ Wilcoxon rank-sum test) for difference between groups. Values are the means and the standard deviations of the diet quality indicators adjusted for the total energy content of the selected daily basket.

induced a decrease in purchasing of neutral products. This is an unwanted effect, which may indicate that the increase in subsidized products is not only to the detriment of charged products. (ii) The policies had hardly any effect on SFA, sodium and free sugars.

Some limitations of the method used in the present study must be noted. Even though the participants were not informed of the nutritional objectives of the experiment, some of them may have behaved as they thought they ought to, in order to please the experimentalist, by avoiding unhealthy products and preferring healthy ones. The incentive mechanisms of experimental economics, i.e. the obligation to buy the products chosen at the end of the session, were expected to limit the social desirability bias. The second limitation may stem from the constitution of the samples, which are convenience samples and not representative samples. However, beyond the major eligibility criterion (income level), these samples highlight the expected socioeconomic differences in terms of education, occupation, and the practice of sport. The third limitation stems from the experimental context itself. This enables us to reach the objective of controlling the environment and reducing noise in the lab, but in doing so we may also highlight the (single) change of context. In addition, whereas wide-ranging taxes and subsidies were selected in this study, it is unlikely that actual policies would use such high rates, which could be judged politically unacceptable.

In spite of such methodological limitations, the present results about fruit and vegetable subsidies, i.e. an increase in their consumption and improvements in diet, are convergent with studies showing an increase in fruit and vegetable purchases when they are subsidized in the literature [20, 21]. Many simulation studies using price elasticity data derived from econometric calculations have shown that taxing unhealthy foods has negligible effects on the nutritional quality of the whole diet [9, 22–24]. Yet, food tax combined with appropriate subsidies could be more efficient [25, 26]. The present results confirm the effectiveness of a policy that consists of simultaneously subsidizing healthy products and taxing unhealthy ones. Combining food taxes with subsidies was also considered as a good method for alleviating potential regressivity 'by enabling consumers to switch to more healthy products without incurring additional costs' [27]. However, we have shown here that such a price manipulation may increase income disparities in financial and nutritional benefits. From this point of view, our results converge with Nordström and Thunström's [28] modeling showing that tax reforms aimed at improving dietary quality seem to have a positive health effect across all income groups, except the lowest income group.

The present results do not converge with the conclusions of two studies that stated that the beneficial nutritional effects of food tax reforms are more pronounced for LI earners [6, 26]. Two reasons may explain the discrepancy between the present experimental study and these econometric studies. First, in this study, LI earners were among the poorest deciles of incomes of the French population and were therefore probably poorer than people from the lowest social class (among five) in the Danish study [6] and people from the lowest income quintile in the British study [26]. Second, these studies considered an aggregate representative consumer and did not take into account all differences in individual preferences. Nnoaham et al. [26] assumed that price elasticities are the same for all income groups. Both studies did not consider that some individuals do not consume one or more of the foods. In the present study, food choices were recorded for each individual and for each price condition. Therefore, the heterogeneity of preferences among consumers and individual food substitutions in response to price changes were directly observed, whereas in econometric studies they are dependent on assumptions.

Overall, the present study shows that price policies that attempt to alter individual food behaviors are not effective in reducing social inequalities in nutrition. The present results are consistent with the findings of Frohlich and Potvin [29] showing that improving the health of the overall population may increase health disparities between social groups: those who were formerly at a lower exposure to risk derive more benefits than those who were formerly at a greater exposure to risk. Given the widening gap in socioeconomic inequalities in health in Europe [30], including in France [31], more research is needed on the possible differential impacts of a food tax reform on individuals, depending on their socioeconomic positions and incomes.

References

1 WHO Regional Office for Europe: The challenge of obesity in the WHO European Region and the strategies for response. Branca F, Nikogosian H, Lobstein T (eds). 2007. http://www.euro.who.int/document/E89858.pdf (accessed February 6, 2016).

2 Darmon N, Drewnowski A: Contribution of food prices and diet cost to socioeconomic disparities in diet quality: a systematic review and analysis. Nutr Rev 2015;73:643–660.

3 Darmon N, Drewnowski A: Does social class predict diet quality? Am J Clin Nutr 2008;87:1107–1117.

4 Wall J, Mhurchu CN, Blakely T, Rodgers A, Wilton J: Effectiveness of monetary incentives in modifying dietary behavior:a review of randomized, controlled trials. Nutr Rev 2006;64:518–531.

5 Schroeter C, Lusk J, Tyner W: Determining the impact of food price and income changes on body weight. J Health Econ 2008;27:45–68.

6 Smed S, Jensen JD, Denver S: Socio-economic characteristics and the effect of taxation as a health policy instrument. Food Policy 2007;32:624–639.

7 Mytton O, Gray A, Rayner M, Rutter H: Could targeted food taxes improve health? J Epidemiol Community Health 2007;61:689–694.

8 Smed S, Robertson A: Are taxes on fatty foods having their desired effects on health? BMJ 2012;345:e6885.

9 Allais O, Bertail P, Nichèle V: The effects of a fat tax on French households purchases: a nutritional approach. Am J Agric Econ 2010;92:228–245.

10 Franck C, Grandi SM, Eisenberg MJ: Taxing junk food to counter obesity. Am J Public Health 2013; 103:1949–1953.

11 Andreyeva T, Long MW, Brownell KD: The impact of food prices on consumption: a systematic review of research on the price elasticity of demand for food. Am J Public Health 2010;100:216–222.

12 Dallongeville J, Dauchet L, de Mouzon O, Requillart V, Soler LG: Increasing fruit and vegetable consumption: a cost-effectiveness analysis of public policies. Eur J Public Health 2011;21:69–73.

13 Davis DD, Holt CA: Experimental Economics. Princeton, Princeton University Press, 1993.

14 Plott C, Smith V: Handbook of Experimental Economics Results. Amsterdam, North Holland, 2008.

15 Friedman D, Sunder S: Experimental Methods: A Primer for Economists. New York, Cambridge University Press, 1994.

16 Darmon N, Vieux F, Maillot M, Volatier JL, Martin A: Nutrient profiles discriminate between foods according to their contribution to nutritionally adequate diets: a validation study using linear programming and the SAIN, LIM system. Am J Clin Nutr 2009;89:1227–1236.

17 Ledikwe JH, Blanck HM, Khan LK, Serdula MK, Seymour JD, Tohill BC, Rolls BJ: Low-energy-density diets are associated with high diet quality in adults in the United States. J Am Diet Assoc 2006;106:1172–1180.

18 Guthrie HA, Scheer JC: Validity of a dietary score for assessing nutrient adequacy. J Am Diet Assoc 1981; 78:240–245.

19 Darmon N, Darmon M, Maillot M, Drewnowski A: A nutrient density standard for vegetables and fruits: nutrients per calorie and nutrients per unit cost. J Am Diet Assoc 2005;105:1881–1887.

20 Herman DR, Harrison GG, Afifi AA, Jenks E: Effect of a targeted subsidy on intake of fruits and vegetables among low-income women in the Special Supplemental Nutrition Program for Women, Infants, and Children. Am J Public Health 2008;98:98–105.

21 Epstein LH, Jankowiak N, Nederkoorn C, Raynor HA, French SA, Finkelstein E: Experimental research on the relation between food price changes and food-purchasing patterns: a targeted review. Am J Clin Nutr 2012;95:789–809.

22 Caraher M, Cowburn G: Taxing food: implications for public health nutrition. Public Health Nutr 2005; 8:1242–1249.

23 Chouinard HH, Davis DE, LaFrance JT, Perloff JM: Fat taxes: big money for small change. Forum Health Econ Policy 2007;10:article 2.

24 Kuchler F, Tegene A, Harris JM: Taxing snack foods: manipulating diet quality or financing information programs? Rev Agric Econ 2005;27:4–20.

25 Jensen JD, Smed S: Cost-effective design of economic instruments in nutrition policy. Int J Behav Nutr Phys Act 2007;4:10.

26 Nnoaham KE, Sacks G, Rayner M, Mytton O, Gray A: Modelling income group differences in the health and economic impacts of targeted food taxes and subsidies. Int J Epidemiol 2009;38:1324–1333.
27 Thow A, Jan S, Leeder S, Swinburn B: The effect of fiscal policy on diet, obesity and chronic disease: a systematic review. Bull World Health Organ 2010; 88:609–614.
28 Nordström J, Thunström L: Can targeted food taxes and subsidies improve the diet? Distributional effects among income groups. Food Policy 2011;36: 259–271.
29 Frohlich KL, Potvin L: Transcending the known in public health practice: the inequality paradox: the population approach and vulnerable populations. Am J Public Health 2008;98:216–221.
30 Mackenbach JP, Bos V, Andersen O, Cardano M, Costa G, Harding S, Reid A, Hemström O, Valkonen T, Kunst AE: Widening socioeconomic inequalities in mortality in six Western European countries. Int J Epidemiol 2003;32:830–837.
31 LeClerc A, Chastang JF, Menvielle G, Luce D: Socioeconomic inequalities in premature mortality in France: have they widened in recent decades? Soc Sci Med 2006;62:2035–2045.

Nicole Darmon
UMR NORT (Nutrition, Obésité et Risque Thrombotique)
INRA1260, INSERM 1062, Aix-Marseille Université
Faculté de Médecine de la Timone, 27 Bd Jean Moulin
FR–13385 Marseille Cedex 05 (France)
E-Mail nicole.darmon@univ-amu.fr

Biesalski HK, Black RE (eds): Hidden Hunger. Malnutrition and the First 1,000 Days of Life: Causes, Consequences and Solutions. World Rev Nutr Diet. Basel, Karger, 2016, vol 115, pp 46–53
DOI: 10.1159/000442070

Income Inequality and Child Mortality in Wealthy Nations

David Collison

Accounting and Finance, School of Business, University of Dundee, Dundee, UK

Abstract

This chapter presents evidence of a relationship between child mortality data and socio-economic factors in relatively wealthy nations. The original study on child mortality that is reported here, which first appeared in a UK medical journal, was undertaken in a school of business by academics with accounting and finance backgrounds. The rationale explaining why academics from such disciplines were drawn to investigate these issues is given in the first part of the chapter. The findings related to child mortality data were identified as a special case of a wide range of social and health indicators that are systematically related to the different organisational approaches of capitalist societies. In particular, the so-called Anglo-American countries show consistently poor outcomes over a number of indicators, including child mortality. Considerable evidence has been adduced in the literature to show the importance of income inequality as an explanation for such findings. An important part of the chapter is the overview of a relatively recent publication in the epidemiological literature entitled *The Spirit Level: Why Equality Is Better for Everyone*, which was written by Wilkinson and Pickett.

The author of this chapter is an academic in a business school with a background in accounting and finance. This is not a common background for a contributor to the Hidden Hunger conference on which this book is based. Therefore, the first part of this chapter will try to explain how the author's interest in this area developed and how such a perspective may be relevant to child health (and that of wider society).

Child mortality is, of course, an issue whose main focus is on the unacceptably high figures in poor countries. However, it is also a social indicator that is reported for developed industrial countries, and within these countries, systematic variations exist. These variations correlate very closely to different 'varieties of capitalism', and it is the contention of this chapter that these variations amount to a serious indictment of one form of capitalism in particular.

What has been termed the 'Anglo-American' or 'stock-market' form of capitalism can be contrasted with what has been called 'welfare' or 'stakeholder capitalism' [1–4]. Alternative and largely equivalent descriptions of these broad classifications are given by Hall and Soskice [5] and Hall and Gingerich [6]. These authors used the terms 'liberal market economies' (LMEs) and 'co-ordinated market economies'. The former group, the LMEs, comprises Australia, Canada, Ireland, New Zealand, the UK and the USA. Amongst this group, the UK and the USA have been identified as relatively 'pure' cases. Amongst the co-ordinated market economies, Germany, Austria, the Nordic countries and Japan are cited as being particularly characteristic of this type, although the term arguably covers all advanced economies that are not in the LME group. These two groups of countries have also been distinguished by reference to their legal origins, with a 'common law' framework being identified with Anglo-American socio-economic traditions and variations of a 'civil law' approach being identified with those of the other countries.

What lies at the heart of the differences between these groups of countries is, it has been argued, the way that corporations operate within the legal frameworks and cultural traditions of the countries concerned. In particular, the question 'In whose interests should companies be run?' is key to the fundamental distinction between the two broad forms of capitalism discussed above. Indeed, Hall and Soskice, in a study [5] intended to link comparative political economy with business studies, stated that they regard 'companies as the crucial actors in a capitalist economy' (p. 6).

This important difference between corporate philosophies can be simply described: the Anglo-American tradition is that companies should be run in the interests of shareholders (in other words, they should be run to maximise shareholder value). By contrast, the social market tradition is based on balancing the interests of a range of stakeholders. Which of these two approaches is in the best interests of society as a whole may be seen as a political question, but it is also a question that can be very clearly answered by empirical evidence, as discussed later in this chapter.

However, in the author's experience, this question is rarely considered or even acknowledged in the Anglo-American business culture. Instead, the maximisation of shareholder value is taken for granted in the teaching of accounting and finance as the incontestable objective of corporations.

Variations in accounting traditions reflect these traditional differences. In broad terms, the German accounting tradition, for example, emphasises prudent valuations, protection for creditors, consequent limitations on dividends to shareholders and the retention of funds for reinvestment in the company. Anglo-American accounting practices emphasise the provision of 'decision useful information' to investors in order to help them maximise the returns from their share ownership. Typically, these characteristics are accompanied by more distributions of funds to investors with commensurately less reinvestment in companies.

The claimed superiority of the Anglo-American approach extends to international accounting standards. In a report by a UK professional body of accountants [7], it was argued that politicians should 'agree to give up their sovereignty over accounting standards in favour of an international but essentially private sector body' (p. 16). The private sector body in question is the International Accounting Standards Board (IASB), which evolved from its predecessor, the International Accounting Standards Committee (IASC). The formation of the IASC took place in 1973, the same year that the UK joined the European Economic Community (the forerunner of the European Union), and it has been claimed in the academic accounting literature that the IASC was formed in order to resist the possible spread of a European accounting culture to the UK.

Both the IASC and the IASB are widely perceived as spreading an Anglo-American accounting culture through their standards. In 2005, the chair of the European Parliament's Economics and Monetary Affairs Committee stated that the role of the US-dominated IASB could lead to 'the financialisation of the [world] economy', which could itself result in 'management boards being more concerned about financial markets than about the true economic well-being of the company' [8].

The unquestioned superiority of the Anglo-American version of capitalism, and its approach to corporate governance in particular, has been a regular feature of the business media in LMEs. Continental European countries have been described as 'overburdened by social security commitments ... [and where] shareholder value cannot be released as aggressively ... as in the US' [9]. Financial Times (FT) editorials have prescribed for Japan 'the discipline of modern management and accounting' [10] and noted 'social barriers' to 'widespread restructuring' [11]. A report in the FT [12] described deregulation of European labour markets continuing at a 'snail's pace' as 'treasured social cohesion' impeded 'a more robust, Anglo-Saxon style of capitalism'. An FT feature on the Japanese economy chastised Japan for its 'cherished social contract', noting that it was no longer viable and calling for 'a more flexible labour market' [13].

The dismissive tone of such media commentary regarding social criteria prompted the author and colleagues to make a comparative investigation into social outcomes. The particular metric investigated was child mortality, as the ability to nurture children seemed to be as good a single measure as any for assessing the health of a society. Additionally, relevant data were also readily available from the United Nation's Children's Fund (UNICEF). The resulting study of under-5 child mortality in the 24 richest member countries of the Organisation for Economic Co-Operation and Development was published in the *Journal of Public Health* [14].

There were three key findings in that paper. First, when ranked by child mortality, the worst countries were the six above-described Anglo-American LMEs. The worst of all were the two countries described (see above) as being the most pure LME cases:

these were the USA (8 deaths per 1,000 up to the age of 5) and the UK (with a figure of 6.5). The best six countries were the Nordic countries and Japan (Sweden was the best with a figure of 3.25). The next 12 countries with respect to performance comprised continental European countries and the Republic of Korea, with rates ranging from 5 to 5.5. These figures were 4-year averages for the years 2001–2004 based on UNICEF surveys published in the years 2003–2006.

The second main finding was that there was a very strong correlation (significant at the 0.1% level) between child mortality figures and measures of income inequality.

Third, the relative ranking of the LMEs had deteriorated over time. The UNICEF figures allowed a longitudinal analysis to be made, and it was clear that, several decades earlier, the Anglo-American countries had occupied middle or upper positions in the equivalent relative ranking (it should be noted that all countries had improved their absolute performance). This period of worsening relative performance has seen the development of neo-liberalism and the increasingly shrill Anglo-American emphasis on maximising returns to shareholders.

More Correlations between Income Inequality and Poor Health and Social Indicators

During the course of the work reported in the *Journal of Public Health* [14], it became apparent to the authors that child mortality was a special case of a much more general phenomenon amongst relatively wealthy countries, whereby income inequality had been shown to be strongly correlated with a wide range of social indicators. In this context, the work of the social epidemiologist Richard Wilkinson has been particularly important and influential. In their recent book entitled *The Spirit Level: Why Equality Is Better for Everyone* [15], Wilkinson and Pickett summarise much of the work that has been conducted in this area by themselves and others. As with the child mortality study reported above, the correlations they report concern the relatively rich developed economies. In addition to child mortality, they show 'a strong relationship between inequality and many different health outcomes'. These outcomes include life expectancy, teenage births, obesity, mental illness, drug and alcohol addiction, homicides, imprisonment levels, trust, attainment in maths and literacy, and social mobility. Figure 1 reports the relationships between income inequality and an index based on each of these indicators.

It should be noted that, amongst the countries studied, neither health nor social problems are correlated to national income per head – see figure 2. Social and health outcomes are indeed related to per capita income as it rises from poverty levels to those of the developed countries, but there comes a point, beyond the 'epidemiological transition', when further increases in income have no observable effect. Beyond that point, what matters is the income distribution within countries rather than be-

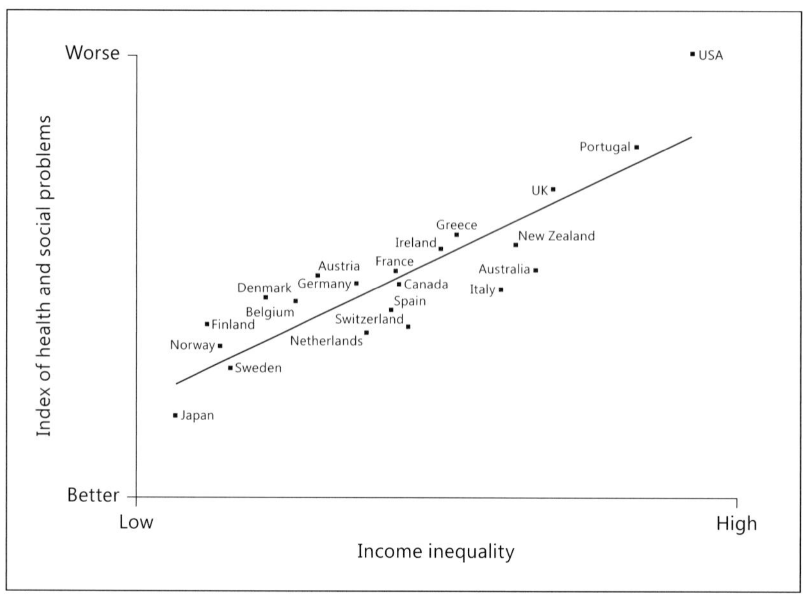

Fig. 1. Adapted from Wilkinson and Pickett [15, p. 20].

tween countries. The USA provide a clear example of a country with a very high level of per capita income but with particularly poor health and social outcomes.

Another key point, emphasised by Wilkinson and Pickett, is demonstrated in figure 3 below. The research summarised in figure 3 exemplifies a common finding that relatively better indicators in less unequal countries are not only found amongst the least well-off levels of society but also can persist across all levels. This finding is reflected in the subtitle of the work by Wilkinson and Pickett [15], which reads *Why Equality Is Better for Everyone.*

Evidence on Causation

Differing health outcomes that have been correlated with income inequality (typically based on international comparisons and also on comparisons of different states within the USA) might immediately lead to the inference that differences in material well-being are the fundamental cause. However, the evidence of poorer outcomes occurring at all levels of society in more unequal countries and the lack of correlations with per capita incomes point to a less obvious, but perhaps even more important, source of causation. Wilkinson and Pickett [15] argue that the 'biology of chronic stress is a plausible pathway which helps us to understand why unequal societies are almost always unhealthy societies' (p. 87).

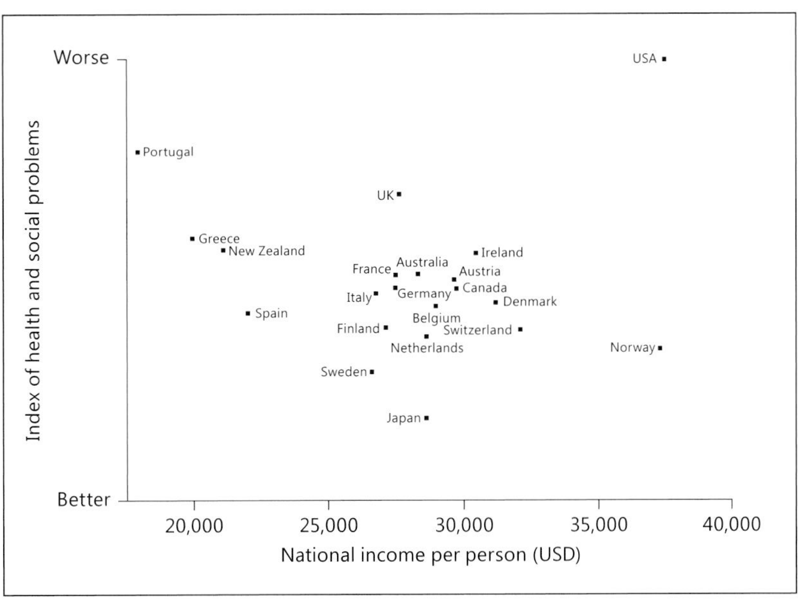

Fig. 2. Adapted from Wilkinson and Pickett [15, p. 21].

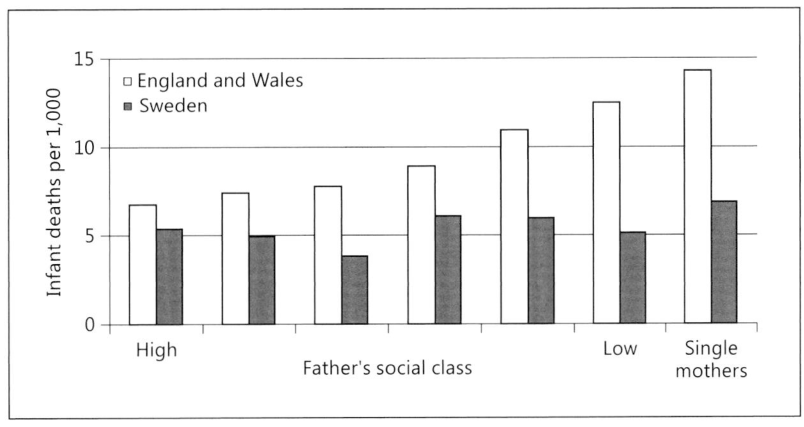

Fig. 3. Adapted from Wilkinson and Pickett [15, p. 179].

The details of their findings regarding causation go beyond the scope of this chapter, but Wilkinson and Pickett cite a range of studies from different cultural contexts to support their argument. Physiological evidence is also adduced, whereby psychosocial factors affect, in turn, the psyche, the neural system and the immune system. In particular, significant evidence is based on the effects of two hormones, cortisol and oxytocin.

This chapter was motivated by an investigation into child mortality, and it seems appropriate to return to that issue to update the evidence on the relative figures that were reported by Collison et al. [14]. The most recent equivalent data based on averaging UNICEF's figures for 2011 and 2012 still show a similar picture to those for 2001–2004, with five of the bottom six places occupied by Anglo-American countries. The exception to this ranking is Ireland, which has improved its relative position. The top places are still occupied by mainly Nordic countries, together with Japan and now also Luxembourg. Again, it should be emphasised that all 24 countries have improved in absolute terms. The complete listing in ascending order of the average 2011–2012 child mortality figures is as follows: Iceland (2.25), Luxembourg (2.6), Sweden (2.9), Finland (2.95), Norway (3.05), Japan (3.20), Portugal (3.7), Denmark (3.85), Italy (3.85), Germany (4.00), Ireland (4.00), the Netherlands (4.00), France (4.05), Austria (4.10), Belgium (4.15), Switzerland (4.20), Republic of Korea (4.25), Spain (4.60), Greece (4.7), Australia (4.9), the UK (5.05), Canada (5.3), New Zealand (5.95), and the USA (7.25).

In light of the evidence cited above, one might ask why the Anglo-American business culture is held up as an example to follow. Arguably, this is simply because of the influence of dominant vested interests, as reflected in some of the examples drawn from the FT. Such influence is not new; indeed, Adam Smith, who has been called the 'father of economics', stated in his famous work *The Wealth of Nations* [16] that 'the clamour and sophistry of merchants and manufacturers easily persuade ... that the private interest of a part, and of a subordinate part of the society is the general interest of the whole' (Bk. I, Ch. X, Pt. II, p. 101).

Finally, and I would argue regrettably, there is evidence to suggest that of the two kinds of capitalism outlined above, it is the Anglo-American version that is spreading to other societies, rather than vice versa. A review of that evidence is beyond the scope of this chapter; however, to cite one example, a 2003 study by Lane [17] concluded that Germany 'is in the process of converging towards the Anglo-American model' (p. 79), which would have 'far-reaching practical consequences ... increasing the level of social inequality in German society' (p. 98). She also argued that such change is not inevitable. I hope that greater awareness of the social evidence will not only make such a process less likely in Germany and elsewhere but also help to reverse it.

References

1 Albert M: Capitalism against Capitalism (transl. by Paul Haviland). London, Whurr Publishers, 1993.
2 Coates D: Models of Capitalism. Cambridge, Polity Press, 2000.
3 Dore R: Stock Market Capitalism: Welfare Capitalism. Oxford, Oxford University Press, 2000.
4 Hutton W: The World We're In. London, Abacus, 2003.
5 Hall PA, Soskice D: Varieties of Capitalism: The Institutional Foundations of Comparative Advantage. New York, Oxford University Press, 2001.
6 Hall PA, Gingerich DW: Varieties of capitalism and institutional complementarities in the political economy: an empirical analysis. Br J Political Science 2009;39:449–482.

7 ICAS (Institute of Chartered Accountants of Scotland): Principles Not Rules: A Question of Judgement. Edinburgh, Technical Policy Board, ICAS, 2006.
8 Wolfe J: Pointing the finger. Accounting and Business, June 2006, pp 44–46.
9 Riley B: Shareholder value revives in Germany's graveyard. Financial Times, Nov 21, 1996, p 21.
10 Mori's regret. Editorial. Financial Times, Aug 1, 2000, p 18.
11 Japan Inc. Editorial. Financial Times, Oct 19, 1999, p 22.
12 Plender J: When capital collides with labour. Financial Times, Oct 24, 1997, p 18.
13 Nakamoto M: Revolution coming, ready or not. Financial Times, Oct 24, 1997, p 18.
14 Collison DJ, Dey CR, Hannah G, Stevenson LA: Income inequality and child mortality in wealthy nations. J Public Health 2007;29:114–117.
15 Wilkinson R, Pickett K: The Spirit Level: Why Equality Is Better for Everyone. London, Penguin Books, 2010.
16 Smith A: An Inquiry into the Nature and Causes of the Wealth of Nations ('The Wealth of Nations'). London/New York, George Routledge & Sons, 1776/1880.
17 Lane C: Changes in corporate governance of German corporations: convergence to the Anglo-American model? Competition Change 2003;7:79–100.

Prof. David Collison
School of Business
University of Dundee
Dundee, DD1 4HN, Scotland (UK)
E-Mail d.j.collison@dundee.ac.uk

Biesalski HK, Black RE (eds): Hidden Hunger. Malnutrition and the First 1,000 Days of Life: Causes, Consequences and Solutions. World Rev Nutr Diet. Basel, Karger, 2016, vol 115, pp 54–60
DOI: 10.1159/000442072

Understanding Food Insecurity in the USA and Canada: Potential Insights for Europe

Craig Gundersen

Department of Agricultural and Consumer Economics, University of Illinois, Urbana, IL, USA

Abstract

Food insecurity is a leading nutrition-related health care issue in the USA due to the magnitude of the problem (almost 50 million Americans are food insecure) and its association with a wide array of negative health and other outcomes. Alongside this interest in the USA, there has also been growing interest in Canada. In contrast, food insecurity has received less attention in Europe. Nevertheless, there is both direct and indirect evidence that food insecurity and its attendant consequences are present in Europe. Given the similarities between the USA, Canada, and Europe, previous research can offer numerous insights into the causes and consequences of food insecurity in Europe and possible directions to address these through measurement and public policies. I first cover the methods used to measure food insecurity in the USA and Canada. In both countries, a series of 18 questions in the Core Food Security Module are used to identify whether a household is food insecure. I then briefly cover the current extent of food insecurity in each country along with some discussion of the recent history of food insecurity. A central advantage to using the Core Food Security Module in Europe is that the measure has been proven useful in other high-income countries, and using a standardized measure would allow for cross-country comparisons. I next cover two large-scale food assistance programs from the USA, the Supplemental Nutrition Assistance Program (formerly known as the Food Stamp Program) and the National School Lunch Program. For each, I summarize how the program is structured, how eligibility is established, and how participation proceeds. Europe has generally used income-based assistance programs to improve the well-being of low-income households; I consider a couple of reasons for why food assistance programs may also be worth considering.

Introduction

Food insecurity (i.e., a household-level economic and social condition of limited access to food) has arguably emerged as the leading nutrition-related health care issue in the USA for two central reasons. First, the magnitude of the problem is enormous. The extent of food insecurity is at an all-time high, and despite the end of the Great Recession, rates have not returned to the levels of 2007. In 2013, 15.8% of all persons (49.1 million) lived in food-insecure households and 20.0% of children in America (15.8 million) lived in food-insecure households [1]. Second, extensive evidence shows that food insecurity is associated with many negative health consequences [for a review, see 2]. There has also been growing recognition of food insecurity and its consequences in Canada (http://nutritionalsciences.lamp.utoronto.ca/).

Unlike the USA and Canada, less attention has been paid to this issue across Europe, nor have there been concerted policy interventions to alleviate food insecurity. One reason might be that food insecurity does not exist across Europe or, if it does, it is of too small of a magnitude to register as an important issue. This seems unlikely as a reason insofar as, at least judging from average income levels and poverty rates, there should be nontrivial levels of food insecurity in Europe with high levels in some countries. Alongside this indirect evidence, there is some direct evidence, discussed below, which is consistent with food insecurity in Europe.

If there is to become an increased awareness of food insecurity in Europe, there are some insights that can be drawn from US and Canadian food insecurity literature that are likely to be relevant. In this paper, I cover two of these. First, I describe how food insecurity is measured in the USA and Canada. Within this discussion, I briefly describe the extent and distribution of food insecurity. Second, I review the extensive literature demonstrating the success of the largest food assistance programs in the USA, the Supplemental Nutrition Assistance Program (SNAP, formerly known as the Food Stamp Program) and the National School Lunch Program (NSLP) in alleviating food insecurity.

Measuring Food Insecurity

The measurement of food insecurity in the USA and Canada is based on the same set of questions from the Core Food Security Module (CFSM). The measure consists of 18 questions for households with children and a subset of 10 of these for households without children, with each condition owing to financial constraints. Some of the conditions are as follows: 'I worried whether our food would run out before we got money to buy more' (the least severe item); 'Did you or the other adults in your household ever cut the size of your meals or skip meals because there wasn't enough money for food'; 'Were you ever hungry but did not eat because you couldn't afford enough food', and 'Did a child in the household ever not eat for a full day because you couldn't afford enough food' (the most severe item for households with children).

Using these 18 questions, households are delineated into the following categories: (a) food secure (defined as cases in which all household members had access at all times to enough food for an active, healthy life), (b) low food secure (cases in which at least some household members were uncertain of having, or unable to acquire, enough food because they had insufficient money and other resources for food), and (c) very low food secure (cases in which one or more household members were hungry, at least some time during the year, because they could not afford enough food). Households responding negatively to 2 or fewer questions are food secure, those responding affirmatively to 3–7 questions are classified as low food secure (3–5 questions for households without children), and those responding affirmatively to 8 or more questions are classified as very low food secure (6 or more for households without children). In most research and policy discussions, the latter two categories of low and very low food secure are combined and called food insecure. In some applications, however, a broader measure of food insecurity is implemented, which classifies households as marginally food insecure if they answer affirmatively to at least 1 question.

In Canada, the same set of questions is used, but the cutoffs for the different food insecurity categories are, in general, less strict. The moderate food insecurity category (roughly similar to low food security in the USA) occurs when there are 2–5 affirmative responses to the adult questions or 2–4 affirmative responses to the child questions, and the severe food insecurity category (roughly very low food security in the USA) occurs when there are 6 or more affirmative responses to the adult questions or 5 or more positive responses to the child questions. The marginal food insecurity category is the same in Canada as in the USA; one affirmative response to either the adult or child questions means a household is in this category.

In the USA, a consistent measure of food insecurity with respect to questions and timing has been available since 2001. From 2001 to 2007, the food insecurity rate for all households was relatively steady at about 12%, and for households with children it was about 17% [1]. For both groups, these rates increased dramatically in 2008. For all households, there was an over 30% increase (from 11.1 to 14.6%), and for households with children, this increased a similar amount (from 16.9 to 22.5%) [1]. Despite the end of the Great Recession in 2009, these rates have remained high for all households and for households with children. As might be expected, there is a great deal of variation across demographic groups with respect to food insecurity rates [for more on these and a broader discussion of the determinants of food insecurity see, e.g., 3, 4].

In Canada, a measure of the extent of food insecurity based on nationally representative data has only been available since 2007. In 2012, the most recent year for which data are available, the food insecurity rate was 8.6%, and the food insecurity among households with children was 10.1% [5]. As in the USA, there was a marked increase due to the Great Recession, but there was not the sharp increase from 2007 to 2008 that was seen in the USA.

There have been uses of the CFSM, or shorter versions, in some European countries, including the UK [6], Ireland [7], and Portugal [8]. While the CFSM has not been widely used, a related measure of food hardship, sometimes called 'food poverty', has been used in some surveys across Europe. This question inquires whether a household is able to afford meat (or a vegetarian equivalent) at least every other day. Those responding negatively are deemed as being in food poverty [9]. Each of these studies demonstrates that food insecurity exists in Europe at nontrivial levels.

Food Assistance Programs in the USA

All European countries have some form of a social safety net that provides temporary or longer-term assistance to those who are poor or in danger of being poor [see 10 for an overview]. These generally take the form of providing cash transfers to families or individuals. The USA also has some programs that are in the form of cash (e.g., the Earned Income Tax Credit), but food assistance programs constitute the central component of the social safety net against hunger. In contrast, in Europe, there is no program like SNAP, although some European countries do have school meal programs. For example, Finland (http://www.oph.fi/download/47657_school_meals_in_finland.pdf) and Portugal [11] have universal school meal programs. Most countries in Europe, however, do not have school meal programs and, in particular, do not have subsidized or free school meals for low-income children.

Supplemental Nutrition Assistance Program

SNAP began with the Food Stamp Act of 1964, and in 1974 it became a national program. Since becoming a national program, SNAP has undergone numerous changes, but its basic structure has stayed the same. It is the largest food assistance program in the USA; in 2013, over 47 million people received SNAP, with benefits totaling almost USD 80 billion (http://www.fns.usda.gov/sites/default/files/pd/SNAPsummary.pdf) [for a broader review of SNAP, see 12].

SNAP benefits can be used to buy food in authorized retail food outlets, which includes virtually all food stores. To receive SNAP benefits, households must both be eligible for and choose to enter the program. To be eligible for SNAP, households first have to meet a monthly gross income test – the household's income (before any deductions) must be under 130% of the poverty line (although some states have set higher thresholds). There are exceptions; for instance, households with at least one elderly member or one disabled member do not have to meet this test. Households then must have a net income below the poverty line, even for states that have set a higher gross income threshold. Net income is calculated as gross income minus certain deductions, including, for example, a 20% earned income deduction and a dependent care deduction. The final SNAP test is that a household's total assets must be less than USD 2,000. Even though some resources are not counted, such as a home, this is often seen as too strict a criterion, and most states now elect to waive this test.

For those who pass the eligibility tests, the amount of SNAP benefits is calculated by multiplying the household's net income by 0.3. The multiplied value is then subtracted from the value of the Thrifty Food Plan, a low-cost, nutritionally adequate food plan, which varies by household size and composition. Though states have discretion over various aspects of SNAP, including the gross income test and the asset test, all benefits are funded by the federal government.

Extensive literature has demonstrated that SNAP leads to reductions in food insecurity [see 13 and references therein] and improvements over other dimensions [e.g., poverty 14]. Despite these benefits, many eligible households do not participate. Nonparticipation reflects three main factors. First, receiving SNAP may carry a stigma due to a person's own distaste for receiving aid, fear of disapproval from others when redeeming SNAP, and/or possible negative reactions from caseworkers [e.g., 15]. Second, transaction costs can diminish the attractiveness of participation, including time spent in or traveling to a SNAP office, the burden of transporting children to the office or paying for childcare, and the cost of transportation. Third, the benefit level can be quite small – for some families, it is as low as USD 10 per month. Given the inverse relationship between income and SNAP benefit levels, this explains why, all else equal, households with incomes closer to the SNAP eligibility threshold are less likely to participate.

National School Lunch Program

The NSLP is a federal assistance program that operates in over 100,000 public and nonprofit private schools across the USA (http://www.fns.usda.gov/sites/default/files/EliMan.pdf). It began in 1946 under the National School Lunch Act and has seen relatively minor changes since. In 2012, more than 31 million students participated in the NSLP. Of these, nearly 17 million received free lunches and slightly over 3 million received reduced-price lunches (the rest paid full price). Along with free food, the federal government gave schools over USD 11 billion in 2012 to reimburse them for the cost of providing these meals.

Eligibility for the NSLP begins at the individual level, insofar as any child at a participating school is potentially eligible (children who are home schooled or who no longer attend school are not). Among children in participating schools, families with incomes at or below 130% of the poverty level are eligible for free meals, and children with household incomes between 130 and 185% of the poverty level are eligible for reduced-price meals, which cannot cost more than 40 cents. In high-poverty areas, the Community Eligibility Option allows schools to provide universal school meals.

The benefits associated with receiving free or reduced-price meals through the NSLP are not trivial. At least as defined by the reimbursement costs to schools, lunch for one child every day for a week is worth about USD 15 [16], and participation in NSLP leads to reductions in food insecurity [17]. Still, a high proportion of eligible children do not participate in the NSLP. This can be ascribed to two main factors. First, as with SNAP, receiving free or reduced-price meals can carry a stigma, so some children or their parents may not want to participate. Second, despite being enrolled, some children, for a myriad of reasons, do not always eat the meals provided. For example, a child might not want the meal served or a parent might decide a meal is not healthy enough. This differs from SNAP – recipients spend virtually all their SNAP benefits because they can decide what foods to purchase.

Conclusion

Food insecurity and its attendant consequences have generated a great deal of interest among researchers, policymakers, and program administrators in the USA and Canada. To date, there has been much more limited interest in these topics in Europe despite some evidence that food insecurity is a problem there as well.

In this paper, I first covered how food insecurity is measured in the USA and Canada. After being appropriately translated, these measures should be applicable to all European countries across different income levels. One advantage to using a standard measure is that it has been widely vetted elsewhere, and this would enable comparisons across Europe.

I next reviewed two food assistance programs that are at the forefront of efforts to reduce food insecurity in the USA. Given the extensive income-based social safety net in many European countries, additional food assistance programs may not be needed in these countries. There are, however, two reasons why these programs may be worth considering. First, at least historically, SNAP has received political support from farmers because it encourages food consumption. Similar support could be generated in Europe by farmers, especially if a food assistance program, for example, provided subsidies for food produced by farmers within a country. Second, in the USA there is always a concern that some children may not be getting enough food to eat, even when their families seemingly have enough money for food. This is one of the justifications for school meal programs – at least then the children have 5 meals a week (10 if breakfast is also supplied) during the school year. If similar concerns exist in Europe about children not getting enough food despite sufficient cash assistance being provided to parents, school meal programs may be one way to address this problem.

Acknowledgments

The work in this paper is supported, in part, by the US Department of Agriculture, National Institute of Food and Agriculture, Hatch project No. ILLU-470-331. I also thank Erin McKee for excellent research assistance.

References

1 Coleman-Jensen A, Gregory C, Singh A: Household Food Security in the United States in 2013. Economic Research Report No. 173. Washington, USDA, Economic Research Service, 2014.
2 Gundersen C, Ziliak J: Food insecurity and health outcomes. Health Aff 2015;34:1830–1839.
3 Gundersen C, Kreider B, Pepper J: The economics of food insecurity in the United States. Appl Econ Perspect Policy 2011;33:281–303.
4 Gundersen C, Ziliak J: Childhood Food Insecurity in the US: Trends, Causes, and Policy Options. Princeton, The Future of Children, 2014.
5 Tarasuk V, Mitchell A, Dachner N: Household Food Insecurity in Canada, 2012. Toronto, Research to Identify Policy Options to Reduce Food Insecurity (PROOF), 2014.
6 Belsky D, Moffitt T, Arseneault L, Melchior M, Caspi A: Context and sequelae of food insecurity in children's development. Am J Epidemiol 2010;172:809–818.
7 Molcho M, Gabhainn S, Kelly C, Friel S, Kelleher C: Food poverty and health among schoolchildren in Ireland: findings from Health Behaviour in School-aged Children (HBSC) study. Public Health Nutr 2007;10:364–370.
8 Alvares L, Amaral T: Food insecurity and associated factors in the Portuguese population. Food Nutr Bull 2014;35:395–402.
9 Looopstra R, Reeves A, Stuckler D: Rising food insecurity in Europe. Lancet 2015;385:2041.
10 Marx I, Nelson K (eds): Minimum Income Protection in Flux. London, Palgrave Macmillan, 2012.
11 Truninger M, Teixeira J, Horta A, da Silva V, Alexandre S: Schools' health education in Portugal: a case study on children's relations with school meals. Educação, Sociedade e Culturas 2013;38:117–133.
12 Bartfeld J, Gundersen C, Smeeding T, Ziliak J (eds): SNAP Matters: How Food Stamps Affect Health and Well Being. Redwood City, Stanford University Press, 2015.
13 Kreider B, Pepper J, Gundersen C, Jolliffe D: Identifying the effects of SNAP (food stamps) on child health outcomes when participation is endogenous and misreported. J Am Stat Assoc 2012;107:958–975.
14 Jolliffe D, Gundersen C, Tiehen L, Winicki J: Food stamp benefits and child poverty. Am J Agric Econ 2005;87:569–581.
15 Stuber J, Schlesinger M: Sources of stigma for means-tested government programs. Soc Sci Med 2006;63:933–945.
16 Bartfeld J: SNAP and the school meal programs; in Bartfeld J, Gundersen C, Smeeding T, Ziliak J (eds): SNAP Matters: How Food Stamps Affect Health and Well Being. Redwood City, Stanford University Press, 2015.
17 Gundersen C, Kreider B, Pepper J: The impact of the National School Lunch Program on child health: a nonparametric bounds analysis. J Econom 2012;166:79–91.

Dr. Craig Gundersen
Department of Agricultural and Consumer Economics
University of Illinois, 324 Mumford Hall
1301 West Gregory Dr., Urbana, IL 61801-3605 (USA)
E-Mail cggunder@illinois.edu

Biesalski HK, Black RE (eds): Hidden Hunger. Malnutrition and the First 1,000 Days of Life:
Causes, Consequences and Solutions. World Rev Nutr Diet. Basel, Karger, 2016, vol 115, pp 61–67
DOI: 10.1159/000444609

Determinants of Child Malnutrition and Infant and Young Child Feeding Approaches in Cambodia

Anika Reinbott • Irmgard Jordan

Institute of Nutritional Sciences, Justus Liebig University Giessen, Giessen, Germany

Abstract

Women's diets often decrease with regard to amounts per meal and day as well as diversity if a household's access to food is limited. The result is a monotonous diet that, in particular, negatively affects women's nutritional status during pregnancy and lactation and, thus, the infant. The infant's diet is of utmost importance, as it needs to meet the nutrient requirements especially during the first 2 years of life, a critical window for the child's healthy development. In Cambodia, infant and young child feeding (IYCF) practices are poor. Preparation of a special complementary meal in addition to breast milk feeds for children aged 6–23 months is often not a common habit. Instead, children eat watery, plain rice porridges that do not meet the nutrient requirements at this young age. A lack of adequate caring practices such as responsive feeding exacerbates the risk of malnutrition. Caregivers are often unaware of the importance of nutrition during the first 2 years of life regarding its effects on children's growth. In 2012, a randomized controlled trial (RCT) was started in two provinces of northern Cambodia: Oddar Meanchey and Preah Vihear. To contribute to reducing child mortality by addressing malnutrition among children 6–23 months of age, the Food and Agriculture Organization of the United Nations (FAO) implemented a nutrition-sensitive agriculture project with nutrition-specific actions, i.e. a nutrition education intervention was embedded in a food security project. Wealth, a child's age, and maternal education were identified as determinants of a child's dietary diversity. The older the child and/or the wealthier the household, the more diverse the child's diet. Maternal education was positively associated with the child's dietary diversity. Household dietary diversity was significantly associated with child dietary diversity in a model including group, child's age, maternal education, and wealth as confounders. The RCT also showed that a 2- to 3-month nutrition education programme carried out by government and community health volunteers as well as local NGOs addressing caregivers with a child between 5 and 18 months of age has great potential to improve IYCF practices. Since no impact on average height-for-age Z-scores could be demonstrated in this RCT, we suggest for Cambodia that (1) more emphasis be put on animal-source food and other protein sources in nutrition education, (2) nutrition education be implemented in the community through trained government and community members including peers as trainers, (3) sessions on family nutrition be included in the curriculum and the continuation of breastfeeding be emphasized, and (4) nutrition education be institutionalized, including continuous in-service training for sustainability.

In the Cambodian context, migration and food insecurity are accepted causes of malnutrition. Additional and increasingly recognized causes are a lack of general knowledge about nutrition and poor awareness of the importance of complementary feeding, with a low educational level as an underlying cause. Insufficient health services and health behaviour contribute to the increased risk of malnutrition [1, 2].

In rural Cambodia, more than 50% of all households do not have access to improved sanitation facilities [1]. All underlying causes, which are subject to seasonal variation, overlap and create a basis for immediate causes. Thus, nutrition-sensitive actions focussing on young child nutrition should include the components of care, food safety, hygiene, and sanitation [3, 4].

The majority of rural Cambodian households live on subsistence farming, producing food mainly for their own consumption rather than for sale. Food security among households in rural Cambodia is highly dependent on seasonal influences; with only one harvest season of the main staple crop (rice) in December, the prevalence of food insecurity rises steadily from March to November [5]. Some families move to the forest for several weeks each year to obtain nourishment from indigenous foods. Sometimes, members of a household migrate to other parts of the country or neighbouring countries to financially support their family. Scenarios like this increase the risk for individual undernutrition: when a household's access to food is limited, women and children are affected the most, i.e. women's diets decrease with regard to amounts per meal and day as well as diversity. Monotonous diets in particular negatively affect women's nutritional status during pregnancy and lactation and, thus, the infant. The infant's diet is of utmost importance, as it needs to meet the nutrient requirements especially during the first 2 years of life, a critical window for the child's healthy development [3, 6, 7].

Infants' Nutritional Status and Infant and Young Child Feeding Practices in Cambodia

Poor nutrition in early infancy leads to undernutrition and is known to be one of the major contributors to stunted growth and child mortality [8]. The reasons for poor nutrition are multifaceted, and so are interventions against it.

According to the 2014 Cambodian Demographic Health Survey (CDHS), 22% of children below 2 years of age are stunted, which is 6% less than in 2010 and 14% less than in 2000 (22% in 2014 vs. 28% in 2010 vs. 36% in 2000) [2, 9, 10]. Thus, stunting remains a major public health issue in Cambodia and is one of the leading causes of morbidity and mortality among children [11]. Its prevalence was found to be less likely among infants younger than 6 months but rapidly increasing until 12–23 months of age [12].

In Cambodia, infant and young child feeding (IYCF) practices are poor. Preparation of a special complementary meal in addition to breast milk feeds for children aged

6–23 months of age is often not a common habit [13, 14]. Instead, children receive watery, plain rice porridges that do not meet the nutrient requirements at this young age. A lack of adequate caring practices such as responsive feeding exacerbates the risk of malnutrition. Caregivers are often unaware of the importance of a nutrious diet during the first 2 years of life regarding its effects on children's growth.

In an analysis of DHS data from 14 low-income countries including Cambodia, a higher dietary diversity was strongly associated with higher height-for-age Z-scores (HAZ) [15]. The same study showed that more than half of Cambodian children aged 18–23 months received foods from 4 or more food groups, which follows the WHO recommendation for minimum dietary diversity (MDD) for children aged 6–23 months of age [15]. If younger children were included, comprising those aged 6–23 months, only 33.5% of the children obtained the MDD[1], 78.6% had an age-appropriate minimum meal frequency (MMF), and only 28.2% received a minimum acceptable diet (MAD) [9, 16].

In 2012, a randomized controlled trial (RCT) was started in two provinces of northern Cambodia: Oddar Meanchey and Preah Vihear. To contribute to reducing child mortality by addressing malnutrition among children 6–23 months of age, the Food and Agriculture Organization of the United Nations (FAO) implemented a nutrition-sensitive agriculture project with nutrition-specific actions, i.e. a nutrition education intervention was embedded in a food security project. In creating market linkages and food security, FAO worked with existing groups of farmers. Besides technical training regarding rice, vegetables, chicken, and cash crops, FAO provided input credits and organized agricultural fairs in the region. After 6 months of agriculture intervention, a nutrition education component was rolled out targeting smallholder farming households with children aged 5–18 months in the villages. Priority was given to those from households already participating in the technical agriculture trainings. Primary caregivers and their children within the respective age range were invited to take part in 7 participatory nutrition education sessions starting in August 2013. A group of 10–15 caregiver-child pairs per village gathered weekly or biweekly and gained knowledge about topics around IYCF including hygiene and sanitation, food safety, preparation of a complementary meal, healthy snacks, dietary diversity, feeding frequency, feeding age-appropriate amounts, and continued breastfeeding.

At baseline, almost all of the 803 children between 0 and 23 months of age had ever been breastfed (99.8%) and were still breastfed at the time of the survey (82%). Breastfeeding was continued for 93% of 186 children aged 12–15 months. Solid, semi-solid, or soft foods were introduced to 94% of 163 children between 6 and 8 months of age. On average, the diet of all children consisted of 3.2 food groups. Overall, the MDD was reached by 44%, the MMF by 70%, and the MAD by 28% only, thus showing rates similar to those of the CDHS 2010 [14].

1 Proportion of children 6–23 months of age who received foods from 4 or more out of 7 food groups; WHO IYCF indicator.

A child feeding index (CFI), an index comprising different IYCF indicators (breastfeeding, bottle feeding, dietary diversity, food, and meal frequency), calculated in the same RCT showed a mean (min., max.) score of 6.7 (1, 10; n = 797) [14]. The mean CFI was highest among the 9- to 11-month-old children (7.9; n = 169), followed by the 6- to 8-month-old (7.5; n = 158). Children between 12 and 23 months of age obtained a mean score of 6.0 (n = 417). Analysing results from an index combining different, important behaviours including weight-scoring, and being disaggregated by age groups, offers the potential to better understand the impact of overall IYCF practices on, for instance, nutritional status. In the RCT, CFI was positively associated with HAZ – but only if the CFI was ≥4. Indicators for the CFI being positively and significantly correlated with age were dietary diversity, food, and meal frequency for the 6- to 8-month-olds. Correlations for older children were either lacking or less strong. Bottle feeding was most prevalent with the 6- to 8-month-olds. Liquids fed in a bottle were mainly water (74%) and infant formula (17%). The number of breastfed children decreased with age ($r = -0.463$, $p < 0.001$) after 1 year of age. In the two younger age groups, the diet mainly consisted of 3 food groups and changed to 3 or 4 food groups for the 12- to 23-month-olds.

Overall, 25% of the children were stunted showing an HAZ below –2 SD, and 4% were severely stunted with an HAZ below –3 SD. Weight-for-age Z-scores below –2 SD were recorded for 23% of the children (n = 803). The prevalence of wasting was 10%, as shown by weight-for-height Z-scores below –2 SD; 1.2% of the cases were severely wasted (n = 802). Five per cent of the children were both stunted and wasted. The mean HAZ scores decreased with age.

Two years after baseline and 1 year after the participatory nutrition education intervention, continued breastfeeding at 12–15 and 20–23 months had decreased in both groups at the community level. In contrast, a higher number of children achieved the MDD and MMF levels and received an MAD in both groups at impact. Consumption of all food groups increased in the intervention group, whereas consumption of β-carotene-rich foods and animal-source food (ASF) decreased in the comparison group.

Overall, consumption of ASF and sugary foods and snacks was high. The children's dietary diversity score (CDDS; 0–7) increased by 0.2 points in the comparison group and by 0.6 in the intervention group. The mean CDDS increased with age in both the intervention and the control group. Children 10–18 months of age in the intervention group showed a higher mean CDDS than did children of the same age in the comparison group. However, this was only significant for 10- to 11-month-olds ($R = 0.23$, $p = 0.007$) and 12- to 13-month-olds ($R = 0.21$, $p = 0.03$). Children 18–23 months of age in both groups showed nearly the same mean CDDS, or those in the comparison group showed higher scores.

The mean (SD) HAZ at baseline was –1.24 (1.03) for the comparison group and –1.27 (1.17) for the intervention group. At impact, the mean (SD) HAZ was –1.25 (1.12) and –1.32 (1.12), respectively, for the comparison and the intervention group.

A vast majority of the infants and young children were growing well or within the lower normal range. The median HAZ did not vary much between the intervention and the comparison group. The average prevalence of stunting at impact was 23.5 and 24.7%, respectively, in the comparison and the intervention group.

Determinants of Children's Dietary Diversity and HAZ

Wealth, a child's age, and maternal education were determinants of a child's dietary diversity. The older the child and/or the wealthier the household, the more diverse the child's diet. Maternal education was positively associated with the child's dietary diversity. Household dietary diversity was significantly associated with child dietary diversity in a model including group, child's age, maternal education, and wealth as confounders. However, although this study revealed associations between a composite CFI and HAZ in infants and young children, more research is required for an assessment of IYCF practices with regard to nutrition education.

Existing Programmes and Health Services in Cambodia

Basic health services are provided by every health centre, and they include immunization, vitamin A supplementation and provision of deworming tablets, as well as antenatal care. Each health centre offered general information and services regarding nutrition for children as well as pregnant or lactating women. Nutrition activities in the respective health centres were mainly dependent on support from NGOs in terms of training, provision of materials, and coordination.

Each health centre in the region received support from an NGO. In total, 4 different NGOs rolled out nutrition education in the above-mentioned research area of the RCT. As part of the government's behaviour change campaign, multiple micronutrient powders were provided to caregivers of children aged 6–23 months.

Nowadays, this represents a common situation in developing countries. The importance for NGOs to function as a facilitator rather than taking over a key role should be stressed. Development projects are usually limited with regard to time and budget as well as human resources. A frequent challenge is related to the fact that after projects have been concluded, government resources and capacities are too meagre to take over and continue their implementation. With regard to nutrition education, the current attention and international support should be used as an opportunity to facilitate the inclusion of nutrition counselling as a basic health service independent of financial resources. This, however, involves larger capacities at the health centre and government level. Thus, the integration of nutrition into the curricula of nursing schools is recommended.

FAO Intervention as an Example of a Nutrition Education Project and Conclusions

Programmes to address the different causes of undernutrition according to the UNICEF conceptual framework ideally include the components of agriculture, nutrition, and hygiene [17]. According to the 2013 *Lancet* series on child and maternal nutrition, appropriate complementary feeding is one of 10 core interventions which even have the potential to reduce child mortality by 15% [4]. Starting points for addressing malnutrition can be either nutrition specific or nutrition sensitive [18]. Nutrition education linked to an agriculture intervention could be one solution to improve complementary feeding practices and prevent malnutrition.

The FAO project's nutrition education addressed different aspects of IYCF. Improvements in children's dietary diversity after 1 year of nutrition education were assessed. There was no impact on HAZ, and changes in children's dietary diversity score proved to not be linked to HAZ either. Other indicators such as meal frequency and continued breastfeeding did not show significant changes. Only a set of indicators was associated with HAZ, which is not surprising. A positive change in one child feeding indicator only does not necessarily lead to improvements in growth. It has to be taken into account that even where local resources allow for adequate IYCF, nutritional knowledge and awareness as well as factors such as a mother's available time are crucial to improving the nutritional status of children.

Nevertheless, the RCT showed that a 2- to 3-month nutrition education programme carried out by government and community health volunteers as well as local NGOs addressing caregivers with a child between 5 and 18 months of age has great potential to improve IYCF practices. As no impact on average HAZ could be demonstrated in the RCT, we suggest for Cambodia that (1) more emphasis be put on ASF and other protein sources in nutrition education, (2) nutrition education be implemented in the community through trained government and community members including peers as trainers, (3) sessions on family nutrition be included in the curriculum and the continuation of breastfeeding be emphasized, and (4) nutrition education be institutionalized, including continuous in-service training for sustainability.

References

1 National Institute of Statistics, Directorate General for Health, ICF International: Cambodia Demographic Health Survey 2014. Phnom Penh, National Institute of Statistics; Phnom Penh, Directorate General for Health; Rockville, ICF International, 2015.

2 Ikeda N, Irie Y, Shibuya K: Determinants of reduced child stunting in Cambodia: analysis of pooled data from three demographic and health surveys. Bull World Health Organ 2013;91:341–349.

3 Victora CG, de Onis M, Hallal PC, et al: Worldwide timing of growth faltering: revisiting implications for interventions. Pediatrics 2010;125:e473–e480.

4 Bhutta ZA, Das JK, Rizvi A, et al: Evidence-based interventions for improvement of maternal and child nutrition: what can be done and at what cost? Lancet 2013;382:452–477.

5 FAO: AQUASTAT – FAO's Information System on Water and Agriculture. 2015. http://www.fao.org/nr/water/aquastat/countries_regions/khm/index.stm (accessed January 5, 2016).

6 Dewey KG, Adu-Afarwuah S: Systematic review of the efficacy and effectiveness of complementary feeding interventions in developing countries. Matern Child Nutr 2008;4(suppl 1):24–85.
7 Prentice AM, Ward KA, Goldberg GR, et al: Critical windows for nutritional interventions against stunting. Am J Clin Nutr 2013;97:911–918.
8 Black RE, Allen LH, Bhutta ZA, et al: Maternal and child undernutrition: global and regional exposures and health consequences. Lancet 2008;371:243–260.
9 National Institute of Statistics, Directorate General for Health, ICF Macro: 2010 Cambodia Demographic and Health Survey: key findings. Phnom Penh, National Institute of Statistics; Phnom Penh, Directorate General for Health; Calverton, ICF Macro, 2011.
10 National Institute of Statistics, Directorate General for Health, DHS Program: Cambodia Demographic and Health Survey 2014: key indicators report. Phnom Penh, National Institute of Statistics; Phnom Penh, Directorate General for Health; Calverton, DHS Program, 2015.
11 Sunil TS, Sagna M: Decomposition of childhood malnutrition in Cambodia. Matern Child Nutr 2015; 11:973–986.
12 Hong R, Mishra V: Effect of wealth inequality on chronic under-nutrition in Cambodian children. J Health Popul Nutr 2006;24:89–99.
13 Jacobs B, Roberts E: Baseline assessment for addressing acute malnutrition by public-health staff in Cambodia. J Health Popul Nutr 2004;22:212–219.
14 Reinbott A, Kuchenbecker J, Herrmann J, et al: A child feeding index is superior to WHO IYCF indicators in explaining length-for-age Z-scores of young children in rural Cambodia. Paediatr Int Child Health 2015;35:124–134.
15 Marriott BP, White A, Hadden L, et al: World Health Organization (WHO) infant and young child feeding indicators: associations with growth measures in 14 low-income countries. Matern Child Nutr 2012;8: 354–370.
16 WHO: Indicators for assessing infant and young child feeding practices. Part 2. Measurement. Geneva, WHO, 2010.
17 UNICEF: Strategy for improved nutrition of children and women in developing countries. A UNICEF policy review. New York, UNICEF, 1990.
18 World Bank: Improving nutrition through multisectoral approaches. Washington, World Bank, 2013, p 172.

Dr. Irmgard Jordan
Institute of Nutritional Sciences, Justus Liebig University Giessen
Wilhelmstrasse 20
DE–35392 Giessen (Germany)
E-Mail Irmgard.Jordan@ernaehrung.uni-giessen.de

Biesalski HK, Black RE (eds): Hidden Hunger. Malnutrition and the First 1,000 Days of Life: Causes, Consequences and Solutions. World Rev Nutr Diet. Basel, Karger, 2016, vol 115, pp 68–81
DOI: 10.1159/000442073

Nutrition Transition in Rural Tanzania and Kenya

Gudrun Keding

Institute of Nutritional Sciences, Justus-Liebig-Universität Giessen, Giessen, Germany;
World Vegetable Center (AVRDC), Arusha, Tanzania; Bioversity International, Nairobi, Kenya

Abstract

All three types of malnutrition – underweight, overweight and micronutrient deficiency – are experienced in countries undergoing a nutrition transition, and they can occur in parallel in one community or even one household. To combat this triple burden of malnutrition, a combination of different strategies will be necessary, including a focus on food-based strategies that promote the consumption of a wide range of foods across nutritionally distinct food groups. In addition to a literature review, data from our own nutrition studies in both Tanzania and Kenya are presented in this paper. The literature review revealed an average of 10% of children in urban areas of Kenya and Tanzania with overweight and obesity, which is an alarming trend, and it is suggested that interventions need to start not only at school but also with adolescent girls and pregnant women to target the '1,000-day window'. From own study data, dietary patterns were generated that included a 'purchase' pattern dominated by bought and processed foods, indicating a possible nutrition transition even in the rural areas of both countries. Vegetable and especially fruit consumption was low in both countries. In addition, in Kenya, study participants exceeded the suggested maximum level of sugar consumption per day, which will most likely contribute to increasing levels in overweight and obesity prevalence and other noncommunicable diseases in general. As sugar was mainly consumed in combination with black tea, next to eating habits, changing drinking habits is also an important part of the nutrition transition and needs to receive more attention. A 'healthy eating at school and at home strategy' is suggested, which needs the support of both schools and parents/caregivers. In general, to take countermeasures against the negative trends of nutrition transition, joint efforts from all players in the field – not only those in nutrition, health and medicine, but also those in education and agriculture – will be essential.

Background

When thinking about malnutrition, most people have in mind the figures of an estimated 840 million people who suffer worldwide from malnutrition or the nearly 2 billion people who are affected by so called hidden hunger, also known as micronutrient deficiency [1]. Still, overweight and obesity are a third form of malnutrition, next to undernutrition and micronutrient deficiency, and are becoming an increasing public health nutrition challenge in developing countries [2, 3], being rated as the 5th leading cause of global mortality [4]. All three types of malnutrition are experienced in countries undergoing a nutrition transition, and they can occur in parallel in one community and even in one household.

Nutrition Transition in Sub-Saharan Africa

There is a need to better characterise the nutrition transition in African countries [5]. It is suggested that most countries in Sub-Saharan Africa (SSA) are in Stage One dietary transition, which is characterised by a diet low in both calories and micronutrients [6]. However, at least in urban areas, several SSA countries have moved already to Stage Two, with a diet that provides adequate basic energy for most people but an inadequate balance of nutrients. Some have even moved to Stage Three, which is marked by an affluent diet that begins to provide excessive calorie energy, which can lead to health problems linked to obesity [6] and which can be observed in urban centres of Kenya and Tanzania [7–9].

According to Popkin [10], there are not only three stages but also five different patterns of nutrition transition that can be distinguished, which are listed in table 1 in comparison to the three stages. The nutrition transition that is discussed for developing countries occurs between pattern No. 3 and 4 through a shift towards low variety and highly processed foods that are high in energy in addition to engaging in low physical activity [10].

Some of the most recent publications describe the nutrition transition in reviews for different areas of SSA. In southern Africa, for example, as reported by Nnyepi et al. [11], nutrition-related noncommunicable diseases explain 20–31% of mortality for Botswana, South Africa, Swaziland, Mozambique and Zambia. It is emphasised that the prevalence of overweight/obesity and hypertension in many southern Africa countries exceeds that of HIV, and they often occur concurrent with stunting in children. In western Africa, most countries are at the early stages of nutrition transition; however, the countries Cape Verde, Ghana and Senegal are at later stages [12]. For this region, adult obesity rates have increased by 115% in 15 years. Also, here, the challenge especially for urban areas is highlighted by children in major cities consuming energy-dense foods up to seven times as frequently as fruits and vegetables [12]. Finally, for eastern Africa, no overview regarding the region is available, but single-country studies indicate a nutrition transition in urban areas (e.g. in inhabitants of Nairobi, Kenya), showing associations between greater mean body mass index (BMI),

Table 1. Different patterns and stages of nutrition transition according to Popkin [10] and Paarlberg [6]

Pattern name (Popkin)	Pattern characteristics (Popkin)	Stage characteristics (Paarlberg)	KEN and TZN*
Collecting food	Hunter-gatherer populations, diet high in carbohydrates and fibre and low in fat	Stage One: diet low in both calories and micronutrients	
Famine	Diet less varied, subject to larger variations + periods of acute scarcity of food		Rural popul.
Receding famine	Increased consumption of fruits, vegetables and animal protein; starchy staples less important; inactivity and leisure more common	Stage Two: diet that provides adequate basic energy for most people but an inadequate balance of nutrients	Rural and urban popul.
Nutrition-related non-communicable diseases	Diet high in total fat, cholesterol, sugar, and other refined carbohydrates and low in polyunsaturated fatty acids and fibre; increasingly sedentary life	Stage Three: affluent diet that begins to provide excessive calorie energy	Urban popul.
Behavioural change	New dietary pattern associated with the desire to prevent or delay degenerative diseases and prolong health		

* According to own observations and different studies in Kenya and Tanzania [9, 23, 32] suggesting a trend/pattern that a majority but not all people may follow. KEN = Kenya; TZN = Tanzania; popul. = population.

per cent body fat and waist circumference with higher age, higher socio-economic group, and increased expenditure, among others [13]. Similar data exist for Dar es Salaam, Tanzania, where the prevalence of overweight and obesity among women attending antenatal clinics increased over a period of 10 years by around 10% [14]. In general, a recent review including all African countries confirmed that adult obesity prevalence is on the rise on the whole continent, especially in North African countries and particularly among women [15].

Triple Burden of Malnutrition and Dietary Guidelines

The double or triple burden of malnutrition leads to the co-existence of underweight, overweight and/or micronutrient-deficient people within the same region, village or even household. However, demographic health survey data sets from 26 SSA countries showed that there is still a low prevalence of double-burden households: under 5% of obese mother and underweight, stunted or wasted child pairs were found, while slightly more overweight mothers with children with undernutrition were recorded [5]. World Health Organization data sets from 28 SSA countries have even indicated inverse associations between prevalence of overweight and obesity in adults and underweight, stunting and wasting in children [5]. Still, this can be different for single countries or areas, as in a poor urban setting, such as in Nairobi, Kenya, where it was found that a much higher share of overweight and obese mothers had stunted children, namely 43 and 37%, respectively, from a sample size of 3,335 mother-child pairs [7]. Consequently, different forms of malnutrition co-exist in one region or even one household, and to combat this burden a combination of different strategies will be necessary. Besides others, a focus on food-based strategies that promote the consumption of a wide range of foods across nutritionally distinct food groups will be important.

It is challenging to ascribe nutritional effects to single nutrients or single dietary components only. Therefore, to take a holistic view and to not concentrate on a single nutrient or food alone, dietary patterns of population groups should be generated and evaluated. Dietary patterns are based on the consumption of different food groups, and up to now the number of food groups used varies across studies, often depending on the food culture context. Dietary patterns are exposed to socio-economic and cultural changes [16], which are important factors, as next to a transition in nutrition in developing countries a cultural transition is also taking place, usually concurrently and closely linked with the nutrition transition. In addition, a physical activity transition is taking place in countries undergoing a nutrition transition, with a trend towards increasing inactivity and leisure [10].

To establish the idea of dietary patterns in nutrition education, dietary recommendations should change from nutrient intake to patterns of dietary intake. While the exact nutrient intake needed by different population groups is still important to know, in daily life, people need easy-to-remember and easy-to-understand recommendations that are based on different foods and foods groups to consume and not on single nutrients. While food-based dietary guidelines are available for most developed countries, in SSA, according to the FAO [17], only five countries have published food-based dietary guidelines, namely Benin, Namibia, Nigeria, South Africa and Seychelles. Some countries might hesitate to publish their own guidelines, as it is difficult to generalise across different food cultures. Still, in general, it is important to educate and inform consumers so that they can make good food choices in order to consume healthy and balanced diets [17], for which food-based dietary guidelines can be an important milestone. As an example, a generation of dietary patterns and a comparison of food intakes to dietary recommendations using data from two studies in Kenya and Tanzania will be shown in this paper.

Studies in Tanzania and Kenya

Next to a literature review performed in PubMed and Web of Science using the key words 'nutrition transition Africa', 'nutrition transition Kenya' and 'nutrition transition Tanzania', data from own studies in both Tanzania and Kenya are presented. The data in Tanzania were collected within the framework of a larger project led by the

AVRDC – The World Vegetable Center's Regional Center of Africa, Arusha, Tanzania, in cooperation with the Universities of Giessen and Göttingen in Germany. The project on 'Promotion of Neglected Indigenous Vegetables for Nutritional Health in Eastern and Southern Africa' was carried out next to Tanzania and also in Rwanda, Uganda, and Malawi and aimed to understand the link between available vegetable diversity ('production'), food consumption/dietary diversity in women ('consumption') and nutritional health status of women ('health'). For the particular sub-study in Tanzania reported here, a cross-sectional sequential study was conducted during three different seasons in three different districts of rural Tanzania and included 252 women. Individual interviews on vegetable production, food consumption (i.e. 24-hour recall with a 7-day recall on vegetables) and nutritional knowledge were performed, and height and length were measured for calculating BMI as well as haemoglobin (Hb) to determine iron status. For more details, see the description of methods provided in Keding et al. [18].

The study in Kenya was conducted by the World Agroforestry Centre, Nairobi, Kenya, and Bioversity International, Nairobi, Kenya, and was entitled 'Leveraging fruit value chains for sustainable and healthier diets in Western Kenya'. The major aim was to identify key trends in gender-disaggregated preferences, attitudes and decision-making processes of rural households for fruit consumption and production. For this, a cross-sectional survey was conducted in five different agro-ecological zones along a transect of humidity in western Kenya. On a map, in each agro-ecological zone, three geo-referenced point locations were selected in a random distribution. During a preparatory visit, the villages closest to each of the geo-referenced points were selected as the study villages. A total of 370 households were sampled randomly from household lists in all 15 villages. Between 21 and 26 households per village were selected for inclusion in the study. A quantitative food consumption survey (i.e. 24-hour recall with a 7-day recall on fruits) was undertaken to identify nutritional gaps and the contribution of fruits to the overall diet. This survey was repeated 6 months later with exactly the same participants; however, due to the dropout of several households because of having moved or not being at home, the sample size dropped to 271 participating households [unpubl. data].

Results

Overweight and Obesity

While the nutrition transition has consequences for several areas, including health, environment, culture, society and economy, one major change regarding people's health next to other noncommunicable diseases is the increase in overweight and obesity. Studies from the last 10 years presenting data on the prevalence of overweight and obesity in Kenya and Tanzania were screened. They focused mainly on women and/or children and on urban rather than rural settings (table 2). The preva-

Table 2. Overview of the prevalence of overweight and obesity as reported in different studies (between 2006 and 2015) in Kenya and Tanzania

Author(s) [Ref.], year	Study area	Study participants	Prevalence of overweight and obesity		
			children	women	adults
Kenya					
Waswa et al. [38], 2015	Rural villages in four different districts (Bondo, Mumias, Teso South, Vihiga) of western Kenya	Mothers and caregivers of children 6–23 months of age; n = 426		16.7%	
Kimenju et al. [8], 2015	Small towns (Ol Kalou, Mwea, Njabini) in the Central Province of Kenya	Adults; n = 615 Children/adolescents (5–19 years of age); n = 216	10%		41%
Kimani-Murage et al. [7], 2015	Urban poor setting in Nairobi	Children aged under 5 years and their mothers; n = 3,335 Adults in total; n = 5,190	9%	32%	22% (35% female 13% male)
Steyn et al. [28], 2011	Four regions both urban and rural (Meru, Kisumu, Nakuru, Nairobi)	Nationally representative sample of women aged 15–60 years; n = 1,008		43.3%	
Adamo et al. [23], 2011	Rural and urban Kenya	Comparative study with children aged 9–13 years; n = 179	Rural: 0% Urban: 6.8% (boys) 16.7% (girls)		
Tanzania					
Galvin et al. [39], 2015	Three group ranches (Maasai community), Imbirikani, Eselengei, and Olgulului/Lorashi, in Kajiado County, southern Kenya	Individuals ranging from infants to 66 years of age; n = 534; prevalence found only in two groups: Children (2–6.9 years); n = 120 Adults (18 years +); n = 228	4.6%		8.7%
Keding et al. [32], 2013	Rural (Kongwa, Muheza) and peri-urban (Singida) villages in northeastern and central Tanzania	Women of reproductive age; n = 210		22%	
Mosha and Fungo [9], 2010	Dodoma and Kinondoni municipalities in central Tanzania	Schoolchildren; n = 428 6- to 9-year-old children 10- to 12-year-old children	12.4% (6–9 years) 10.2% (10–12 years)		
Villamor et al. [14], 2006	Dar es Salaam, Tanzania	Women 14–52 years of age attending antenatal clinics in 1995; n = 3,778 2004; n = 35,794		21.4% (1995) 30.9% (2004)	

lence as reported in four studies for children in urban areas is similar for both countries, with around 10% and only half for rural areas. The prevalence of overweight and obesity for women and adults in general in Kenya is nearly twice as high in urban compared to rural areas. In Tanzania, the rural-urban difference is less pronounced; however, the prevalence in rural farming communities is higher than in rural pastoralist communities (table 2). While these studies were the main country studies published and listed in PubMed and/or Web of Science, additional data from reviews comparing different countries have already contributed to the discussion [3, 15, 19, 20].

Dietary Patterns in Tanzania and Kenya

While the physical activity transition plays an important role in the increasing prevalence of overweight and obesity, here, the focus will be on nutrition transition and dietary patterns. The latter captures foods and food groups instead of single nutrients only and reflects a more holistic picture, including cultural and socio-economic influences and changes [16]. Dietary patterns from both Tanzanian and Kenyan data were generated based on participants' consumption of 12 different food groups and based on 24-hour recalls during 3 nonconsecutive days in Tanzania and 2 nonconsecutive days in Kenya. To generate the patterns, principal component analysis with varimax rotation was selected as the factor extraction model, which is explained in detail in Keding et al. [18].

In Tanzania, only one dietary pattern was positively associated with the BMIs of the participants, namely, the so-called purchase pattern, which was characterised by the food groups bread/cakes, which often contain high amounts of oil/fat, sugar and tea (table 3). Two dietary patterns were negatively associated with Hb level, namely, the 'purchase' and the 'traditional-coast' patterns, while the 'animal products' pattern was positively associated with the Hb levels of the participating women. The 'animal products' pattern was also found to be positively associated with the wealth level of the participants [18].

In Kenya, the younger a respondent, the more she consumed food according to the 'purchase' pattern and the 'bread/cake' pattern (table 3). The more wealthy a respondent, the more she consumed food according to the 'fruits' pattern; however, wealth level was also slightly associated with the consumption of all other patterns, except for the 'nuts and fish' pattern. Women consuming food according to the 'fruits' pattern and the 'traditional' pattern had a higher dietary diversity score. The dietary diversity score was also slightly associated with the other patterns, except for the 'purchase' pattern [unpubl. data].

Food-Based Dietary Guidelines

Next to the determination of dietary patterns, the two studies also surveyed the amounts of single-food intake in Tanzania and Kenya. The average intakes of different foods from seven major food groups in grams per day were then compared with

Table 3. Dietary patterns in Tanzania (n = 210) and Kenya (n = 271), dominating food groups and associated variables

Dietary pattern	Dominating food groups	Associated variables		
		variable	correlation coefficient	p value
Tanzania				
Traditional-coast	Fruits, nuts, starchy plants, fish	Hb level	ρ = –0.291	<0.001
Purchase	Breads/cakes, sugar, tea	BMI	ρ = 0.192	0.005
		Hb level	ρ = –0.241	0.001
Traditional-inland	Cereals, oil/fat, vegetables	–		
Pulses	Pulses	–		
Animal products	Animal-source foods	Hb level	ρ = 0.216	0.003
		Wealth level	τ = 0.171	<0.001
Kenya				
Traditional	Vegetables, pulses, cereals, oil/fat	DDS	σ = 0.237	<0.001
Purchase	Tea, sugar, animal-source foods	Age	σ = –0.177	0.003
Fruits	Fruits, oil/fat	Wealth level	σ = 0.191	0.002
		DDS	σ = 0.331	<0.001
Nuts and fish	Nuts, fish	–		
Breads and cakes	Breads/cakes	Age	σ = –0.254	<0.001

Data from Tanzania: Keding et al. [18]; data from Kenya: unpublished data. DDS = Dietary diversity score. Correlation coefficients: ρ = Spearman's rank-order correlation coefficient; τ = Kendall's rank correlation coefficient.

dietary recommendations, which are, however, not available for Tanzania and Kenya; thus, other sources had to be used. These dietary recommendations are usually given in a range of a minimum and maximum amount, and they also depend on the amounts consumed of other food groups with similar nutrient content (e.g. fruits and vegetables or pulses and animal-source foods). Thus, figure 1 can only show a trend for the surveyed population group.

Participants in Tanzania consumed more or less the recommended amounts of starchy staples and pulses/nuts. They even ate far more vegetables than the recommended 200 g/day; however, as fruit consumption was especially low, they did not reach the recommended amount of 400 g of fruits and vegetables per day [21]. Participants consumed only around one third of the recommended animal-source foods; yet, as stated above, this could also be substituted by pulses or other plant-source foods. Sugar consumption was low; however, the recommendation in case of sugar is a maximum value, and of course it is not a recommended value that has to be reached.

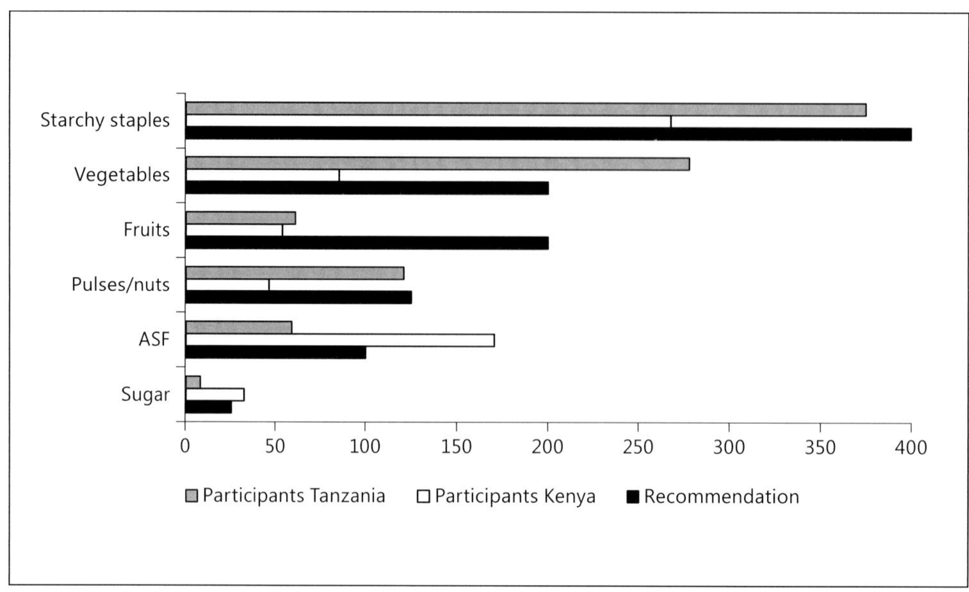

Fig. 1. The mean food intakes in gram per day of participants in Tanzania (n = 210) and in Kenya (n = 370) from different food groups compared to food intake recommendations according to different sources [35–37]. ASF = Animal-source foods.

The Kenyan participants consumed fewer starchy staples than recommended and especially far less vegetables and fruits. They also did not reach the recommended amounts of pulses and nuts, yet, they consumed more animal-source food, which was due to high milk consumption. They also exceeded the suggested maximum level of sugar consumption.

Discussion

Overweight and Obesity

The observed trends in Kenya and Tanzania with higher overweight and obesity rates in urban than in rural areas (table 2) is not surprising. A more comprehensive Tanzanian study surveyed participants before they moved from a rural area (Morogor rural region) to an urban area (Dar es Salaam) and again 12 months later. Vigorous physical activity declined significantly by more than 50% for men and by around 20% for women, and weight increased significantly by 2.3 kg for men and 2.4 kg for women [22]. As highlighted by this Tanzanian study, next to weight status, physical activity level must always be taken into account, such that the 'nutrition-physical activity transition' is what should actually be discussed, as suggested by Adamo et al. [23]. In the latter study, urban Kenyan children were found to have similar anthropometric values to contemporarily living Canadian children; thus, they showed signs of the 'nutrition-physical activity transition'.

Also, in Kenya, the evaluation of data from mother-child pairs from 2003 and 2009 demographic and health surveys revealed that there is geographic variability regarding BMI values and that overweight/obese mothers and children tend to cluster more in urban areas, while underweight mothers and children appear to cluster more in rural regions and in the Northeast area [24]. While these results are not really surprising, from earlier studies, it was learned that the greater prevalence of overweight and obese mothers and children living in urban areas was not linked to socio-economic status and that there must be more specific factors related to urbanisation that contribute to greater food intake and more sedentarism [25–27]. In fact, while some studies still describe overweight and obesity to be a problem of people mainly in high-income groups in urban areas [28], it is also suggested that there is a shift towards lower-income groups having much higher increases in overweight/obesity rates in urban areas [19, 20] in developing countries. This is important to note, especially when developing education materials and activities that need to be adapted to certain population groups (e.g. considering literacy levels) and in determining which locations to use to reach groups or individuals.

Overweight and obesity, as all forms of undernutrition, reflect to a certain extent the enabling or disabling nature of local food environments with regard to appropriate food choice [29]. Next to nutrition education interventions, agriculture interventions are being discussed more and more as an entry point for improving diets. As it is expected that double-burden homes will be a growing problem in SSA [5], agriculture interventions that target households or communities as a whole to improve food availability and accessibility need to also focus on better quality foods in order to prevent a simultaneous increase in obesity rates [5]. This is very much possible, as in most diets, for both underweight and overweight people, similar food groups (namely, fruits and vegetables as well as pulses) are particularly lacking and are at the same time often neglected in agricultural research and development.

In general, the high numbers of children in Kenya and Tanzania with overweight and obesity, which are at an average of 10% (table 2), is alarming and suggest that any intervention needs to start as early as possible, both at school and also for adolescent girls and pregnant women to target the '1,000-day window'.

Dietary Patterns and Guidelines

The generated dietary patterns in Tanzania and Kenya both included a 'purchase' pattern dominated by bought and processed foods, which indicates a possible nutrition transition [18]. While in Tanzania the 'purchase' pattern was even positively associated with BMI, in Kenya, where no nutritional data (i.e. BMI and Hb level) were collected, two patterns indicating a nutrition transition ('purchase' and 'breads/cakes') were generated and were mainly consumed by younger study participants, who are obviously more likely to change their nutritional habits, than by older participants, who stick to traditional dietary patterns. The 'bread/cakes' pattern, referring largely to the consumption of flat breads ('chapatti') or donut-type cakes ('mandazi') prepared with a high amount of oil, can especially be seen as an increased consumption of fast food in terms of street food, which has in fact become an important source of energy for urban Kenyan populations and is a possible contributor to changing diets [30]. The finding that more wealthy participants consumed foods according to the 'fruits' pattern is important for any future intervention targeting low fruit consumption levels and at the same time low fruit production levels and availability during all seasons.

Vegetable and especially fruit consumption was low in both countries. Through urbanisation, it was found in a Tanzanian study that the intake of red meat increased; yet, interestingly, the intake of fresh fruit and vegetables also increased [21], which can be seen as a starting point for changing diets in a nutritiously favourable direction through urbanisation. Study participants in Kenya exceeded the suggested maximum level of sugar consumption, which will most likely contribute to increasing levels in overweight and obesity prevalence and other noncommunicable diseases in general [4]. Here, the physical activity level would need to be taken into account, and a more holistic picture regarding a nutrition-physical activity transition [23] is needed. In addition, the sugar-producing industry, including agriculture, needs to be approached, as the observed sugar intake was mostly derived from sugar in tea and not from sugary soft drinks or other highly processed foods. In general, the increased consumption of energetically sweetened and often caffeinated drinks [31], as well as in the Kenyan and Tanzanian case in which large amounts of sugar were used with black tea as a regular beverage [32], needs to receive more attention, as changing drinking habits are an important part of the nutrition transition in addition to changing eating habits.

Conclusions and Recommendations

The prevalence of the 'purchase' pattern suggests that the nutrition transition – previously reported mainly from urban areas – is on the rise even in rural Tanzania and Kenya. This trend is likely to be accompanied by chronic diseases and probably a loss of local traditional foods and knowledge. It is suggested that generated dietary patterns should be established for additional regions of the countries and incorporated into dietary guidelines as a realistic and acceptable tool for improving nutrition. Also, in rural settings, behavioural factors, including attitudes and activity levels, need to be considered in addition to a balanced diet to address all facets of malnutrition, and the term 'nutrition-physical activity transition' should be employed more regularly. In general, the focus needs to be not only on adults, as it was in many studies in Kenya and Tanzania during the last 10 years, but also – or especially – on children, covering the '1,000-day window'. In order to reduce risks of obesity and chronic diseases later in life, early investment already starting during pregnancy is necessary, primarily to prevent low birth weight and stunting and achieve early initiation of and exclusive breastfeeding [3, 33].

As stated by Paarlberg [6], what is even more important than good governance in each stage of the nutrition transition – and what is often overlooked – is the empowerment of mothers and fathers to provide better care for their children. As has been known for decades already, especially women with better educations follow better feeding practices and have better nourished and healthier children; thus, a key resource needed is education for girls and women. It is even argued that good governance across the different sectors of nutrition, health and agriculture must start with achieving adequate education for young women [6].

Also Onywera [34] summarises strategies to promote active lifestyles among African children as well as a 'healthy eating at school and at home strategy'. Regarding a healthy lifestyle, the author emphasises the various cultural beliefs, local socio-cultural realities and barriers to communication that need to be kept in mind when formulating messages and adapting interventions. A very ambitious suggestion is the 'collaboration with and high visibility in the mass media to enhance publicity, advocacy and awareness campaigns' [34], which so far has not been implemented by the people in power, as shown by the great dominance of advertising for a few large food companies, such as for high-sugar carbonated soft drinks, all over Kenya and Tanzania. Regarding healthy eating strategies, it should be highlighted that not only schools can be asked to encourage the consumption of highly nutritious foods, such as vegetables and fruits, and at the same time discourage the consumption of sugary and fatty foods: parents and caregivers must also be included in the healthy eating plan [34] and can encourage their children to follow healthy eating behaviours and appropriate levels of physical activity [9]. In any case, to counter steer against the negative trends of the nutrition transition, joint efforts from all players in the field – not only nutrition, health and medicine but also education and agriculture – will be essential.

References

1 von Grebmer K, Saltzman A, Birol E, Wiesmann D, Prasai N, Yin S, et al: 2014 Global Hunger Index: The Challenge of Hidden Hunger. Bonn, Washington and Dublin, Welthungerhilfe, International Food Policy Research Institute, and Concern Worldwide, 2014.

2 Popkin BM, Adair LS, Ng SW: Global nutrition transition and the pandemic of obesity in developing countries. Nutr Rev 2012;70:3–21.

3 Black RE, Victora CG, Walker SP, Bhutta ZA, Christian O, de Onis P, et al: Maternal and child undernutrition and overweight in low-income and middle-income countries. Lancet 2013;382:427–451.

4 WHO: Global health risks: mortality and burden of disease attributable to selected major risks. 2009. http://who.int/healthinfo/global_burden_disease/GlobalHealthRisks_report_full.pdf (accessed August 31, 2015).

5 Wojcicki JM: The double burden household in sub-Saharan Africa: maternal overweight and obesity and childhood undernutrition from the year 2000: results from World Health Organization Data (WHO) and Demographic Health Surveys (DHS). BMC Public Health 2014;14:1124.

6 Paarlberg R: Governing the dietary transition: linking agriculture, nutrition, and health; in Leveraging Agriculture for Improving Nutrition & Health: Highlights from an International Conference: 10–12 February 2011, New Delhi, India. Washington, International Food Policy Research Institute, 2011.

7 Kimani-Murage EW, Muthuri SK, Oti SO, Mutua MK, van de Vijver S, Kyobutungi C: Evidence of a double burden of malnutrition in urban poor settings in Nairobi, Kenya. PLoS One 2015;10:e0129943.

8 Kimenju SC, Rischke R, Klasen S, Qaim M: Do supermarkets contribute to the obesity pandemic in developing countries? Public Health Nutr 2015;15: 1–10.

9 Mosha TC, Fungo S: Prevalence of overweight and obesity among children aged 6–12 years in Dodoma and Kinondoni municipalities, Tanzania. Tanzan J Health Res 2010;12:6–16.

10 Popkin BM: An overview on the nutrition transition and its health implications: the Bellagio meeting. Public Health Nutr 2002;5(1A):93–103.

11 Nnyepi MS, Gwisai N, Lekgoa M, Seru T: Evidence of nutrition transition in Southern Africa. Proc Nutr Soc 2015;17:1–9.

12 Bosu WK: An overview of the nutrition transition in West Africa: implications for non-communicable diseases. Proc Nutr Soc 2015;22:1–12.

13 Mbochi RW, Kuria E, Kimiywe J, Ochola S, Steyn NP: Predictors of overweight and obesity in adult women in Nairobi Province, Kenya. BMC Public Health 2012;12:1471–2458.

14 Villamor E, Msamanga G, Urassa W, Petraro P, Spiegelman D, Hunter DJ, et al: Trends in obesity, underweight, and wasting among women attending prenatal clinics in urban Tanzania, 1995–2004. Am J Clin Nutr 2006;83:1387–1394.

15 Norris SA, Wrottesley S, Mohamed RS, Micklesfield LK: Africa in transition: growth trends in children and implications for nutrition. Ann Nutr Metab 2014;64(suppl 2):8–13.

16 Wandel M, Raberg M, Kumar B, Holmboe-Ottesen G: Changes in food habits after migration among South Asians settled in Oslo: the effect of demographic, socio-economic and integration factors. Appetite 2008;50:376–385.

17 FAO: Food-based dietary guidelines – Africa. 2016. http://www.fao.org/nutrition/education/food-dietary-guidelines/regions/africa/en/ (accessed February 10, 2016).

18 Keding GB, Msuya JM, Maass BL, Krawinkel MB: Dietary patterns and nutritional health of women: the nutrition transition in rural Tanzania. Food Nutr Bull 2011;32:218–226.

19 Popkin BM, Adair LS, Ng SW: Global nutrition transition and the pandemic of obesity in developing countries. Nutr Rev 2012;70:3–21.

20 Ziraba AK, Fotso JC, Ochako R: Overweight and obesity in urban Africa: a problem of the rich or the poor? BMC Public Health 2009;9:465.

21 WHO: WHO fruit and vegetable promotion initiative – report of the meeting. Geneva, Switzerland, 25–27 August, 2003.

22 Unwin N, James P, McLarty D, Machybia H, Nkulila P, Tamin B, et al: Rural to urban migration and changes in cardiovascular risk factors in Tanzania: a prospective cohort study. BMC Public Health 2010; 10:1471–2458.

23 Adamo KB, Sheel AW, Onywera V, Waudo J, Boit M, Tremblay MS: Child obesity and fitness levels among Kenyan and Canadian children from urban and rural environments: a KIDS-CAN Research Alliance Study. Int J Pediatr Obes 2011;6:e225–e232.

24 Pawloski LR, Curtin KM, Gewa C, Attaway D: Maternal-child overweight/obesity and undernutrition in Kenya: a geographic analysis. Public Health Nutr 2012;15:2140–2147.

25 Deleuze Ntandou Bouzitou G, Fayomi N, Delisle H: Child malnutrition and maternal overweight in same households in poor urban areas of Benin (in French). Sante 2005;15:263–270.

26 Pawloski LR, Kitsantas P: Classification tree analysis of stunting in Malian adolescent girls. Am J Hum Biol 2008;20:285–291.

27 Gewa CA: Childhood overweight and obesity among Kenyan pre-school children: association with maternal and early child nutritional factors. Public Health Nutr 2010;13:496–503.

28 Steyn NP, Nel JH, Parker WA, Ayah R, Mbithe D: Dietary, social, and environmental determinants of obesity in Kenyan women. Scand J Public Health 2011;39:88–97.

29 UNSCN: Nutrition and the Post-2015 Sustainable Development Goals. A Technical Note. Geneva, Switzerland, United Nations Standing Committee on Nutrition, 2014.

30 van't Riet H, den Hartog AP, van Staveren WA: Non-home prepared foods: contribution to energy and nutrient intake of consumers living in two low-income areas in Nairobi. Public Health Nutr 2002;5: 515–522.

31 Popkin BM: Contemporary nutritional transition: determinants of diet and its impact on body composition. Proc Nutr Soc 2011;70:82–91.

32 Keding GB, Msuya JM, Maass BL, Krawinkel MB: Obesity as a public health problem among adult women in rural Tanzania. Glob Health Sci Pract 2013;1:359–371.

33 Adair LS, Fall CH, Osmond C, Stein AD, Martorell R, Ramirez-Zea M, et al: Associations of linear growth and relative weight gain during early life with adult health and human capital in countries of low and middle income: findings from five birth cohort studies. Lancet 2013;382:525–534.

34 Onywera VO: Childhood obesity and physical inactivity threat in Africa: strategies for a healthy future. Glob Health Promot 2010;17(2 suppl):45–46.
35 FAO: Agriculture, Food and Nutrition for Africa. A Resource Book for Teachers of Agriculture. Rome, Food and Nutrition Division, FAO, 1997.
36 DGE: DGE-Ernährungskreis – Lebensmittelmengen. Beratungspraxis 05/2004. 2012. http://ernaehrungsdenkwerkstatt.de/fileadmin/user_upload/EDW-Text/TextElemente/PHN-Texte/Dietary_Goals/DGE_Lebensmittelmengen_Ernaehrungskreis.pdf (accessed December 10, 2012).
37 USDA/USDHHS: Dietary Guidelines for Americans, 2010, ed 7. Washington, US Government Printing Office, 2010.
38 Waswa LM, Jordan I, Herrmann J, Krawinkel MB, Keding GB: Community-based educational intervention improved the diversity of complementary diets in western Kenya: results from a randomized controlled trial. Public Health Nutr 2015;18:3406–3419.
39 Galvin KA, Beeton TA, Boone RB, BurnSilver SB: Nutritional status of Maasai pastoralists under change. Hum Ecol Interdiscip J 2015;43:411–424.

Dr. Gudrun Keding
Bioversity International/University of Göttingen
Department of Crop Sciences, Quality of Plant Products
Carl-Sprengel-Weg 1, DE–37075 Göttingen (Germany)
E-Mail gkeding@gwdg.de

Biesalski HK, Black RE (eds): Hidden Hunger. Malnutrition and the First 1,000 Days of Life: Causes, Consequences and Solutions. World Rev Nutr Diet. Basel, Karger, 2016, vol 115, pp 82–97
DOI: 10.1159/000442075

The Role of Breastfeeding in the Prevention of Childhood Malnutrition

Veronika Scherbaum[a, b] · M. Leila Srour[c]

[a]Institute for Biological Chemistry and Nutrition, 140, and [b]Food Security Center, University of Hohenheim, Stuttgart, Germany; [c]Health Frontiers, Vientiane, Laos

Abstract

Breastfeeding has an important role in the prevention of different forms of childhood malnutrition, including wasting, stunting, over- and underweight and micronutrient deficiencies. This chapter reviews research that demonstrates how improved breastfeeding rates have the potential to improve childhood nutrition, with associated impacts on infectious and noninfectious disease prevention. The unique composition of breastmilk, the importance of breastfeeding in infectious disease prevention, the iron status of breastfed infants, and breastfeeding's protective effect on overweight and obesity are discussed based on currently available research. Early and tailored dietary counseling is needed to improve maternal diets, which can affect the nutritional status of breastmilk. Promotion and support of breastfeeding are important to prevent childhood morbidity and mortality. A review of the literature reveals key factors shown to be effective in improving breastfeeding rates, especially including legislation to control the marketing of breastmilk substitutes. In conclusion, breastfeeding is shown to be the best natural resource to improve childhood nutrition throughout the world.

Introduction

For several decades, studies have shown that promotion of exclusive and long-term breastfeeding is one of the most effective interventions to improve child health and survival throughout the world [1–3]. However, global breastfeeding rates remain persistently low, as currently only 38% of infants worldwide are being exclusively breastfed for the first 6 months of life [4]. At the same time, suboptimal breastfeeding practices have been estimated to be responsible for more than 11% of deaths and 10% of disability-adjusted life years among children under 5 years of age worldwide [5, 6]. Recent calculations in Mexico and the USA reveal the substantially high costs of inadequate breastfeeding [7–9]. In the USA, annually, over 900 infant and child deaths and USD 13 billion in US health care costs could be saved by exclusive breastfeeding for the first 6 months of life [9].

With respect to the preventive effects of breastfeeding on different forms of undernutrition, large-scale longitudinal studies are still rare [3, 10–13]. From a public health perspective, this information gap is very critical, considering the high global prevalence of stunting (25%), underweight (15%), wasting (8%), and iron deficiency anemia (47%) among children under 5 years of age [14, 15]. Apart from the direct and indirect impact of malnutrition on child mortality [5], the consequences of undernutrition for the growth, development and health of individuals are substantial, often perpetuating across generations [6, 16]. Regarding the intermediate and long-term effects of breastfeeding in the prevention of overweight, obesity and associated illnesses [17–20], investigations have primarily been conducted in high- and middle-income countries. Meanwhile, the rates of childhood obesity, often associated with stunting [21, 22], are reaching epidemic levels in many countries. Therefore, prevention of childhood obesity is seen as one of today's most serious challenges [23–25].

This chapter aims to review current knowledge about the potential role of breastfeeding in the prevention of different forms of child malnutrition. Due to the critical interrelationship between infection and malnutrition [26], the impact of breastfeeding on infectious disease prevention will also be discussed.

Properties of Breastfeeding and Human Milk

The composition of human milk is unique, dynamically and actively adapting to the individual infant's nutritional needs, with modification according to prematurity and postnatal age. Breastmilk composition changes during each feeding session, for while the foremilk is rich in micronutrients and watery, quenching thirst, the hind milk is rich in fat, satisfying the energy demands of the fast-growing infant. Hormones in the hind milk signal satiety to the child [27]. Breastmilk contributes to the child's health, growth and development due to its unique composition of macro- and micronutrients; digestive enzymes; hormones; anti-inflammatory substances; growth modulators, and prebiotics, such as bifidus factors, which enhance the maturation of the gastrointestinal tract and stimulate the growth of bifidobacteria. The bioactive compounds in human milk, which have been only partially elucidated, include specific and nonspecific antimicrobial factors contributing to protection against infectious diseases [28, 29].

The macro- and micronutrients in breastmilk are best suited to meet the recommended dietary allowance for infants up to 6 months of age. Breastmilk, in contrast to infant formula, contains relatively low levels of protein and a high whey-to-casein fraction of approximately 90% during the first days of life. This high whey fraction is particularly beneficial in the support of antimicrobial activity. The casein fraction of breastmilk protein facilitates the absorption of calcium, iron, and zinc [30]. The micronutrients in human milk have high bioavailability [31]. Up to 80% of breastmilk iron is absorbed compared to the absorption of heme iron, which is usually between 12 and 25%, and of nonheme iron, which is below 5% [32].

During the first month of life, breastmilk composition changes daily, beginning with colostrum, then via transitional milk becoming mature milk, meeting the specific needs of the newborn for optimal growth, gastrointestinal function and host defense [27]. The initial breastmilk produced by mothers of premature babies is different in composition: higher in protein and minerals and with fats that are easier to digest [29]. The first breast fluid, or colostrum, is particularly high in protein and fat-soluble vitamins like vitamin A as well as in growth factors and immunological components. Due to its important role in disease prevention, colostrum is often considered to be the infant's first immunization. In order to ensure its full advantage, breastfeeding should start as soon as possible. Recent meta-analyses have demonstrated that neonatal deaths in low- and middle-income countries can be prevented in up to 50% of infants when breastfeeding is started in the first hour of life. Exclusively breastfed neonates have a significantly lower risk of sepsis, diarrhea and respiratory infections when compared to partially breastfed infants [33, 34]. Furthermore, surveys in India and Haiti showed an association between initiation of breastfeeding within the first hour of life and a reduced risk of stunting in children <5 years of age [35, 36].

Due to its high protein content, the consistency of colostrum appears creamy, and the color is yellowish. Unfortunately, due to its different appearance compared to mature milk, colostrum is widely believed to be dirty and is consequently discarded and often replaced by prelacteal feedings [37–39]. Studies in Ethiopia, Indonesia, and China revealed that many newborns did not receive colostrum within the first hour of life. Breastfeeding was delayed for up to 5 days after delivery, during which time prelacteal feedings were frequently offered [37, 38, 40]. Studies in urban and rural areas of the Sichuan province of China revealed that there was a significant association between cesarean births and delayed offering of breastmilk by more than 2 days, which is particularly concerning because 67% of newborns were delivered by cesarean section [38, 40].

Delayed onset of breastfeeding, discarding of colostrum and replacement with prelacteal fluids or foods are practices that lead to suboptimal breastfeeding and can contribute to undernutrition and increased morbidity and mortality. Therefore, nutrition educators must understand cultural practices and family factors, like the role of grandmothers [38, 41], to effectively improve breastfeeding promotion and encourage parents to choose the best nutrition for their infant. This also applies to infants with low birth weight (<2,500 g), who, according to World Health Organization [42] recommendations, should be put to the breast as soon as possible, supported by intensive skin-to-skin contact and exclusively breastfed until 6 months of age.

Infectious Diseases and Malnutrition

There is plenty of evidence that breastfeeding is associated with a lower risk of infectious diseases in industrialized countries [43], and particularly low-income countries [44], where breastfeeding can play an important role in interrupting the vicious cycle of malnutrition and infection. Acute-phase responses induced by infectious diseases generally lead to concomitant anabolic and catabolic reactions, which, on the one hand, help to stimulate immunity and, on the other hand, can have negative consequences for the nutritional status [45] due to loss of appetite, consequently lowering dietary intake. At the same time, macro- and micronutrients are diverted for immune responses, while the basal metabolic rate, including the energy and nutrient requirements, is generally increased [32]. Similarly, during gastroenteritis, nutritional deficiencies are aggravated by malabsorption, urinary nitrogen losses and nutrient losses, with particularly high risks during severe, persistent or repeated infections [46, 47].

As a key child survival strategy, multiple studies have shown that breastfeeding is the number-one preventive intervention to reduce child deaths [1–3]. While it can reduce the incidence and severity of infectious diseases, the protective effect varies with the degree of breastfeeding [48]. The risk of infectious disease morbidity and mortality is lowest in exclusively breastfed infants, slightly increases in predominantly breastfed infants, further rises in partially breastfed infants and is highest in children who were never breastfed [49, 50].

Regarding mortality, infants who are not breastfed compared to those who are exclusively breastfed are approximately 10 times more likely to die from diarrheal disease and 15 times more likely to die from pneumonia [51].

Exclusive breastfeeding for the first 6 months and continued for the first 2 years is critical to reduce the burden of pneumonia [50], the leading cause of child mortality, which resulted in the deaths of 1.4 million children less than 5 years of age in 2010, with the majority of morbidity and mortality in developing countries occurring among the poorest and most vulnerable children [52].

Similarly, breastfeeding protects infants against diarrheal morbidity and mortality through immunological mechanisms and by reducing exposure to contaminated fluids and foods [49]. There is clear evidence that no or suboptimal breastfeeding is associated with increased diarrheal incidence and duration. Additionally, the recurrence of diarrheal episodes within short time periods as well as persistent gastrointestinal diseases poses significant risks of a lack of weight gain and failure to catch up in growth, which subsequently can result in stunting [49, 51]. The higher risk of malnutrition associated with artificial feeding becomes particularly obvious under conditions of poor environmental hygiene in low-income countries but can be found worldwide, especially in the context of emergencies [53, 54]. There is evidence that continued breastfeeding during and after illness is conducive to recovery. It is suggested that the favorable energy and nutrient content of breastmilk, its immunological properties and its easy digestibility as well as psycho-emotional effects are beneficial factors that can counteract the adverse nutritional outcomes of infectious diseases [55]. It has been demonstrated that during infections, most breastfed children can maintain close-to-normal energy intake from breastmilk, while energy intake from breastmilk substitutes has been shown to decrease by about 20% during illness [56].

Besides gastroenteritis and pneumonia, there are a number of other infectious diseases, like otitis media, *Haemophilus influenzae* meningitis, urinary tract infections and respiratory syncytial virus infections, in which an association of a lower incidence and/or severity with breastfeeding has been demonstrated [57–61]. Although plausible explanations for certain preventive mechanisms exist, further research in nutritional immunology and studies on the correlation of infection and nutrition are needed to fully understand the immunoprotective role of breastfeeding.

Prevention of Different Forms of Undernutrition

In a Cochrane meta-analysis, no evidence that full-term, exclusively breastfed infants suffer from growth deficits during the first 6 months of life was found [13]. More recently, in low- and middle-income countries, an association between exclusive breastfeeding and a reduced risk of undernutrition has been found. While most small-scale studies revealed that exclusively breastfed infants were less likely to develop stunting and/or to be underweight [12, 62, 63], a large-scale study in Brazil showed that height and weight gain among exclusively breastfed infants is similar to or greater than the US National Center for Health Statistics (1977) and the World Health Organization (2006) reference curves, with a greater mean weight between the 4th and the 6th months of life in particular [64]. Analyses of large-scale demographic and health surveys in Bangladesh and Zambia have shown that exclusively breastfed infants were significantly less likely to experience wasting [65]. Compared to stunting, wasting is considered to be a more sensitive indicator of inadequate growth in early infancy [66]. As cumulative growth deficits leading to stunting are more pronounced in later childhood, the potential impact of exclusive breastfeeding on the prevention of stunting is difficult to assess. In addition, a lack of consistent assessments of breastfeeding patterns and utilization of these assessments by researchers has hampered the interpretation and comparison of study results [67, 68], contributing to partly inconsistent findings and generalizations in previous publications [3, 6, 69]. Apart from potential biases due to various confounding variables [13], it is also difficult to differentiate the specific impact of breastfeeding on a child's nutritional status from the quality and quantity of complementary foods and/or dietary supplements [69].

Worldwide, the peak incidence of growth faltering and micronutrient deficiencies usually occurs during the period of complementary feeding, which is defined as being from 6 to 23 months [57]. While studies on the interplay between breastfeeding and complementary feeding are rare, continuing breastfeeding together with complementary foods is critical in terms of providing all the nutrients with the high bioavailability needed for linear growth [70]. This is of particular importance under conditions of poor-nutritional-quality complementary foods, ranging from monotonous, watery porridges, as prepared in many socially deprived households [71], to commercially marketed complementary foods lacking essential nutrients [25, 72]. Thus, the continued intake of breastmilk by on-demand nursing during the infant's first 2 years of life contributes to the prevention of child malnutrition [73].

Regarding the reports of slower growth trajectories among young breastfed children [74–76], there is a controversial discussion of a suspected biased relationship due to reverse causality [77–79]. In low-income countries, small and more slowly growing infants are usually more likely to be breastfed for a longer period of time, leading to the erroneous conclusion that breastfeeding is associated with poor growth [79, 80]. In industrialized countries, a mother's confidence in her ability to breastfeed adequately may be challenged if her infant is smaller, leading to early supplementation and premature weaning [77].

Undernutrition in infants may also be the consequence of overdilution of commercial infant formula. In low-income countries, 20% of mothers who used formula were found to have overdiluted breastmilk substitutes by more than 40% [81, 82]. In contrast, underdilution may cause damage to organs like the kidneys due to the high osmolality of improperly reconstituted infant formulas. These problems are particularly relevant when caregivers cannot read product labels and/or fully understand instructions, which are often not written in the local language [83, 84].

Regarding the iron status of breastfed infants, there has been controversy about the adequacy of breastmilk for maintaining an optimum iron status in babies who are exclusively breastfed. Earlier research showed iron deficiency and anemia with exclusive breastfeeding and recommended supplementation via complementary foods at 4–6 months of age [85–88]. Currently, no internationally agreed-upon guidelines regarding iron exist for exclusively breastfed infants. Commonly referenced research has major methodological limitations due to a lack of control for confounders. Delayed cord clamping may enhance iron endowment at birth. Breastmilk iron and lactoferrin are efficiently absorbed in the gut, and as a result of this together with adequate body iron stores, the infant's iron supply is usually sufficient to maintain normal iron metabolism during the first 6 months of life for appropriate-for-gestational-age babies. Therefore, there is no need to routinely add therapeutic iron for exclusively breastfed term infants until 6 months of age [89–91].

Prevention of Overweight and Obesity

Concerning childhood obesity, the protective effect of breastfeeding has been demonstrated in several studies, primarily in the industrialized world, showing a 15–38% obesity risk reduction through breastfeeding [18, 19, 92, 93]. Besides the preventive role of breastfeeding during the critical period of metabolic programming [92, 94, 95], there are multiple biologically plausible explanations for obesity prevention related to breastmilk's properties. Breastmilk contains moderate amounts of calories and changes as the infant grows compared to infant formula, which remains static and contains, for example, higher levels of protein. The potential consequences of a high protein intake during early infancy have been recently studied in Europe under the label of the 'Early Protein Hypothesis' [96]. During a follow-up study in 6-year-olds, the prevalence of obesity was 10% in children who had received standard infant formula with a high protein content, 4.4% in children who had received formula with a lower protein content and 2.9% in the breastfed control group [97]. The reduced energy metabolism of breastfed infants may lead to lower insulin levels and lower deposition of fat [98]. In comparison to formula-fed infants, less growth acceleration and less upward centile crossing have been observed in breastfed children, leading to a decreased risk of overweight-obesity, even as early as 2 years of age [98, 99]. Other plausible explanations concern the level of bioactive substances in breastmilk that influence the proliferation of adipocytes. In addition, breastfed infants have the capacity to self-regulate their energy intake, influencing appetite regulation [98, 100]. Therefore, bottle-fed infants are more likely to be overfed because they are fully under parental control and consume up to 30% more milk than breastfed infants [100]. Moreover, breastmilk contains a variety of flavors, reflecting the maternal diet, which influences food choices later in life [101, 102].

With respect to the growing public health concern regarding childhood obesity throughout the world, a recent meta-analysis was conducted on populations in 12 countries. The risk of childhood obesity was found to be 22% lower in breastfed infants compared to infants who were never breastfed. Further, this meta-analysis showed a dose-response relationship between breastfeeding and childhood obesity. Breastfeeding for <3 months provided minor childhood obesity protection, and 7 months or more of breastfeeding was linked to significantly higher protection [103]. Simultaneously, genetic and environmental determinants, parental obesity, smoking, birth weight and the velocity of weight gain are considered to supersede infant feeding patterns as risk factors for childhood obesity [104].

Effects of Maternal Diet and Nutritional Status on Breastmilk

Maternal factors can influence lactation. However, even among mothers with a marginal nutritional status combined with heavy physical activity, the volume capacity of breastmilk production remains relatively stable, probably due to compensatory increases in prolactin secretion [105–107]. The volume of breastmilk is increased by the infant's frequency of suckling. Stress, smoking and feeding supplementary formula decrease the volume of breastmilk. Mothers' age, parity and body mass index (BMI) have no impact on breastmilk volume [105]. Significantly, the volume of breastmilk produced is negatively affected by a mother's lack of confidence in her ability to adequately satisfy her child's needs with breastmilk alone [108, 109], emphasizing the importance of maternal support to breastfeed successfully. Mothers' perception of inadequate breastmilk production is also an important reason for offering prelacteal or supplementary feedings, which leads to less suckling and consequently less milk production. This is a vicious cycle and can be the beginning of the end of the breastfeeding relationship.

With increased maternal age, obesity and insulin resistance, the onset of lactation has been shown to be delayed and the duration shortened [110–112]. While there is no association between maternal diet and the protein content of human milk, the quality of the fatty acids correlates with maternal dietary intake [113] and the quantity is endogenously regulated [114]. More recently, it has also been shown that the milk of obese mothers contains higher amounts of unsaturated fatty acids and a higher level of trans-fatty acids [115]. During pregnancy and lactation, dietary counseling, appropriate weight gain and physical activity are important aspects of medical supervision, particularly for overweight women [116].

Concerning micronutrients, maternal nutrition does affect the content of breastmilk. It is likely that water-soluble vitamins are more affected than fat-soluble vitamins. For example, infantile beriberi is a major cause of mortality among infants breastfed by mothers with inadequate thiamine (vitamin B_1) intake in Laos, where pregnant and lactating mothers often follow strict food taboos, eating primarily milled rice and consuming food containing thiaminases. Culturally appropriate public health education and perhaps vitamin supplementation are needed to prevent thiamine deficiency, especially in vulnerable populations [117].

Selenium and iodine levels in breastmilk depend on maternal dietary intake [118, 119]. In contrast, calcium, iron, zinc, magnesium and copper appear to be independent of maternal nutritional status [120–122]. It appears to be important to improve maternal dietary intake as early as possible in the life cycle, ideally before pregnancy and at the latest during lactation [123, 124]. Promotion of food-based strategies, including food fortifications and supplementations, is important, especially for women in food-insecure areas and with low BMIs [125]. When nutrient levels in breastmilk are suboptimal, which can be the case in women with a very high or very low BMI, the woman's nutritional status should be improved as early as possible. Tailored dietary counseling during pregnancy and lactation is particularly important [116].

Protection, Promotion and Support of Breastfeeding

In view of the fact that 13% of child deaths could be prevented by 100% exclusive breastfeeding, appropriate promotion programs are of utmost importance [126]. Meta-analyses and randomized controlled trials in various countries have shown that appropriate counseling and educational interventions, ideally with ongoing personal contact, lead to early initiation of nursing, improve breastfeeding rates and prolong lactation duration [127]. In primary health care settings with a low prevalence of timely initiation and limited breastfeeding duration, structured programs showed a greater benefit compared to unstructured programs [128]. Higher effectiveness was found when individual counseling and group counseling were combined and supported by peer groups and follow-up visits [129–131]. In high-income countries, health education and peer support interventions were effective to improve initiation of breastfeeding, especially among lower-income families [132]. Women with known risk factors for premature cessation of breastfeeding, such as maternal smoking, a low education level, and preterm and/or low-birth-weight babies, should be identified early in order to offer specific lactation support [133]. The support should include guidance on important information gaps, like milk supply management, the frequency and duration of feeds, proper feeding positions, and nipple care, among others [134].

Key factors for the significant increase, from 2.5 to 38.6%, in exclusive breastfeeding in Brazil during the past 20 years included legislation to control the marketing of breastmilk substitutes, improvements in socioeconomic status and female education. As shown by several intervention studies, antenatal education regarding the nutrition/health properties of breastmilk and the benefits of breastfeeding as well as postnatal contact and mothers' support groups have effectively contributed to higher breastfeeding rates [132, 135]. A prospective birth cohort followed up 30 years later in Brazil showed the long-term benefits of breastfeeding, including improved intelligence, increased educational attainment and increased income in adulthood [136, 137]. Publicity about these research findings can encourage parents to choose exclusive breastfeeding and to continue nursing until at least 2 years of age. A rise in exclusive breastfeeding, from 11 to 74%, was achieved in Cambodia between 2000 and 2010, supported by an innovative media campaign, extensive training of health workers and support groups for mothers, which contributed to significant reductions in infant and child morbidity and mortality [126]. Similarly, the PROMISE-EBF study demonstrated the feasibility and positive effect of peer counselor promotion of exclusive breastfeeding in countries of sub-Saharan Africa, more than doubling the proportion of mothers reporting exclusive breastfeeding [131]. In recent small-scale trials, innovative approaches addressing cultural beliefs during pregnancy, lactation and the complementary feeding period have demonstrated effectiveness. Creative support in terms of higher self-efficacy is needed to address the unfounded belief that many mothers are unable to produce enough milk for their infants [138–140].

Despite the large number of intervention studies evaluating the effectiveness of promotion programs in increasing breastfeeding rates, the nutritional outcomes of the concerned children have rarely been assessed [3, 130].

There is sufficient evidence that a supportive environment is a key factor for successful breastfeeding. However, breastfeeding promotion lacks both sufficient public health support and implementation of effective programs. Compared to the global investments in ready-to-use food, micronutrient supplementation and fortified complementary foods, very little attention is paid to culturally sensitive breastfeeding protection, support and promotion. In sharp contrast to the very limited public health investment in breastfeeding promotion, the infant formula industry is increasingly spending millions of dollars on formula promotion [141–144]. In this context, Cattaneo [145] proposed the need for a paradigm shift. Instead of investing increased resources into research to continuously prove the benefits of a natural way of infant feeding, those who propose alternative ways of infant feeding should demonstrate, by scientifically sound studies, that their option is not harmful and/or is at least equivalent to breastfeeding.

In order to protect breastfeeding and to ensure appropriate use of breastmilk substitutes in situations of need (e.g. mothers' death), the International Code of Marketing of Breastmilk Substitutes (the Code) was adopted in 1981. Stronger enforcement of the Code and the associated World Health Assembly resolutions are necessary to control aggressive advertising practices of the formula industry. Additional regulations and public health efforts are needed to restrict adverse marketing of energy-rich and nutrient-poor foods and beverages used during the stage of complementary feeding and later childhood periods [25]. Due to increasingly globalized problems of marketing of breastmilk substitutes and processed foods, a new optional protocol on infant nutrition needs to be designed, adopted and amended as part of the International Convention on the Rights of the Child [143]. Implementation of existing legislation protecting maternity leave and breastfeeding-friendly workplaces are urgently required to better support lactating mothers [146]. More systematic studies could help to find ways to enable working mothers to continue breastfeeding in the workplace [147, 148].

Conclusions

There is compelling evidence that breastfeeding is beneficial for children's health, growth and development and that it has an important role in the prevention of malnutrition in both under- and overnourished children. However, current scientific evidence shows a wide degree of preventive effects, varying with the size of the study, the age group, socioeconomic factors and the nutritional status of the children. Well-designed research with clear and consistent definitions is needed to clarify the impact of breastfeeding in the prevention of childhood malnutrition.

Concerning the development of overweight/obesity and associated illnesses, risks seem to be reduced when children are breastfed during the critical periods of early metabolic programming and behavioral imprinting. Regarding the prevention of different forms of undernutrition, exclusive breastfeeding until 6 months and continued on-demand nursing during the period of complementary feeding are known to be beneficial. Simultaneously, breastfeeding contributes to protection from infectious diseases and their adverse nutritional effects. There is particularly strong evidence that the risk of persistent and/or recurrent episodes of gastroenteritis and the potential negative impact on weight gain and catch-up growth are reduced by breastfeeding, which is particularly important during child illness.

With respect to maternal undernutrition, lactation performance and the quantity and nutritional quality of breastmilk seem to be relatively stable, even among women with a marginal nutritional status. However, provision of dietary supplements should be considered for women at risk of undernutrition as early as possible, best before conception. Meanwhile, maternal obesity is associated with impaired lactogenesis, increased insulin resistance, and higher amounts of unsaturated fatty acids and trans-fatty acids in breastmilk, which demands close medical and nutritional supervision.

The impact of maternal diet and nutritional status and the effect of nutritional supplements on the quality of breastmilk as well as on the child's health, growth and development need to be studied in more detail.

Within a life cycle perspective, strategies of breastfeeding promotion have strong potential to improve maternal and child health worldwide. National and international legislation and effective implementation to control the inappropriate marketing of breastmilk substitutes are urgently needed. Working mothers require adequate maternity leave and support to continue breastfeeding when they return to work. Freely available across economic and cultural divides, breastfeeding is the best natural resource to improve infant and young child nutrition, support maternal health, and save the lives of children throughout the world.

References

1 Jones G, Steketee RW, Black RE, Bhutta ZA, Morris SS: How many child deaths can we prevent this year? Lancet 2003;362:65–71.

2 Lassi ZS, Mallick D, Das JK, Mal L, Salam RA, Bhutta ZA: Essential interventions for child health. Reprod Health 2014;11(suppl 1):S4.

3 Bhutta ZA, Ahmed T, Black RE, Cousens S, Dewey K, Giugliani E, Haider BA, Kirkwood B, Morris SS, Sachdev HP, Shekar M: What works? Interventions for maternal and child undernutrition and survival. Lancet 2008;371:417–440.

4 UNICEF: Adopting optimal feeding practices is fundamental to a child's survival, growth and development, but too few children benefit. New York, UNICEF, 2015.

5 Black RE, Allen LH, Bhutta ZA, Caulfield LE, de Onis M, Ezzati M, Mathers C, Rivera J: Maternal and child undernutrition: global and regional exposures and health consequences. Lancet 2008;371:243–260.

6 Black RE, Victora CG, Walker SP, Bhutta ZA, Christian P, de Onis M, Ezzati M, Grantham-McGregor S, Katz J, Martorell R, Uauy R: Maternal and child undernutrition and overweight in low-income and middle-income countries. Lancet 2013;382:427–451.

7 Colchero MA, Contreras-Loya D, Lopez-Gatell H, Gonzalez de Cosio T: The costs of inadequate breastfeeding of infants in Mexico. Am J Clin Nutr 2015; 101:579–586.

8 Ma P, Brewer-Asling M, Magnus JH: A case study on the economic impact of optimal breastfeeding. Matern Child Health J 2013;17:9–13.

9 Bartick M, Reinhold A: The burden of suboptimal breastfeeding in the United States: a pediatric cost analysis. Pediatrics 2012;125:e1048–e1056.

10 Engebretsen IM, Jackson D, Fadnes LT, Nankabirwa V, Diallo AH, Doherty T, Lombard C, Swanvelder S, Nankunda J, Ramokolo V, Sanders D, Wamani H, Meda N, Tumwine JK, Ekström EC, Van de Perre P, Kankasa C, Sommerfelt H, Tylleskär T: Growth effects of exclusive breastfeeding promotion by peer counsellors in sub-Saharan Africa: the cluster-randomised PROMISE EBF trial. BMC Public Health 2014;14:633.

11 Arpadi S, Fawzy A, Aldrovandi GM, Kankasa C, Sinkala M, Mwiya M, Thea DM, Kuhn L: Growth faltering due to breastfeeding cessation in uninfected children born to HIV-infected mothers in Zambia. Am J Clin Nutr 2009;90:344–353.

12 Kuchenbecker J, Jordan I, Reinbott A, Herrmann J, Jeremias T, Kennedy G, Muehlhoff E, Mtimuni B, Krawinkel MB: Exclusive breastfeeding and its effect on growth of Malawian infants: results from a cross-sectional study. Paediatr Int Child Health 2015;35: 14–23.

13 Kramer MS, Kakuma R: Optimal duration of exclusive breastfeeding. Cochrane Database Syst Rev 2012;8:CD003517.

14 UNICEF: The State of the World's Children Report 2015. New York, UNICEF, 2014.

15 Benoist B, McLean E, Egli I, Cogswell M: Worldwide prevalence of anaemia 1993–2005. WHO global database on Anaemia. Genf, WHO, 2008.

16 Martorell R, Zongrone A: Intergenerational influences on child growth and undernutrition. Paediatr Perinat Epidemiol 2012;26(suppl 1):302–314.

17 Rossiter MD, Colapinto CK, Khan MK, McIsaac JL, Williams PL, Kirk SF, Veugelers PJ: Breast, formula and combination feeding in relation to childhood obesity in Nova Scotia, Canada. Matern Child Health J 2015;19:2048–2056.

18 Arenz S, Ruckerl R, Koletzko B, von Kries R: Breast-feeding and childhood obesity – a systematic review. Int J Obes Relat Metab Disord 2004;28:1247–1256.

19 Owen CG, Martin RM, Whincup PH, Smith GD, Cook DG: Effect of infant feeding on the risk of obesity across the life course: a quantitative review of published evidence. Pediatrics 2005;115:1367–1377.

20 Owen CG, Whincup PH, Kaye SJ, Martin RM, Davey Smith G, Cook DG, Bergström E, Black S, Wadsworth ME, Fall CH, Freudenheim JL, Nie J, Huxley RR, Kolacek S, Leeson CP, Pearce MS, Raitakari OT, Lisinen I, Viikari JS, Ravelli AC, Rudnicka AR, Strachan DP, Williams SM: Does initial breastfeeding lead to lower blood cholesterol in adult life? A quantitative review of the evidence. Am J Clin Nutr 2008; 88:305–314.

21 Sawaya AL, Dallal G, Solymos G, de Sousa MH, Ventura ML, Roberts SB, Sigulem DM: Obesity and malnutrition in a Shantytown population in the city of Sao Paulo, Brazil. Obes Res 1995;3(suppl 2):107s–115s.

22 Le Nguyen BK, Le Thi H, Nguyen Do VA, Tran Thuy N, Nguyen Huu C, Thanh Do T, Deurenberg P, Khouw I: Double burden of undernutrition and overnutrition in Vietnam in 2011: results of the SEANUTS study in 0.5–11-year-old children. Br J Nutr 2013;110(suppl 3):S45–S56.

23 Sahoo K, Sahoo B, Choudhury AK, Sofi NY, Kumar R, Bhadoria AS: Childhood obesity: causes and consequences. J Family Med Prim Care 2015;4:187–192.

24 Daniels SR: The consequences of childhood overweight and obesity. Future Child 2006;16:47–67.

25 Lobstein T, Jackson-Leach R, Moodie ML, Hall KD, Gortmaker SL, Swinburn BA, James WP, Wang Y, McPherson K: Child and adolescent obesity: part of a bigger picture. Lancet 2015;385:2510–2520.

26 Dewey KG, Mayers DR: Early child growth: how do nutrition and infection interact? Matern Child Nutr 2011;7(suppl 3):129–142.

27 Riordan JM: The biological specifity of breast milk; in Wambach K, Riordan JM (eds): Breastfeeding and Human Lactation. Burlington, Jones and Bartlett Learning, 2014, pp 117–151.

28 Newton ER: Breastmilk: the gold standard. Clin Obstet Gynecol 2004;47:632–642.

29 Ballard O, Morrow AL: Human milk composition: nutrients and bioactive factors. Pediatr Clin North Am 2013;60:49–74.

30 Lubetzky R, Mandel D, Mimouni FB: Vitamin and mineral supplementation of term infants: are they necessary? World Rev Nutr Diet 2013;108:79–85.

31 Davidsson L, Kastenmayer P, Yuen M, Lönnerdal B, Hurrell RF: Influence of lactoferrin on iron absorption from human milk in infants. Pediatr Res 1994; 35:117–124.

32 Bailey RL, West KP Jr, Black RE: The epidemiology of global micronutrient deficiencies. Ann Nutr Metab 2015;66(suppl 2):22–33.

33 Khan J, Vesel L, Bahl R, Martines JC: Timing of breastfeeding initiation and exclusivity of breast-feeding during the first month of life: effects on neonatal mortality and morbidity-a systematic review and meta-analysis. Matern Child Health J 2014;19: 468–479.

34 Debes AK, Kohli A, Walker N, Edmond K, Mullany LC: Time to initiation of breastfeeding and neonatal mortality and morbidity: a systematic review. BMC Public Health 2013;13(suppl 3):S19.

35 Kumar D, Goel NK, Mittal PC, Misra P: Influence of infant-feeding practices on nutritional status of under-five children. Indian J Pediatr 2006;73:417–421.

36 MEASURE DHS: Haiti. DHS 2012. Enquête Mortalité, Morbidité et Utilisation des Services: IHE – Haitian Childhood Institute, 2013.

37 Getahun Z, Scherbaum V, Taffese Y, Teshome B, Biesalski HK: Breastfeeding in Tigray and Gonder, Ethiopia, with special reference to exclusive/almost exclusive breastfeeding beyond six months. Breastfeed Rev 2004;12:8–16.

38 Inayati DA, Scherbaum V, Purwestri RC, Hormann E, Wirawan NN, Suryantan J, Hartono S, Bloem MA, Pangaribuan RV, Biesalski HK, Hoffmann V, Bellows AC: Infant feeding practices among mildly wasted children: a retrospective study on Nias Island, Indonesia. Int Breastfeed J 2012;7:3.

39 de Sa J, Bouttasing N, Sampson L, Perks C, Osrin D, Prost A: Identifying priorities to improve maternal and child nutrition among the Khmu ethnic group, Laos: a formative study. Matern Child Nutr 2013;9: 452–466.

40 Gao H, Wang Q, Stütz W, Hormann E, Biesalski HK, Scherbaum V: Birth outcomes and breastfeeding practices in urban and rural areas of Deyang regions, Sichuan Province, China. Int Breastfeed J, in process.
41 Aubel J: The role and influence of grandmothers on child nutrition: culturally designated advisors and caregivers. Matern Child Nutr 2012;8:19–35.
42 WHO: Guidelines on optimal feeding of low birth-weight infants in low- and middle-income countries. Geneva, WHO, 2011.
43 AHRQ: Breastfeeding and Maternal and Infant Health Outcomes in Developed Countries. Evidence Report. Rockville, Agency for Healthcare Research and Quality (AHRQ), 2007.
44 Solomons NW: Malnutrition and infection: an update. Br J Nutr 2007;98(suppl 1):S5–S10.
45 Beisel WR: Herman Award Lecture, 1995: infection-induced malnutrition – from cholera to cytokines. Am J Clin Nutr 1995;62:813–819.
46 Schaible UE, Kaufmann SH: Malnutrition and infection: complex mechanisms and global impacts. PLoS Med 2007;4:e115.
47 Keusch GT: The history of nutrition: malnutrition, infection and immunity. J Nutr 2003;133:336S–340S.
48 Ladomenou F, Moschandreas J, Kafatos A, Tselentis Y, Galanakis E: Protective effect of exclusive breastfeeding against infections during infancy: a prospective study. Arch Dis Child 2010;95:1004–1008.
49 Lamberti LM, Fischer Walker CL, Noiman A, Victora C, Black RE: Breastfeeding and the risk for diarrhea morbidity and mortality. BMC Public Health 2011;11(suppl 3):S15.
50 Lamberti LM, Zakarija-Grkovic I, Fischer Walker CL, Theodoratou E, Nair H, Campbell H, Black RE: Breastfeeding for reducing the risk of pneumonia morbidity and mortality in children under two: a systematic literature review and meta-analysis. BMC Public Health 2013;13(suppl 3):S18.
51 Richard SA, Black RE, Gilman RH, Guerrant RL, Kang G, Lanata CF, Mølbak K, Rasmussen ZA, Sack RB, Valentiner-Branth P, Checkley W: Catch-up growth occurs after diarrhea in early childhood. J Nutr 2014;144:965–971.
52 Field CJ: The immunological components of human milk and their effect on immune development in infants. J Nutr 2005;135:1–4.
53 Howie PW, Forsyth JS, Ogston SA, Clark A, Florey CD: Protective effect of breast feeding against infection. BMJ 1990;300:11–16.
54 Kramer MS, Chalmers B, Hodnett ED, Sevkovskaya Z, Dzikovich I, Shapiro S, Collet JP, Vanilovich I, Mezen I, Ducruet T, Shishko G, Zubovich V, Mknuik D, Gluchanina E, Dombrovskiy V, Ustinovitch A, Kot T, Bogdanovich N, Ovchinikova L, Helsing E: Promotion of Breastfeeding Intervention Trial (PROBIT): a randomized trial in the Republic of Belarus. JAMA 2001;285:413–420.
55 Coates MM, Riordan J: Breastfeeding during maternal or infant illness. NAACOGS Clin Issu Perinat Womens Health Nurs 1992;3:683–694.
56 Brown KH, Stallings RY, de Kanashiro HC, Lopez de Romana G, Black RE: Effects of common illnesses on infants' energy intakes from breast milk and other foods during longitudinal community-based studies in Huascar (Lima), Peru. Am J Clin Nutr 1990;52:1005–1013.
57 WHO: Infant and Young Child Feeding. Geneva, WHO, 2009.
58 Abrahams SW, Labbok MH: Breastfeeding and otitis media: a review of recent evidence. Curr Allergy Asthma Rep 2011;11:508–512.
59 Silfverdal SA, Bodin L, Olcén P: Protective effect of breastfeeding: an ecologic study of *Haemophilus influenzae* meningitis and breastfeeding in a Swedish population. Int J Epidemiol 1999;28:152–156.
60 Mårild S, Hansson S, Jodal U, Odén A, Svedberg K: Protective effect of breastfeeding against urinary tract infection. Acta Paediatr 2004;93:164–168.
61 Nishimura T, Suzue J, Kaji H: Breastfeeding reduces the severity of respiratory syncytial virus infection among young infants: a multi-center prospective study. Pediatr Int 2009;51:812–816.
62 Nakamori M, Nguyen XN, Nguyen CK, Cao TH, Nguyen AT, Le BM, Vu TT, Bui TN, Nakano T, Yoshiike N, Kusama K, Yamamoto S: Nutritional status, feeding practice and incidence of infectious diseases among children aged 6 to 18 months in northern mountainous Vietnam. J Med Invest 2010;57:45–53.
63 Kamudoni P, Maleta K, Shi Z, Holmboe-Ottesen G: Exclusive breastfeeding duration during the first 6 months of life is positively associated with length-for-age among infants 6–12 months old, in Mangochi district, Malawi. Eur J Clin Nutr 2015;69:96–101.
64 Marques R, Taddei JA, Konstantyner T, Lopez FA, Marques ACV, de Oliveira CS, Braga JAP: Anthropometric indices and exclusive breastfeeding in the first six months of life: a comparison with reference standards NCHS, 1977 and WHO, 2006. Int Breastfeed J 2015;10:20.
65 Zongrone A, Winskell K, Menon P: Infant and young child feeding practices and child undernutrition in Bangladesh: insights from nationally representative data. Public Health Nutr 2012;15:1697–1704.

66 Golden MH: Proposed recommended nutrient densities for moderately malnourished children. Food Nutr Bull 2009;30(3 suppl):S267–S342.
67 Labbok MH, Starling A: Definitions of breastfeeding: call for the development and use of consistent definitions in research and peer-reviewed literature. Breastfeed Med 2012;7:397–402.
68 Noel-Weiss J, Taljaard M, Kujawa-Myles S: Breastfeeding and lactation research: exploring a tool to measure infant feeding patterns. Int Breastfeed J 2014;9:5.
69 Jones AD, Ickes SB, Smith LE, Mbuya MN, Chasekwa B, Heidkamp RA, Menon P, Zongrone AA, Stoltzfus RJ: World Health Organization infant and young child feeding indicators and their associations with child anthropometry: a synthesis of recent findings. Matern Child Nutr 2014;10:1–17.
70 Greiner T: Speakers' Corner: a new theory: breastmilk displacement may be the major cause of nutritional stunting. SCN News 2004;28:63–64.
71 Dewey KG: Guiding Principles for Complementary Feeding of the Breastfed Child. Washington, PAHO, WHO, 2003.
72 WHO: First meeting of the WHO Scientific and Technical Advisory Group on Inappropriate Promotion of Foods for Infants and Young Children. Geneva, WHO, 2013.
73 Dewey KG, Brown KH: Update on technical issues concerning complementary feeding of young children in developing countries and implications for intervention programs. Food Nutr Bull 2003;24:5–28.
74 Dewey KG: Growth characteristics of breast-fed compared to formula-fed infants. Biol Neonate 1998; 74:94–105.
75 Haschke F, van't Hof MA: Euro-Growth references for breast-fed boys and girls: influence of breastfeeding and solids on growth until 36 months of age. Euro-Growth Study Group. J Pediatr Gastroenterol Nutr 2000;31(suppl 1):S60–S71.
76 Kramer MS, Guo T, Platt RW, Vanilovich I, Sevkovskaya Z, Dzikovich I, Michaelsen KF, Dewey K: Feeding effects on growth during infancy. J Pediatr 2004;145:600–605.
77 Kramer MS, Moodie EE, Dahhou M, Platt RW: Breastfeeding and infant size: evidence of reverse causality. Am J Epidemiol 2011;173:978–983.
78 Adair LS, Guilkey DK: Age-specific determinants of stunting in Filipino children. J Nutr 1997;127:314–320.
79 Marquis GS, Habicht JP, Lanata CF, Black RE, Rasmussen KM: Association of breastfeeding and stunting in Peruvian toddlers: an example of reverse causality. Int J Epidemiol 1997;26:349–356.
80 Simondon KB, Simondon F: Mothers prolong breastfeeding of undernourished children in rural Senegal. Int J Epidemiol 1998;27:490–494.
81 Potur AH, Kalmaz N: An investigation into feeding errors of 0–4-month-old infants. J Trop Pediatr 1996;42:173–175.
82 Meier BM, Labbok M: From the bottle to the grave: realizing a human right to breastfeeding through global health policy. Case West Reserve Law Rev 2010;60.
83 Scherbaum V: Säuglingsernährung in Nordirak. Ernährungsumschau 2003;50:476–480.
84 Ho TF, Yip WC, Tay JS, Wong HB: Variability in osmolality of home prepared formula milk samples. J Trop Pediatr 1985;31:92–94.
85 Cohen RJ, Brown KH, Canahuati J, Rivera LL, Dewey KG: Effects of age of introduction of complementary foods on infant breast milk intake, total energy intake, and growth: a randomised intervention study in Honduras. Lancet 1994;344:288–293.
86 Torres MA, Braga JA, Taddei JA, Nóbrega FJ: Anemia in low-income exclusively breastfed infants. J Pediatr (Rio J) 2006;82:284–287.
87 Chantry CJ, Howard CR, Auinger P: Full breastfeeding duration and risk for iron deficiency in US infants. Breastfeed Med 2007;2:63–73.
88 Dube K, Schwartz J, Mueller MJ, Kalhoff H, Kersting M: Iron intake and iron status in breastfed infants during the first year of life. Clin Nutr 2010;29:773–778.
89 Pisacane A, De Vizia B, Valiante A, Vaccaro F, Russo M, Grillo G, Giustardi A: Iron status in breast-fed infants. J Pediatr 1995;127:429–431.
90 Meinzen-Derr JK, Guerrero ML, Altaye M, Ortega-Gallegos H, Ruiz-Palacios GM, Morrow AL: Risk of infant anemia is associated with exclusive breastfeeding and maternal anemia in a Mexican cohort. J Nutr 2006;136:452–458.
91 Raj S, Faridi M, Rusia U, Singh O: A prospective study of iron status in exclusively breastfed term infants up to 6 months of age. Int Breastfeed J 2008; 3:3.
92 Koletzko B, Brands B, Chourdakis M, Cramer S, Grote V, Hellmuth C, Kirchberg F, Prell C, Rzehak P, Uhl O, Weber M: The power of programming and the EarlyNutrition project: opportunities for health promotion by nutrition during the first thousand days of life and beyond. Ann Nutr Metab 2014;64: 187–196.
93 McCrory C, Layte R: Breastfeeding and risk of overweight and obesity at nine-years of age. Soc Sci Med 2012;75:323–330.
94 Koletzko B, Chourdakis M, Grote V, Hellmuth C, Prell C, Rzehak P, Uhl O, Weber M: Regulation of early human growth: impact on long-term health. Ann Nutr Metab 2014;65:101–109.
95 Lucas A: Programming by early nutrition in man; in Bock GR, Whelan J (eds): The Childhood Environment and Adult Disease. Chichester, Wiley, 1991, pp 38–55.

96 Koletzko B, Beyer J, Brands B, Demmelmair H, Grote V, Haile G, Gruszfeld D, Rzehak P, Socha P, Weber M: Early influences of nutrition on postnatal growth. Nestle Nutr Inst Workshop Ser 2013;71: 11–27.
97 Weber M, Grote V, Closa-Monasterolo R, Escribano J, Langhendries JP, Dain E, Giovannini M, Verduci E, Gruszfeld D, Socha P, Koletzko B: Lower protein content in infant formula reduces BMI and obesity risk at school age: follow-up of a randomized trial. Am J Clin Nutr 2014;99:1041–1051.
98 Oddy W, McHugh MF: The impact of infant feeding on later metabolic health; in Watson RR, Grimble G, Preedy VR, Zibadii S (eds): Nutrition in Infancy Nutrition and Health. New York, Springer Science & Business Media, 2013, pp 221–237.
99 de Sa J, Bouttasing N, Sampson L, Perks C, Osrin D, Prost A: Identifying priorities to improve maternal and child nutrition among the Khmu ethnic group, Laos: a formative study. Matern Child Nutr 2015;9: 452–466.
100 Li R, Fein SB, Grummer-Strawn LM: Do infants fed from bottles lack self-regulation of milk intake compared with directly breastfed infants? Pediatrics 2010;125:e1386–1393.
101 Beauchamp GK, Mennella JA: Early flavor learning and its impact on later feeding behavior. J Pediatr Gastroenterol Nutr 2009;48(suppl 1):S25–S30.
102 Disantis KI, Collins BN, Fisher JO, Davey A: Do infants fed directly from the breast have improved appetite regulation and slower growth during early childhood compared with infants fed from a bottle? Int J Behav Nutr Phys Act 2011;8:89.
103 Yan J, Liu L, Zhu Y, Huang G, Wang PP: The association between breastfeeding and childhood obesity: a meta-analysis. BMC Public Health 2014;14: 1267.
104 Butte NF: Impact of infant feeding practices on childhood obesity. J Nutr 2009;139:412S–416S.
105 Brown KH, Akhtar NA, Robertson AD, Ahmed MG: Lactational capacity of marginally nourished mothers: relationships between maternal nutritional status and quantity and proximate composition of milk. Pediatrics 1986;78:909–819.
106 Dewey KG, Heinig MJ, Nommsen LA, Lönnerdal B: Maternal versus infant factors related to breast milk intake and residual milk volume: the DARLING study. Pediatrics 1991;87:829–837.
107 Villalpando SF, Butte NF, Wong WW, Flores-Huerta S, Hernandez-Beltran MJ, Smith EO, Garza C: Lactation performance of rural Mesoamerindians. Eur J Clin Nutr 1992;46:337–348.
108 Peters E, Wehkamp KH, Felberbaum RE, Krüger D, Linder R: Breastfeeding duration is determined by only a few factors. Eur J Public Health 2006;16:162–167.
109 Xu F, Qiu L, Binns CW, Liu X: Breastfeeding in China: a review. Int Breastfeed J 2009;4:6.
110 Nommsen-Rivers LA, Dolan LM, Huang B: Timing of stage II lactogenesis is predicted by antenatal metabolic health in a cohort of primiparas. Breastfeed Med 2012;7:43–49.
111 Matias SL, Dewey KG, Quesenberry CP Jr, Gunderson EP: Maternal prepregnancy obesity and insulin treatment during pregnancy are independently associated with delayed lactogenesis in women with recent gestational diabetes mellitus. Am J Clin Nutr 2014;99:115–121.
112 Wojcicki JM: Maternal prepregnancy body mass index and initiation and duration of breastfeeding: a review of the literature. J Womens Health (Larchmt) 2010;20:341–347.
113 Kim J, Friel J: Lipids and human milk. Lipid Technol 2012;24:103–105.
114 Hachey DL, Silber GH, Wong WW, Garza C: Human lactation. II: Endogenous fatty acid synthesis by the mammary gland. Pediatr Res 1989;25:63–68.
115 Anderson AK, McDougald DM, Steiner-Asiedu M: Dietary trans fatty acid intake and maternal and infant adiposity. Eur J Clin Nutr 2010;64:1308–1315.
116 Kruger HS, Butte NF: Nutrition in pregnancy and lactation. World Rev Nutr Diet 2015;111:64–70.
117 Barennes H, Sengkhamyong K, Rene JP, Phimmasane M: Beriberi (thiamine deficiency) and high infant mortality in northern Laos. PLoS Negl Trop Dis 2015;9:e0003581.
118 Gushurst CA, Mueller JA, Green JA, Sedor F: Breast milk iodide: reassessment in the 1980s. Pediatrics 1984;73:354–357.
119 Mannan S, Picciano MF: Influence of maternal selenium status on human milk selenium concentration and glutathione peroxidase activity. Am J Clin Nutr 1987;46:95–100.
120 Prentice A: Calcium supplementation during breast-feeding. N Engl J Med 1997;337:558–559.
121 Dallman PR: Iron deficiency in the weanling: a nutritional problem on the way to resolution. Acta Paediatr Scand Suppl 1986;323:59–67.
122 Kraemer K, de Pee S, Badham J: Evidence in multiple micronutrient nutrition: from history to science to effective programs. J Nutr 2012;142:138S–142S.
123 PMNCH: A global review of the key interventions related to reproductive, maternal, newborn and child health (RMNCH). Geneva, The Partnership for Maternal, Newborn and Child Health, 2011.
124 Persson LA, Arifeen S, Ekström EC, Rasmussen KM, Frongillo EA, Yunus M: Effects of prenatal micronutrient and early food supplementation on maternal hemoglobin, birth weight, and infant mortality among children in Bangladesh: the MINIMat randomized trial. JAMA 2012;307:2050–2059.

125 Chapman DJ, Nommsen-Rivers L: Impact of maternal nutritional status on human milk quality and infant outcomes: an update on key nutrients. Adv Nutr 2012;3:351–352.
126 UNICEF, WHO, World Bank: Joint Child Malnutrition Estimates – Levels and Trends. New York, Geneva, Washington, UNICEF, WHO, World Bank, 2012.
127 Ibanez G, de Reynal de Saint Michel C, Denantes M, Saurel-Cubizolles MJ, Ringa V, Magnier AM: Systematic review and meta-analysis of randomized controlled trials evaluating primary care-based interventions to promote breastfeeding in low-income women. Fam Pract 2012;29:245–254.
128 Beake S, Pellowe C, Dykes F, Schmied V, Bick D: A systematic review of structured compared with non-structured breastfeeding programmes to support the initiation and duration of exclusive and any breastfeeding in acute and primary health care settings. Matern Child Nutr 2012;8:141–161.
129 Ingram L, MacArthur C, Khan K, Deeks JJ, Jolly K: Effect of antenatal peer support on breastfeeding initiation: a systematic review. CMAJ 2010;182: 1739–1746.
130 Haroon S, Das JK, Salam RA, Imdad A, Bhutta ZA: Breastfeeding promotion interventions and breastfeeding practices: a systematic review. BMC Public Health 2013;13(suppl 3):S20.
131 Tylleskar T, Jackson D, Meda N, Engebretsen IM, Chopra M, Diallo AH, Doherty T, Ekström EC, Fadnes LT, Goga A, Kankasa C, Klungsoyr JI, Lombard C, Nankabirwa V, Nankunda JK, Van de Perre P, Sanders D, Shanmugam R, Sommerfelt H, Wamani H, Tumwine JK: Exclusive breastfeeding promotion by peer counsellors in sub-Saharan Africa (PROMISE-EBF): a cluster-randomised trial. Lancet 2011;378:420–427.
132 Dyson L, McCormick F, Renfrew MJ: Interventions for promoting the initiation of breastfeeding. Cochrane Database Syst Rev 2005:CD001688.
133 Quinlivan J, Kua S, Gibson R, McPhee A, Makrides MM: Can we identify women who initiate and then prematurely cease breastfeeding? An Australian multicentre cohort study. Int Breastfeed J 2015;10: 16.
134 Dietrich Leurer M, Misskey E: 'Be positive as well as realistic': a qualitative description analysis of information gaps experienced by breastfeeding mothers. Int Breastfeed J 2015;10:10.
135 Bhandari N, Kabir AK, Salam MA: Mainstreaming nutrition into maternal and child health programmes: scaling up of exclusive breastfeeding. Matern Child Nutr 2008;4(suppl 1):5–23.
136 Victora CG, Horta BL, Loret de Mola C, Quevedo L, Pinheiro RT, Gigante DP, Goncalves H, Barros FC: Association between breastfeeding and intelligence, educational attainment, and income at 30 years of age: a prospective birth cohort study from Brazil. Lancet Glob Health 2015;3:e199–e205.
137 Mortensen EL: Life course consequences of breastfeeding. Lancet Glob Health 2015;3:e179–e180.
138 SCF: Superfood for Babies. How Overcoming Barriers to Breastfeeding Will Save Children's Lives. London, Save the Children, 2013.
139 Perez-Escamilla R: Can experience-based household food security scales help improve food security governance? Glob Food Sec 2012;1:120–125.
140 Entwistle F, Kendall S, Mead M: Breastfeeding support – the importance of self-efficacy for low-income women. Matern Child Nutr 2010;6:228–242.
141 Holla-Bhar R, Iellamo A, Gupta A, Smith JP, Dadhich JP: Investing in breastfeeding – the world breastfeeding costing initiative. Int Breastfeed J 2015;10:8.
142 Rouw E, Hormann E, Scherbaum V: The high cost of half-hearted breastfeeding promotion in Germany. Int Breastfeed J 2015;9:22.
143 Kent G: Global infant formula: monitoring and regulating the impacts to protect human health. Int Breastfeed J 2015;10:6.
144 Smith JP: Markets, breastfeeding and trade in mothers' milk. Int Breastfeed J 2015;10:9.
145 Cattaneo A: The benefits of breastfeeding or the harm of formula feeding? J Paediatr Child Health 2008;44:1–2.
146 Kimani-Murage EW, Madise NJ, Fotso JC, Kyobutungi C, Mutua MK, Gitau TM, Yatich N: Patterns and determinants of breastfeeding and complementary feeding practices in urban informal settlements, Nairobi Kenya. BMC Public Health 2011; 11:396.
147 Abdulwadud OA, Snow ME: Interventions in the workplace to support breastfeeding for women in employment. Cochrane Database Syst Rev 2012; 10:CD006177.
148 Hirani SA, Karmaliani R: Evidence based workplace interventions to promote breastfeeding practices among Pakistani working mothers. Women Birth 2013;26:10–16.

Dr. Veronika Scherbaum
Institute for Biological Chemistry and Nutition, 140
University of Hohenheim
Garbenstrasse 30, DE–70593 Stuttgart (Germany)
E-Mail veronika.scherbaum@uni-hohenheim.de

Biesalski HK, Black RE (eds): Hidden Hunger. Malnutrition and the First 1,000 Days of Life: Causes, Consequences and Solutions. World Rev Nutr Diet. Basel, Karger, 2016, vol 115, pp 98–108
DOI: 10.1159/000442076

A Vitamin on the Mind: New Discoveries on Control of the Brain by Vitamin A

Patrick N. Stoney · Peter McCaffery

Institute of Medical Sciences, School of Medical Sciences, University of Aberdeen, Aberdeen, UK

Abstract

Vitamin A is essential for many physiological processes and is particularly crucial during early life, when vitamin A deficiency increases mortality through elevated rates of infection. This deadly aspect of vitamin A deficiency masks other effects that, while not lethal, may nevertheless cause significant issues if vitamin A insufficiency reoccurs during later childhood or in the adult. One such effect is on the brain. Vitamin A is essential for several regions of the brain, and this chapter focuses on two regions: the hippocampus, needed for learning and memory, and the hypothalamus, necessary to maintain the body's internal physiological balance. Vitamin A, through its active metabolite retinoic acid, is required to support neuroplasticity in the hippocampus, and vitamin A deficiency has a dramatic effect on depressing learning and memory. The effects of vitamin A deficiency on the hypothalamus may lead to depression of appetite and growth. Much of this research has relied on animal studies, and it will be essential in the future to determine the full role of vitamin A in the human brain.

The importance of vitamin A for the central nervous system (CNS) was first evident with the discovery that vitamin A is required for the function of the eye [1]. A lack of vitamin A leads to decline and loss of vision, as this vitamin has a fundamental role in retinal function and visual transduction. The rods and cones of the retina respond to light via their expression of proteins of the opsin family. Each opsin protein is bound to a form of vitamin A called retinaldehyde, which undergoes a light-induced shape change (photoisomerization) [2]. This is key to triggering a G protein-activated pathway that eventually leads to a signal sent to the brain to allow visual perception. The earliest sign of vitamin A deficiency is xerophthalmia, which can start with night-blindness, reflecting a decline in the retina's capacity for light detection [3]. Night-blindness is reversible with restoration of vitamin A, but the vitamin is also necessary for the health of the cornea, the transparent structure in the front of the eye. Later stages of xerophthalmia resulting from vitamin A deficiency can include ulceration of the cornea and finally corneal melting, causing irreversible blindness [3]. Vitamin A is even necessary for the development of the eye in the foetus, and vitamin A deficiency can cause severe malformation of this structure [4].

The major consequences of vitamin A deficiency in man, blindness and immune deficiency leading to susceptibility to infection, have prompted large-scale schemes to prevent deficiency in the young. Effects on regions of the CNS other than the eye, including the brain, which do not cause an immediate hazard to health have, quite reasonably, been considered less of an issue. However, new evidence from studies of animal models suggests that vitamin A is essential for a number of key functions of the brain [5], and these may be affected by even relatively mild vitamin A deficiency or can be problematic when combined with a genetic susceptibility to vitamin A deficiency, such as in individuals who cannot make efficient use of carotenes [6]. Administration of vitamin A during infancy may reduce mortality rates, although the case remains open [7–9]. Much less investigated, however, are the problems that may arise from vitamin A deficiency in older children or adults as a result of effects on, for instance, cognition and body homeostasis under CNS control. This chapter will describe some of the recent advances in understanding the function of vitamin A in the brain and the potential consequences of vitamin A deficiency based on studies of animal models. The focus is on two regions of the brain: the hippocampus, essential for cognition, and the hypothalamus, which regulates body homeostasis.

The brain's requirement for vitamin A is not driven by a need for the vitamin per se, but instead for a molecule derived from vitamin A. The molecule is an active form of vitamin A called retinoic acid and is generated in two steps by enzymes [retinol dehydrogenases and retinaldehyde dehydrogenases (RALDHs)] present in those cells that activate vitamin A [10]. These pathways are summarized in figure 1. Once retinoic acid is synthesized, it binds to receptors present in the nucleus of cells. These retinoic acid receptors (RARs), once triggered by retinoic acid, can bind to the genomic promoter regions that activate specific genes, leading to expression of protein to control cell function. A common action of retinoic acid is to control proliferating cells, generally directing their differentiation into particular cell types and inhibiting their capacity to divide. This role accounts for many of the functions of vitamin A in the epithelium of the eye and gut, the keratinocytes of the skin and the proliferating cells of the immune system. A second route exists by which the RARs can control the expression of proteins by binding directly to the mRNA used as a template by the ribosomes to assemble the proteins (fig. 1). These are the two main routes by which vitamin A acts in the brain, while the system is turned off by breakdown of retinoic acid by a set of enzymes known as CYP26s (fig. 1).

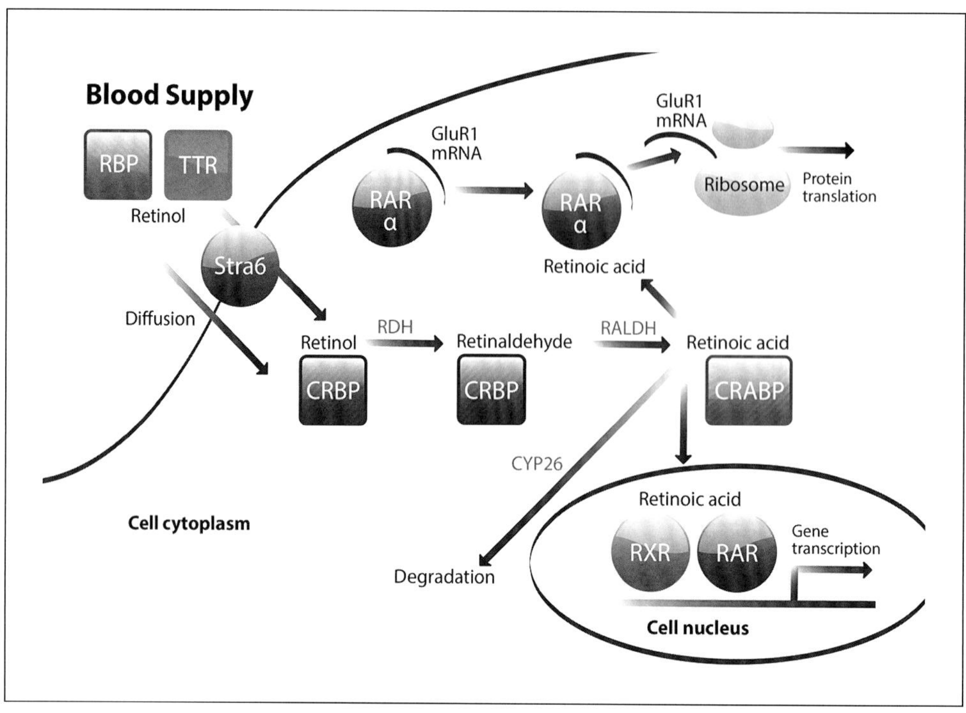

Fig. 1. How vitamin A signals in the cell via its metabolite retinoic acid. Retinol is carried in the blood supply by the proteins retinol-binding protein (RBP) and transthyretin (TTR). Retinol is unloaded at the cell and crosses the plasma membrane either through passive diffusion or, in some cells, transport by the protein stimulated by retinoic acid 6 (Stra6). Now in the cytoplasm, retinol is bound by cellular retinol-binding protein (CRBP) and is oxidized to retinaldehyde, while still bound to the protein, by the enzyme retinol dehydrogenase (RDH). RALDH enzymes can then further oxidize retinaldehyde to produce retinoic acid, which is bound by cellular retinoic acid-binding protein (CRABP). Retinoic acid induces changes in the cell by binding to specific RARs. In the nucleus, these receptors bind to the retinoid X receptor (RXR) to form a heterodimer, and together, bound to retinoic acid, they induce expression of target genes. Alternatively, retinoic acid can bind to cytoplasmic RARα, which is associated with certain mRNA species, such as GluR1, blocking their translation into protein. On binding to retinoic acid, RARα releases the mRNA, allowing it to be translated into protein, in this case the α-amino-3-hydroxy-5-methyl-4-isoxazolepropionic acid (AMPA) receptor subunit GluR1. Finally, vitamin A signalling can be switched off by degradation of retinoic acid by the enzyme CYP26.

The functions of vitamin A and retinoic acid in controlling cell proliferation and differentiation had previously suggested only minor functions for this vitamin in the brain, given that neurons are nonproliferative. However, vitamin A is essential for neuroplasticity, which is a group of mechanisms that allow neurons to alter their connections with other cells and the strength of the signal that passes along them. The rule that cell division is absent in the brain is broken in a few restricted areas, and vitamin A is in control of these processes in such regions.

The hippocampus is a region of the brain in which neuroplasticity is essential for function and is one of the best-studied regions regarding the roles of vitamin A and retinoic acid; it is part of the limbic system and essential for long-term memory, including the emotional responses that can be linked with these. The hippocampus' role in spatial memory is crucial for mapping the world around us and for navigation. Long-term potentiation (LTP) and long-term depression (LTD) are forms of neuroplasticity required for hippocampus-dependent memory and are the processes by which synaptic strength is altered [11]. The receptor RARα is present in the hippocampus [12]. When vitamin A is depleted, there is a significant reduction of LTP in the hippocampus and almost complete loss of LTD in the CA1 subfield [13]. This can be restored by addition of retinoic acid to the hippocampus, indicating that vitamin A is required as a source of retinoic acid and that it acts directly on the hippocampus. A study blocking the action of endogenous RARs in transgenic mice using a dominant negative receptor verified the role of retinoic acid in learning and memory and in LTP in the hippocampus [14]. The involvement of a specific RAR was studied in mice lacking the gene encoding RARβ. In these mice, there was an almost complete loss of hippocampal LTP and LTD, and their ability to navigate through a maze was significantly impaired [15]. Vitamin A deficiency in the rat during postnatal development resulted in significant impairment in performance in learning and memory tasks and a decline in hippocampal LTP. One potential mechanism for this decline was a reduction in the expression of the N-methyl-D-aspartate (NMDA) receptor subunit NR1 [16], with this receptor being a glutamate receptor and voltage-dependent ion channel essential for neuroplasticity. The authors of this study have also shown that RARα has a central role to play in NR1 expression and suggest that one mechanism of hippocampal dysfunction and learning and memory impairment in vitamin A deficiency is through epigenetic change, with a decline in histone acetylation mediated through RARα's control of cyclic AMP response element-binding protein-binding protein [17]. These studies are dependent on rodent animal models, but a study of the nonhuman primate brain has found that genes mediating retinoic acid signalling are amongst the unique gene expression 'signatures' of the hippocampus [18].

A further intriguing action for retinoic acid in the hippocampus is its role in the daily (circadian) rhythm of gene expression [19]; such day/night oscillations occur in all tissues and, in the hippocampus, are important for the persistence of long-term memory [20]. The retinoid signalling pathway shows a daily oscillation of expression in the hippocampus [21]. Vitamin A deficiency interferes with the daily pattern of expression of the genes *Bmal1* and *Per1*, 'clock' genes that encode key components of the mechanism that drives the daily oscillation of gene expression [21, 22]. Retinoic acid itself is known to change the rhythmic expression of another clock gene, *Per2*, in the vasculature [23]. Downstream of these daily rhythms of retinoic acid in the hippocampus may be the gene encoding brain-derived neurotrophic factor *(Bdnf)*, a growth factor that supports neuron survival [22] and promotes neuronal growth and synaptogenesis. Other rhythmically expressed genes that may be downstream of retinoic acid are *Cat* and *Gpx*, encoding catalase and glutathione peroxidase respectively, factors that protect against the damaging effects of oxidizing molecules in the brain [24].

Retinoic acid also plays an essential role in another form of plasticity in the hippocampus, known as homeostatic plasticity, which gives stability to networks of neurons and prevents, for instance, uncontrolled positive feedback loops. Retinoic acid can be synthesized in activated excitatory neurons to control the expression of the α-amino-3-hydroxy-5-methyl-4-isoxazolepropionic acid (AMPA) receptor subunit GluR1 and, through this, to limit the extent of activity across neural circuits. The mechanism by which retinoic acid controls this process is via direct regulation of protein translation, as illustrated in figure 1.

The receptor RARα binds directly to sequences in the *GluR1* mRNA [25, 26], preventing translation of the corresponding protein by the ribosome. Retinoic acid binding to RARα results in release of the mRNA and allows *GluR1* to be translated. This effect of retinoic acid to promote the expression of GluR1 in excitatory neurons parallels the capacity of retinoic acid to *reduce* the number of γ-aminobutyric acid A receptors in *inhibitory* neurons [27].

The last type of neuroplasticity in the hippocampus to be described as regulated by vitamin A and retinoic acid is the birth of new neurons, a process called neurogenesis. The hippocampus is one of the few regions in the postnatal brain where new neurons are born, which is necessary for certain types of memory formation [28]. Neurogenesis occurs in the dentate gyrus of the hippocampus, giving rise to new granule neurons [29]. In general, retinoic acid stimulates the process of neuronal differentiation and can, for instance, induce NeuroD and p21 in cultured stem cells [30]. Postnatal animals treated with retinoic acid show an increase in the thickness of the layer of granule neurons in the dentate gyrus, suggesting that retinoic acid may also promote neurogenesis in vivo [31]. Given these findings, it is unsurprising that depletion of vitamin A in mice results in a decline in hippocampal neurogenesis [32]. The effects of vitamin A deficiency are not on cell division but instead reduce the ability of newborn cells to differentiate into neurons and survive. The same study identified *Wnt7b*, a member of the secreted Wnt protein signalling system that is known to regulate neurogenesis [33], as a gene likely to be regulated by vitamin A in the hippocampus. Interestingly, a set of genes were also identified as being involved in cholesterol and fatty acid homeostasis, including *ABCa1*, *SREBP1a*, *ApoE*, and *cd36*, and the authors proposed that these genes prepare cells for changes in energy requirements and a future need for lipids. Later studies on the influence of vitamin A deficiency on hippocampal neurogenesis confirmed that retinoic acid mediates the effects of vitamin A on neurogenesis and identified the neurotrophin receptor tropomyosin receptor kinase A (TrkA) to also be a potential mediator of retinoic acid function [34].

Cell division is distributed unevenly in the dentate gyrus [35], with a higher rate of proliferation in the upper part of the dentate gyrus, and this asymmetric distribution is likely to be controlled by a gradient of retinoic acid that spreads across the area [36].

This asymmetric pattern of neurogenesis in the dentate gyrus supports the pattern separation function of the hippocampus; this allows similar patterns of neural activity to be made more distinct, allowing separation of memories that may be generally similar to each other [37]. The way in which retinoic acid regulates this pattern of neurogenesis is very similar to the way in which retinoic acid controls the growth of the embryonic CNS in a patterned fashion [38, 39]. It is of note, though, that the correct local concentration of retinoic acid is essential to support neurogenesis, as a deficiency in retinoic acid results in decreased neuronal differentiation, while an excess will inhibit the proliferation of neuronal precursors [40]. This has strong parallels to the corticosteroid hormones, as a minimal level of these hormones is necessary to maintain plasticity, but excess amounts will inhibit the same processes [41, 42].

The second region of the brain where vitamin A has been studied in detail is the hypothalamus. The hypothalamus controls many autonomic functions of the peripheral nervous system and is the command centre for hormonal regulation. It is the site by which the brain controls body homeostasis, regulating, for instance, appetite and thirst. Its integrative function places the hypothalamus at the crossroads between body and brain, controlling the body through its command of the pituitary gland and circulating hormone balance.

All the components necessary for vitamin A are present in the hypothalamus. Retinoic acid is present in the arcuate nucleus and dorsolateral hypothalamus [43]. The tanycytes that line the third ventricle, whose long processes permeate the hypothalamus, express cellular retinol-binding protein [12] as well as the retinoic acid-synthesizing enzyme RALDH1 (fig. 2a, b) [44]. The RARs are present in the dorsomedial posterior arcuate nucleus [45]. Further, in the paraventricular nucleus of the human hypothalamus, the receptor RARα is expressed in a subset of cells, where it may regulate expression of corticotropin-releasing hormone [46]. The relationship between retinoic acid signalling and depression proposed in this last study suggests retinoic acid signalling as a potential target for the treatment of affective disorders.

Amongst the first indications that vitamin A was necessary for the hypothalamus were studies in which rats were deprived of vitamin A but kept healthy with a constant supply of retinoic acid [47]. Retinoic acid is metabolized very quickly (within hours), which means that once the retinoic acid supplement was removed, the animals were almost immediately deficient in this active form of vitamin A, and since they had already been depleted of vitamin A reserves, they had no ability to make retinoic acid. It was found in such studies that the animals showed an almost immediate decrease in body weight and food intake (fig. 2c, d). As the hypothalamus is the control centre for these processes, the findings hinted at an effect in this brain region.

The second indication of a function for vitamin A in the hypothalamus, and particularly the control of body weight, growth and appetite, came from studies using animals that change seasonally in body weight and food intake, putting on weight during the summer and limiting appetite to conserve stores during the winter. These changes are precisely regulated by the hypothalamus, and a series of previous studies demonstrated

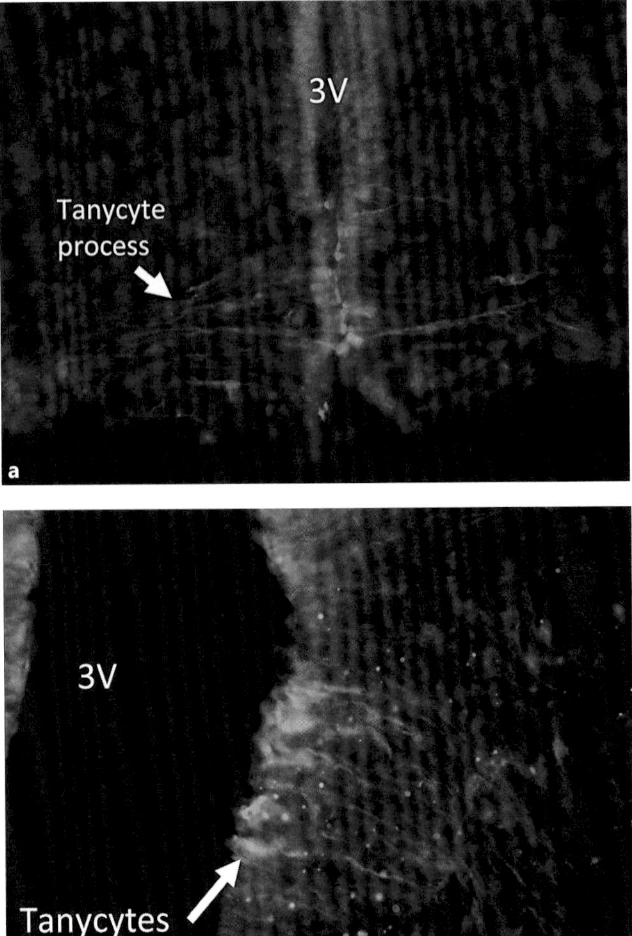

2

(For legend see next page.)

how the hypothalamus uses thyroid hormone to change gene expression in the hypothalamus to stimulate or repress growth and appetite between the seasons [48–50]. More recently, though, it has been shown that vitamin A has a role to play in appetite and growth control by the hypothalamus. The tanycytes, which send their processes into the arcuate nucleus and the dorsomedial hypothalamic nucleus of the hypothalamus, can convert vitamin A into retinoic acid via their expression of RALDH1. The levels of this enzyme, and thus retinoic acid synthesis, change greatly between the seasons, with much higher hypothalamic retinoic acid levels in the summer [5, 44, 51, 52]. These changes in hypothalamic RA levels are accompanied by changes in other components of the retinoic acid signalling pathway, which together cause a summertime upregulation of retinoic signalling in regions of the hypothalamus that control appetite and growth.

Fig. 2. Potential roles of vitamin A in the hypothalamus. Immunohistochemistry shows that the rat hypothalamus expresses the enzyme retinaldehyde dehydrogenase 1, which converts vitamin A to active retinoic acid in the tanycytes that line the third ventricle and send their processes into the hypothalamus (**a**). A higher-magnification view shows the cell bodies in the wall of the third ventricle (**b**). The potential effects of vitamin A deficiency on the hypothalamus are shown in illustrations adapted from Anzano et al. [47]. These show body weight as a percentage of T_0 body weight in retinoic acid-supplemented (RA), retinyl palmitate (A^+) control and vitamin A-deficient (A^-) rats fed either an 18% casein vitamin A-free diet (**c**) or force-fed isoenergetic liquid 18% casein (**d**). The numbers in parentheses indicate the number of animals in each group, and values are the mean ± SD. Vitamin A deficiency results in a rapid decline in body weight (**c**). The force feeding (**d**) results in a lesser decrease in body weight, suggesting that the rapid reduction in body weight is in part due to a loss of appetite and may represent an influence of vitamin A deficiency on the hypothalamus.

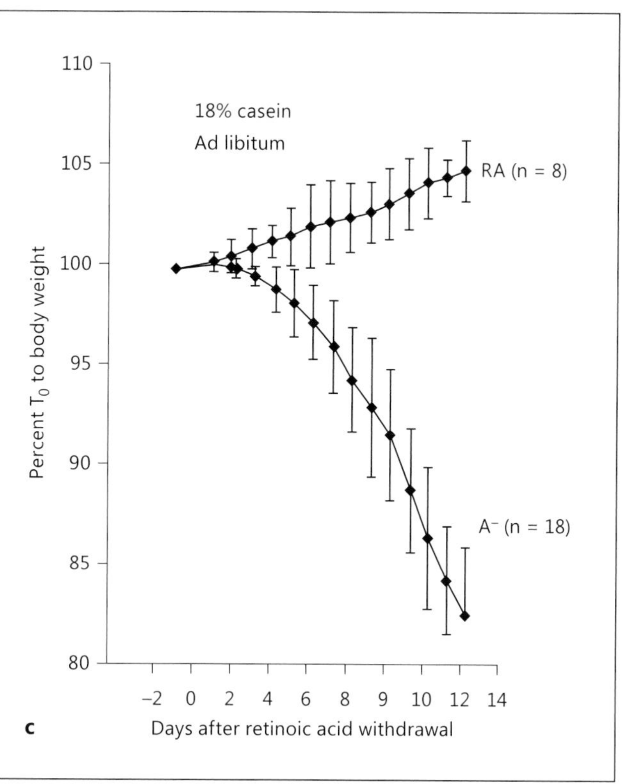

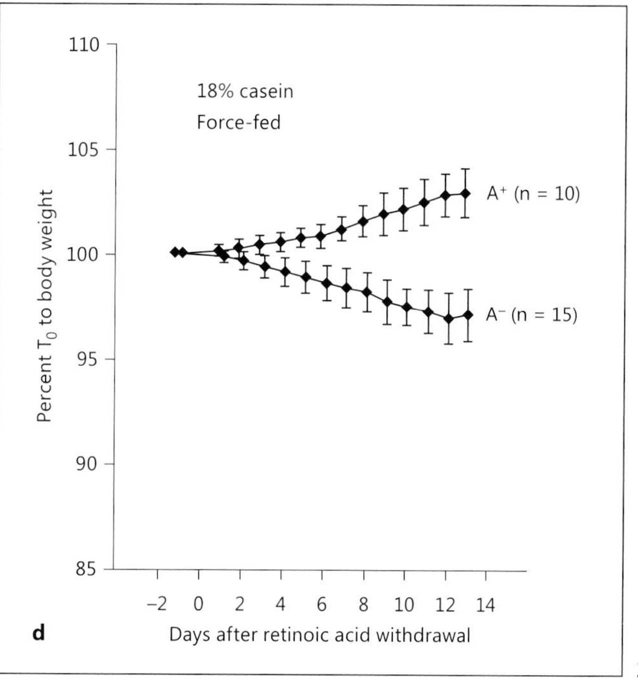

2

The hormones regulated by hypothalamic retinoic acid are not completely understood but may include adrenocorticotropic hormone [44] as well as gonadotrophin-releasing hormone, which contains an RAR-binding site in its promoter region [53]. As in the case of retinoic acid's control of neurogenesis in the hippocampus, the Wnt signalling pathway has been suggested to be regulated by retinoic acid in the hypothalamus [5, 51]. Indeed, the hypothalamus is one of the few regions in which neurogenesis takes place, with the newborn neurons potentially regulating appetite [54]. Retinoic acid is synthesized in the same region of the hypothalamus in which the neural stem cells reside [52], and retinoic acid may regulate cell proliferation in this region [52]. Control of Wnt signalling is perhaps one route by which retinoic acid may regulate hypothalamic neurogenesis.

In summary, the focus in the past has been on the serious and life-threatening effects of vitamin A deficiency. Now, with greater effectiveness in vitamin A delivery to the most vulnerable young children, the effects of vitamin A deficiency on the brain in older children and adults should be considered. The chapter has considered two regions of the brain: the hippocampus and hypothalamus. Abnormal function of the hippocampus will have serious effects on learning and memory, while disruption of the hypothalamus will result in imbalance of body homeostasis. Such changes resulting from human vitamin A deficiency will need to be investigated in greater detail in the future.

References

1 Wald G: Carotenoids and the visual cycle. J Gen Physiol 1935;19:351–371.

2 Saari JC: Retinoids in photosensitive systems; in Sporn MB, Roberts AB, Goodman DS (eds): The Retinoids: Biology, Chemistry, and Medicine. New York, Raven Press, 1984.

3 Sommer A: Xerophthalmia and vitamin A status. Prog Retin Eye Res 1998;17:9–31.

4 See AW, Clagett-Dame M: The temporal requirement for vitamin A in the developing eye: mechanism of action in optic fissure closure and new roles for the vitamin in regulating cell proliferation and adhesion in the embryonic retina. Develop Biol 2009;325:94–105.

5 Shearer KD, Stoney PN, Morgan PJ, McCaffery PJ: A vitamin for the brain. Trends Neurosci 2012;35:733–741.

6 Leung WC, Hessel S, Meplan C, Flint J, Oberhauser V, Tourniaire F, Hesketh JE, von Lintig J, Lietz G: Two common single nucleotide polymorphisms in the gene encoding beta-carotene 15,15′-monoxygenase alter beta-carotene metabolism in female volunteers. FASEB J 2009;23:1041–1053.

7 Edmond KM, Newton S, Shannon C, O'Leary M, Hurt L, Thomas G, Amenga-Etego S, Tawiah-Agyemang C, Gram L, Hurt CN, Bahl R, Owusu-Agyei S, Kirkwood BR: Effect of early neonatal vitamin A supplementation on mortality during infancy in Ghana (Neovita): a randomised, double-blind, placebo-controlled trial. Lancet 2015;385:1315–1323.

8 Mazumder S, Taneja S, Bhatia K, Yoshida S, Kaur J, Dube B, Toteja GS, Bahl R, Fontaine O, Martines J, Bhandari N: Efficacy of early neonatal supplementation with vitamin a to reduce mortality in infancy in Haryana, India (Neovita): a randomised, double-blind, placebo-controlled trial. Lancet 2015;385:1333–1342.

9 Masanja H, Smith ER, Muhihi A, Briegleb C, Mshamu S, Ruben J, Noor RA, Khudyakov P, Yoshida S, Martines J, Bahl R, Fawzi WW: Effect of neonatal vitamin A supplementation on mortality in infants in Tanzania (Neovita): a randomised, double-blind, placebo-controlled trial. Lancet 2015;385:1324–1332.

10 Napoli JL: Physiological insights into all-trans-retinoic acid biosynthesis. Biochim Biophys Acta 2012;1821:152–167.

11 Artola A, Singer W: Long-term depression of excitatory synaptic transmission and its relationship to long-term potentiation. Trends Neurosci 1993;16: 480–487.
12 Zetterström RH, Simon A, Giacobini MMJ, Ericksson U, Olson L: Localization of cellular retinoid-binding proteins suggests specific roles for retinoids in the adult central nervous system. Neuroscience 1994;62:899–918.
13 Misner DL, Jacobs S, Shimizu Y, de Urquiza AM, Solomin L, Perlmann T, De Luca LM, Stevens CF, Evans RM: Vitamin A deprivation results in reversible loss of hippocampal long-term synaptic plasticity. Proc Natl Acad Sci USA 2001;98:11714–11719.
14 Nomoto M, Takeda Y, Uchida S, Mitsuda K, Enomoto H, Saito K, Choi T, Watabe AM, Kobayashi S, Masushige S, Manabe T, Kida S: Dysfunction of the RAR/RXR signaling pathway in the forebrain impairs hippocampal memory and synaptic plasticity. Mol Brain 2012;5:8.
15 Chiang MY, Misner D, Kempermann G, Schikorski T, Giguere V, Sucov HM, Gage FH, Stevens CF, Evans RM: An essential role for retinoid receptors RARbeta and RXRgamma in long-term potentiation and depression. Neuron 1998;21:1353–1361.
16 Jiang W, Yu Q, Gong M, Chen L, Wen EY, Bi Y, Zhang Y, Shi Y, Qu P, Liu YX, Wei XP, Chen J, Li TY: Vitamin A deficiency impairs postnatal cognitive function via inhibition of neuronal calcium excitability in hippocampus. J Neurochem 2012;121:932–943.
17 Hou N, Ren L, Gong M, Bi Y, Gu Y, Dong Z, Liu Y, Chen J, Li T: Vitamin A deficiency impairs spatial learning and memory: the mechanism of abnormal CBP-dependent histone acetylation regulated by retinoic acid receptor alpha. Mol Neurobiol 2015;51: 633–647.
18 Dalgard CL, Jacobowitz DM, Singh VK, Saleem KS, Ursano RJ, Starr JM, Pollard HB: A novel analytical brain block tool to enable functional annotation of discriminatory transcript biomarkers among discrete regions of the fronto-limbic circuit in primate brain. Brain Res 2015;1600:42–58.
19 Ransom J, Morgan PJ, McCaffery PJ, Stoney PN: The rhythm of retinoids in the brain. J Neurochem 2014; 129:366–376.
20 Eckel-Mahan KL, Phan T, Han S, Wang H, Chan GC, Scheiner ZS, Storm DR: Circadian oscillation of hippocampal MAPK activity and cAmp: implications for memory persistence. Nat Neurosci 2008;11: 1074–1082.
21 Navigatore-Fonzo LS, Golini RL, Ponce IT, Delgado SM, Plateo-Pignatari MG, Gimenez MS, Anzulovich AC: Retinoic acid receptors move in time with the clock in the hippocampus. Effect of a vitamin-A-deficient diet. J Nutr Biochem 2013;24:859–867.
22 Golini RS, Delgado SM, Navigatore Fonzo LS, Ponce IT, Lacoste MG, Anzulovich AC: Daily patterns of clock and cognition-related factors are modified in the hippocampus of vitamin A-deficient rats. Hippocampus 2012;22:1720–1732.
23 McNamara P, Seo SB, Rudic RD, Sehgal A, Chakravarti D, FitzGerald GA: Regulation of CLOCK and MOP4 by nuclear hormone receptors in the vasculature: a humoral mechanism to reset a peripheral clock. Cell 2001;105:877–889.
24 Fonzo LS, Golini RS, Delgado SM, Ponce IT, Bonomi MR, Rezza IG, Gimenez MS, Anzulovich AC: Temporal patterns of lipoperoxidation and antioxidant enzymes are modified in the hippocampus of vitamin A-deficient rats. Hippocampus 2009;19:869–880.
25 Poon MM, Chen L: Retinoic acid-gated sequence-specific translational control by RARalpha. Proc Natl Acad Sci USA 2008;105:20303–20308.
26 Chen N, Napoli JL: All-trans-retinoic acid stimulates translation and induces spine formation in hippocampal neurons through a membrane-associated RARalpha. FASEB J 2008;22:236–245.
27 Sarti F, Zhang Z, Schroeder J, Chen L: Rapid suppression of inhibitory synaptic transmission by retinoic acid. J Neurosci 2013;33:11440–11450.
28 Deng W, Aimone JB, Gage FH: New neurons and new memories: how does adult hippocampal neurogenesis affect learning and memory? Nat Rev Neurosci 2010;11:339–350.
29 Alvarez-Buylla A, Lim DA: For the long run: maintaining germinal niches in the adult brain. Neuron 2004;41:683–686.
30 Takahashi J, Palmer TD, Gage FH: Retinoic acid and neurotrophins collaborate to regulate neurogenesis in adult-derived neural stem cell cultures. J Neurobiol 1999;38:65–81.
31 Luo T, Wagner E, Crandall JE, Drager UC: A retinoic-acid critical period in the early postnatal mouse brain. Biol Psychiatry 2004;56:971–980.
32 Jacobs S, Lie DC, Decicco KL, Shi Y, Deluca LM, Gage FH, Evans RM: Retinoic acid is required early during adult neurogenesis in the dentate gyrus. Proc Natl Acad Sci USA 2006;103:3902–3907.
33 Papachristou P, Dyberg C, Lindqvist M, Horn Z, Ringstedt T: Transgenic increase of Wnt7b in neural progenitor cells decreases expression of T-domain transcription factors and impairs neuronal differentiation. Brain Res 2014;1576:27–34.
34 Bonnet E, Touyarot K, Alfos S, Pallet V, Higueret P, Abrous DN: Retinoic acid restores adult hippocampal neurogenesis and reverses spatial memory deficit in vitamin A deprived rats. PLoS One 2008;3:e3487.
35 Jinno S: Topographic differences in adult neurogenesis in the mouse hippocampus: a stereology-based study using endogenous markers. Hippocampus 2011;21:467–480.

36 Goodman T, Crandall JE, Nanescu SE, Quadro L, Shearer K, Ross A, McCaffery P: Patterning of retinoic acid signaling and cell proliferation in the hippocampus. Hippocampus 2012;22:2171–2183.
37 Schmidt B, Marrone DF, Markus EJ: Disambiguating the similar: the dentate gyrus and pattern separation. Behav Brain Res 2012;226:56–65.
38 Maden M: Role and distribution of retinoic acid during CNS development. Int Rev Cytol 2001;209:1–77.
39 McCaffery PJ, Adams J, Maden M, Rosa-Molinar E: Too much of a good thing: retinoic acid as an endogenous regulator of neural differentiation and exogenous teratogen. Eur J Neurosci 2003;18:457–472.
40 Crandall J, Sakai Y, Zhang J, Koul O, Mineur Y, Crusio WE, McCaffery P: 13-cis-retinoic acid suppresses hippocampal cell division and hippocampal-dependent learning in mice. Proc Natl Acad Sci USA 2004; 101:5111–5116.
41 McEwen BS: Plasticity of the hippocampus: adaptation to chronic stress and allostatic load. Ann NY Acad Sci 2001;933:265–277.
42 Sousa N, Almeida OF: Corticosteroids: sculptors of the hippocampal formation. Rev Neurosci 2002;13: 59–84.
43 Stumpf WE, Bidmon HJ, Murakami R: Retinoic acid binding sites in adult brain, pituitary, and retina. Naturwissenschaften 1991;78:561–562.
44 Shearer KD, Goodman TH, Ross AW, Reilly L, Morgan PJ, McCaffery PJ: Photoperiodic regulation of retinoic acid signaling in the hypothalamus. J Neurochem 2010;112:246–257.
45 Ross AW, Bell LM, Littlewood PA, Mercer JG, Barrett P, Morgan PJ: Temporal changes in gene expression in the arcuate nucleus precede seasonal responses in adiposity and reproduction. Endocrinology 2005;146:1940–1947.
46 Chen XN, Meng QY, Bao AM, Swaab DF, Wang GH, Zhou JN: The involvement of retinoic acid receptor-alpha in corticotropin-releasing hormone gene expression and affective disorders. Biol Psychiatry 2009;66:832–839.
47 Anzano MA, Lamb AJ, Olson JA: Growth, appetite, sequence of pathological signs and survival following the induction of rapid, synchronous vitamin A deficiency in the rat. J Nutr 1979;109:1419–1431.
48 Ono H, Hoshino Y, Yasuo S, Watanabe M, Nakane Y, Murai A, Ebihara S, Korf HW, Yoshimura T: Involvement of thyrotropin in photoperiodic signal transduction in mice. Proc Natl Acad Sci USA 2008; 105:18238–18242.
49 Barrett P, Ebling FJ, Schuhler S, Wilson D, Ross AW, Warner A, Jethwa P, Boelen A, Visser TJ, Ozanne DM, Archer ZA, Mercer JG, Morgan PJ: Hypothalamic thyroid hormone catabolism acts as a gatekeeper for the seasonal control of body weight and reproduction. Endocrinology 2007;148:3608–3617.
50 Ross AW, Johnson CE, Bell LM, Reilly L, Duncan JS, Barrett P, Heideman PD, Morgan PJ: Divergent regulation of hypothalamic neuropeptide Y and agouti-related protein by photoperiod in F344 rats with differential food intake and growth. J Neuroendocrinol 2009;21:610–619.
51 Helfer G, Ross AW, Russell L, Thomson LM, Shearer KD, Goodman TH, McCaffery PJ, Morgan PJ: Photoperiod regulates vitamin A and Wnt/beta-catenin signaling in F344 rats. Endocrinology 2012;153:815–824.
52 Shearer KD, Stoney PN, Nanescu SE, Helfer G, Barrett P, Ross AW, Morgan PJ, McCaffery P: Photoperiodic expression of two RALDH enzymes and the regulation of cell proliferation by retinoic acid in the rat hypothalamus. J Neurochem 2012;122:789–799.
53 Cho S, Cho H, Geum D, Kim K: Retinoic acid regulates gonadotropin-releasing hormone (GnRH) release and gene expression in the rat hypothalamic fragments and GT1-1 neuronal cells in vitro. Brain Res Mol Brain Res1998;54:74–84.
54 Kokoeva MV, Yin H, Flier JS: Neurogenesis in the hypothalamus of adult mice: potential role in energy balance. Science 2005;310:679–683.

Prof. Peter McCaffery
Institute of Medical Sciences, University of Aberdeen
School of Medical Sciences
Foresterhill, Aberdeen, Scotland AB25 2ZD (UK)
E-Mail p.j.mccaffery@abdn.ac.uk

Biesalski HK, Black RE (eds): Hidden Hunger. Malnutrition and the First 1,000 Days of Life: Causes, Consequences and Solutions. World Rev Nutr Diet. Basel, Karger, 2016, vol 115, pp 109–117
DOI: 10.1159/000442077

Current Information Gaps in Micronutrient Research, Programs and Policy: How Can We Fill Them?

Lindsay H. Allen

USDA, ARS Western Human Nutrition Research Center, University of California, Davis, CA, USA

Abstract

Micronutrient (MN) interventions have a very positive effect on public health and have been a major focus of nutrition research and policy for over 3 decades. Most MN policies are established by the World Health Organization based on available evidence from well-designed trials. These include recommendations on iron + folic acid supplements for pregnancy, high-dose vitamin A supplementation for children <5 years, multiple MN supplementation in young children, food fortification, and universal salt iodization. However, important gaps remain in the evidence base, some periods of the life span have been paid insufficient attention, and some MN policies are incomplete or inconsistent. Examples include the pending decision about whether to recommend multiple MN supplementation in pregnancy or preconception, a lack of information about whether supplementation of lactating women improves breast milk quality and infant development, uncertainty about when and where fortification of complementary foods or supplements is beneficial to preschoolers, and whether folic acid fortification can be harmful in population groups with a high prevalence of vitamin B_{12} deficiency. The most effective dose of MNs has rarely been tested systematically. MN interventions alone are not very effective for improving the growth and development of young children. Newer methods for the analysis of MNs in breast milk are revealing low concentrations in many populations, so more information is needed on the effects of different interventions on milk nutrient content. We need to improve biomarkers of MN status and should measure multiple biological responses to MN interventions using modern nutritional science methods, including metabolomics, proteomics and epigenetics; these will reveal effects of MNs that are not yet fully appreciated.

Introduction

The fundamental questions underlying micronutrient (MN) intervention policies are which MNs should be delivered, when, how and to whom? This chapter attempts to define some of the gaps in the information needed to answer these questions. MN deficiencies are most commonly caused by inadequate intake of MN-dense foods, and notably animal-source foods (ASFs), which provide the only dietary source of vitamin B_{12}, retinol (preformed vitamin A), bioavailable heme iron, and vitamin D. ASFs are also important sources of riboflavin, vitamin E, iron, bioavailable zinc, calcium and choline. Fruits and vegetables are the main dietary sources of vitamin C, β-carotene, folate and phytonutrients. In resource-limited populations, consumption of ASFs and some fruits and vegetables is low, so that intake of many or all of these MNs is inadequate; the problem is rarely deficiency of one or a few nutrients.

Current World Health Organization (WHO) MN recommendations are as follows: for pregnancy, iron + folic acid, as well as calcium where intake is low; for infants under 6 months of age, breast milk as the sole source of nutrients, with breastfeeding continuing for the first 2 years and beyond; from 6 months to 5 years, nutrient-dense household foods, vitamin-mineral supplements (such as MN powders or lipid-based supplements) or fortified complementary foods; for children and women, iron treatment for anemia and fortification of staples with iron, vitamin A, zinc, folic acid and vitamin B_{12}; and for all, universal salt iodization. Biofortification can increase intake of provitamin A, iron and zinc, but the WHO states that further research is needed before specific recommendations can be made on this strategy [1].

Micronutrient Supplementation in Pregnancy

One of the more important decisions to be made in the near future is whether to replace iron + folic acid supplements with multiple MN (MMN) supplements during pregnancy. A series of studies using the United Nations Children's Fund's 'UNIMMAP' MMN supplement demonstrated that compared to iron + folic acid supplements alone, birthweight was increased by 21.2 g and the prevalence of low birthweight reduced by 7%, which are both significant effects [2]. However, when data from two large studies in Nepal were combined, the investigators found an apparent increase in perinatal and neonatal deaths in the MMN group versus the iron + folic acid group [3], which raised concern about the safety of recommending MMNs in pregnancy. An interesting and still unexplained finding from the UNIMMAP studies was that the relative effect of MMNs versus iron + folic acid increased as maternal body mass index (BMI) increased, i.e. by 7.6 g per unit greater BMI, even across the range of normal BMI values.

In 2012, a meta-analysis of 23 trials including 75,785 women also concluded that MMNs reduced the prevalence of low birthweight and small-for-gestational-age births compared to iron + folic acid alone, but that there were no additional benefits for maternal or infant mortality and that the data were insufficient to evaluate the impact on other pregnancy outcomes [4]. Similar findings were reported in another meta-analysis [5]. A recent trial in Bangladesh added more critically needed information supporting a policy of supplementation with MMNs, rather than only iron + folic acid, in pregnancy [6]. The study participants were 44,567 pregnant women with 28,516 infants enrolled in a randomized clinical trial. MMN or iron + folic acid was provided from the first trimester of pregnancy through 12 weeks postpartum. The relative risk of preterm delivery was 0.85, of lower birthweight, 0.88, and of stillbirth, 0.89, for the MMN group versus the iron + folic acid group. The MMNs increased the duration of pregnancy by 0.3 weeks, which explained the 55 g higher birthweight and the greater length and head circumference of the infants. There was no effect on small-for-gestational-age deliveries, but mortality was lower in female infants.

In 2015, the WHO accepted the evidence that MMN supplements may be more effective for reducing the risk of low birthweight and of a small size for gestational age compared to iron + folic acid supplements but stated that we need further research on the relative advantages of replacement of iron + folic acid supplements with MMNs [1].

In addition to ongoing discussion about the relative efficacy of MMNs versus iron + folic acid for pregnancy outcomes, uncertainty exists about the optimal content and dose of MNs in pregnancy supplements. The UNIMMAP supplement contains the Recommended Dietary Allowance (RDA) of 15 MNs and has been used in most studies, but giving twice the RDA increased birthweight by 177 g more than the RDA did in anemic women in Guinea-Bissau [7]. Even after supplementation with the RDA, a high prevalence of MN deficiencies remains across studies [8]. Another unanswered question is whether the essential fatty acids in lipid-based nutrient supplements (LNSs) confer additional benefits for pregnancy outcome.

Micronutrient Supplements for Young Children

There was considerable optimism that MMN supplements would prevent stunting and improve the growth of stunted young children. However, meta-analyses of the many studies on this question show that providing MMNs compared with no, one or two MNs, whether as supplements or in fortified food, has only a small effect on longitudinal growth [9]. Further confirmation of the marginal effect of MNs on the growth of young children has been forthcoming from recent studies. For example, a large trial in Bangladesh enrolled 5,536 children of 6–18 months of age who were randomized to supplements providing 19–29% of their energy requirements for a year [10]. The supplements were chickpea- and rice- and lentil-based, fortified, ready-to-use local foods, a fortified wheat-soy blend ('WSB++') or Plumpy'doz (a lipid-based MN supplement), all supported by nutrition counselling, or nutrition counselling alone was administered (the control group). Length Z scores fell in all groups, although by –0.02 to –0.04 Z/month less, with the two ready-to-use local foods and Plumpy'doz compared to the controls. At 18 months of age, 44% of the control-group children were stunted, but 5–6% fewer were stunted in the groups given chickpea-based food and Plumpy'doz. The authors concluded that the small amounts of daily fortified complementary foods plus nutrition counselling modestly increased linear growth and reduced stunting at 18 months of age. In Malawi, 640 six-month-old infants were supplemented for a year with nothing or with milk-LNS, soy-LNS or corn-soy blend, providing about 250 kcal/day [11]. There was no conclusive evidence of an effect on stunting, although milk-LNS was more beneficial between 9 and 12 months.

Micronutrient Fortification of Staple Foods

Fortification of staple foods with MNs has seen tremendous growth since the WHO published its Guidelines on Micronutrient Fortification of Foods in 2006 [12]. According to the Flour Fortification Initiative, in 2014, 84 countries had mandatory fortification of at least one flour: 83, plus the Punjab province in Pakistan, required fortification of wheat flour, 14 required fortification of maize, and 6 required fortification of rice. All of these countries require fortification with iron and folic acid, except Australia, which mandates fortification with folic acid alone. About 30% of the world's total milled wheat flour is fortified. In addition, there is voluntary fortification of many foods with a wide range of MNs. The initial incentive for mandatory fortification of flour was to reduce the risk of neural tube defects by increasing folic acid intake, and indeed, the prevalence of neural tube defects has fallen in many countries, especially where the baseline prevalence was highest and the folate status the poorest [13]. However, many countries have implemented folic acid fortification programs without first assessing the folate status of the population or the prevalence of neural tube defects. Many such countries have a high prevalence of vitamin B_{12} deficiency, and there is some concern that high folic acid intake and status may further exacerbate vitamin B_{12} deficiency and the risk of anemia and impaired cognitive function [14]. We still need to better understand the physiological and functional impacts of providing high amounts of folic acid to populations with a range of folate and vitamin B_{12} statuses at baseline. Some guidance on when folic acid fortification is needed has been recently published based on erythrocyte folate concentrations [15]. Unfortunately, few surveys have measured erythrocyte folate, and concentrations in about half of the countries in the world have already been elevated by fortification. Iron fortification of flour only had a small effect on iron status and anemia for many years because the form and/or amount of iron added were incorrect. Newer guidelines have improved this situation, but not enough iron can be added to meet the iron requirements of women of reproductive age where wheat flour intake is <75 g/day. Vitamin A is more commonly added to oils and fats than to flour, and fortified food provides a more sustained supply than high-dose supplements, which improve status for only about 2 months. There has been recent discussion and new guidelines on when to scale back large-dose capsule distribution where there is fortification and/or improved dietary supply of the vitamin [16]. Universal salt iodization has been an enormous success, although recently, more attention has been paid to the benefits of iodine supplements for pregnant and lactating women and their offspring in areas with moderate-to-severe iodine deficiency [17]. A high-dose supplement for the mother immediately postpartum increases iodine in breast milk and is more effective at improving infant iodine status than direct infant supplementation [18].

In general, there has been inadequate evaluation of both the consumption of potentially fortifiable foods and MN status when fortification programs are planned. Such programs are typically planned based on estimates of usual consumption of target foods based on household consumption data collected in national surveys to avoid the more labor- and time-intensive collection of intake data on individuals. However, intake estimated from household surveys can be substantially different from data collected based on 24-hour recall or other methods that measure the intake of individual household members [19]. Another emerging issue is the relative ability of different interventions to achieve effective coverage at the lowest cost. Optimization models offer the potential to answer this question, which is very important for setting population intervention policy and which can help to minimize unnecessary overlap between programs while improving effective coverage [20].

A neglected issue continues to be the high prevalence of deficiencies in other MNs, such as vitamin B_{12}, riboflavin and vitamin D. While these MNs are usually included in vitamin-mineral supplements, they are not often added as fortificants, with the exception being vitamin D addition to dairy products in higher-income countries. Vitamin B_{12} has now been added as a fortificant to wheat flour in Cameroon at levels recommended by the WHO that supply approximately the RDA. This has resulted in a much greater increase in serum and breast milk concentrations of the vitamin than was expected [Engle-Stone, unpubl. data]. Although this is not of concern given the lack of toxicity of this nutrient, it does illustrate the importance of pilot studies to measure efficacy prior to wide-scale fortification; efficacy may be greater when small amounts of vitamin B_{12} are consumed throughout the day in fortified foods than when taken as a larger amount in a supplement once a day.

Need to Improve Biomarkers of Micronutrient Status

A joint report on the 'Indicators and Methods for Cross-Sectional Surveys of Vitamin and Mineral Status of Populations' was published by the Micronutrient Initiative and the Centers for Disease Control and Prevention [21]. The report recognized that iron, vitamin A and iodine deficiencies affect the population in many developing countries to some extent. The indicators and methods recommended in the report were limited to those three MNs: for iron, hemoglobin, ferritin and transferrin receptors were recommended as indicators; for vitamin A, serum retinol, and for iodine, urinary iodine. These indicators are useful but not completely satisfactory. For example, ≈50% of anemia (low hemoglobin) is not due to iron deficiency, but to factors such as hemoglobinopathy and infection; inflammation increases ferritin, and both inflammation and *Plasmodium falciparum* increase transferrin receptors [22]. Serum retinol is lowered by inflammation.

Status indicators for the several other common MN deficiencies were not considered in the joint report and deserve more attention. Erythrocyte folate has emerged as an indicator of a need for folic acid interventions to prevent neural tube defects, but serum folate, the usual biomarker for folate status, is not useful for this purpose, and inter-laboratory variability in analyses has been common but is improving. For vitamin B_{12}, serum B_{12} is the most commonly used status indicator, although three other indicators are also useful: serum holotranscobalamin, serum or urinary methylmalonic acid, and serum homocysteine (which is also affected by folate, riboflavin and vitamin B_6 status). It has been difficult to determine the cut-point(s) to use for each indicator and which of the indicators to choose for estimating the prevalence or risk of deficiency since individually or as ratios, they give different estimates. However, vitamin B_{12} is an example of where some innovative work is in progress to improve assessment of population status. Fedosov et al. [23] developed a formula for combining two, three, or optimally four of the vitamin B_{12} status biomarkers into a combined status indicator ('cB12'), with the option of including factors to correct for poor folate status and age. While the application of cB12 needs further work, it has already demonstrated the effect of high serum folate on vitamin B_{12} status better than any of the single markers alone [24]. Other advances have been the use of thyroglobulin in dried blood spots to assess iodine status [25] and a consensus statement on how to correct for the effects of inflammation on nutritional status biomarkers [26]. The status of many other common MN deficiencies is not usually assessed, in part due to the difficulty of measuring the indicators, e.g. vitamins B_1, B_2, B_6, D, and E and choline and selenium. A method exists for measuring seven water-soluble vitamins concurrently in plasma and urine by high-pressure liquid chromatography [27], but it has not yet been applied in nutritional status surveys or to assess the effect of programmatic interventions.

Breast Milk Micronutrient Concentrations

While we have known for some time that the concentrations of MNs in breast milk are affected by maternal intake and/or status, this has been a neglected issue. Data on milk composition are poor, even in high-income countries, because most investigators have collected relatively few samples from nonrepresentative population subgroups using unknown or invalid collection procedures and/or analytical methods, and with no or insufficient attention to maternal nutritional status or supplementation. This situation has created inaccurate estimates of the average milk MN values used to set recommended intake for infants, young children and lactating women. At the same time, since infants and young children should depend on breast milk to supply most of their MNs during the first 2 years of life, it is critically important to understand whether MN levels in milk are adequate and, if not, how to most effectively improve maternal or infant status during the period of lactation.

One limitation to collecting better information on breast milk MNs has been the inefficient and sometimes inaccurate analysis of MNs in the milk matrix. We have developed and validated an accurate, rapid method for the simultaneous analysis of thiamin, riboflavin, niacin and vitamin B_6 in human milk using ultra-performance liquid chromatography-tandem mass spectrometry [28]. Vitamins A and E can be measured simultaneously by HPLC, and iron, copper and zinc simultaneously by inductively coupled plasma atomic emission spectroscopy. Analytical problems caused by the strong binding of vitamin B_{12} in the human milk matrix have been solved [29]. Using these methods, we have found that there is a very wide variation in the MN concentrations of women in different populations and that these can be considerably below the values assumed for setting dietary intake recommendations for infants. Moreover, levels of some MNs in milk can be readily and substantially increased by maternal supplementation during lactation (e.g. riboflavin), while others are much more difficult to increase (e.g. vitamin B_{12}). We also recently documented that antiretroviral drugs lower some MN levels in human milk and interfere with the beneficial effects of maternal MN supplements on milk vitamins [30].

Need to Better Understand Links between Status Biomarkers and Physiological Functions

There is a need and opportunity to further quantify relationships between biochemical markers of status and functional health outcomes. A recent example of modeling such a relationship is that between erythrocyte folate and the estimated risk of neural tube defects, described above. A recent study used a systematic review of iodine supplementation during pregnancy to model the cost effectiveness of iodine supplementation of pregnant women in the UK [31]. Another example is the improvement in immune function that was seen in Bangladeshi women given vitamin B_{12} supplements during pregnancy and lactation [32]. 'Omics' technologies, including metabolomics, proteomics and genomics, can be applied to identify metabolites and systems most strongly related to impaired function and response, such as those that predict growth response. These technologies may also detect unanticipated metabolic responses that suggest unsuspected benefits or harm, leading to the development of new biomarkers. Epigenetic responses to periconceptional MN supplementation and dietary interventions have become relatively easy to measure. In general, these analytical tools are leading us to a new era of understanding of the biological causes of MN deficiencies and the metabolic effects of and variability in response to MN interventions.

References

1 World Health Organization: E-Library of Evidence for Nutrition Actions (eLENA). Geneva, World Health Organization, 2015.

2 Fall CH, Fisher DJ, Osmond C, Margetts BM: Multiple micronutrient supplementation during pregnancy in low-income countries: a meta-analysis of effects on birth size and length of gestation. Food Nutr Bull 2009;30:S533–S546.

3 Christian P, Osrin D, Manandhar D, Khatry S, de L Costello A, West KJ: Antenatal micronutrient supplements in Nepal. Lancet 2005;366:711–712.

4 Haider BA, Bhutta ZA: Neonatal vitamin A supplementation for the prevention of mortality and morbidity in term neonates in developing countries. Cochrane Database Syst Rev 2011;10:CD006980.

5 Kawai K, Spiegelman D, Shankar AH, Fawzi WW: Maternal multiple micronutrient supplementation and pregnancy outcomes in developing countries: meta-analysis and meta-regression. Bull World Health Organ 2011;89:402–411B.

6 West KP Jr, Shamim AA, Mehra S, Labrique AB, Ali H, Shaikh S, Klemm RD, Wu LS, Mitra M, Haque R, et al: Effect of maternal multiple micronutrient vs iron-folic acid supplementation on infant mortality and adverse birth outcomes in rural Bangladesh: the JiVitA-3 randomized trial. JAMA 2014;312:2649–2658.

7 Kaestel P, Michaelsen KF, Aaby P, Friis H: Effects of prenatal multimicronutrient supplements on birth weight and perinatal mortality: a randomised, controlled trial in Guinea-Bissau. Eur J Clin Nutr 2005;59:1081–1089.

8 Allen LH: Micronutrient research, programs, and policy: from meta-analyses to metabolomics. Adv Nutr 2014;5:344S–351S.

9 Allen LH, Peerson JM, Olney DK: Provision of multiple rather than two or fewer micronutrients more effectively improves growth and other outcomes in micronutrient-deficient children and adults. J Nutr 2009;139:1022–1030.

10 Christian P, Shaikh S, Shamim AA, Mehra S, Wu L, Mitra M, Ali H, Merrill RD, Choudhury N, Parveen M, et al: Effect of fortified complementary food supplementation on child growth in rural Bangladesh: a cluster-randomized trial. Int J Epidemiol 2015;44:1862–1876.

11 Mangani C, Maleta K, Phuka J, Cheung YB, Thakwalakwa C, Dewey K, Manary M, Puumalainen T, Ashorn P: Effect of complementary feeding with lipid-based nutrient supplements and corn-soy blend on the incidence of stunting and linear growth among 6- to 18-month-old infants and children in rural Malawi. Matern Child Nutr 2015;11(suppl 4):132–143.

12 Allen L, de Benoist B, Dary O, Hurrell R: Guidelines on Food Fortification with Micronutrients. Geneva, World Health Organization/Food and Agriculture Organization, 2006.

13 Heseker HB, Mason JB, Selhub J, Rosenberg IH, Jacques PF: Not all cases of neural-tube defect can be prevented by increasing the intake of folic acid. Br J Nutr 2009;102:173–180.

14 Morris MS, Jacques PF, Rosenberg IH, Selhub J: Folate and vitamin B-12 status in relation to anemia, macrocytosis, and cognitive impairment in older Americans in the age of folic acid fortification. Am J Clin Nutr 2007;85:193–200.

15 Cordero AM, Crider KS, Rogers LM, Cannon MJ, Berry RJ: Optimal serum and red blood cell folate concentrations in women of reproductive age for prevention of neural tube defects: World Health Organization guidelines. Morb Mortal Wkly Rep 2015;64:421–423.

16 West KP Jr, Sommer A, Palmer A, Schultink W, Habicht JP: Commentary: vitamin A policies need rethinking. Int J Epidemiol 2015;44:292–294; discussion 294–296.

17 Zimmermann MB: The effects of iodine deficiency in pregnancy and infancy. Paediatr Perinat Epidemiol 2012;26(suppl 1):108–117.

18 Bouhouch RR, Bouhouch S, Cherkaoui M, Aboussad A, Stinca S, Haldimann M, Andersson M, Zimmermann MB: Direct iodine supplementation of infants versus supplementation of their breastfeeding mothers: a double-blind, randomised, placebo-controlled trial. Lancet Diabetes Endocrinol 2014;2:197–209.

19 Engle-Stone R, Brown KH: Comparison of a household consumption and expenditures survey with nationally representative food frequency questionnaire and 24-hour dietary recall data for assessing consumption of fortifiable foods by women and young children in Cameroon. Food Nutr Bull 2015;36:211–230.

20 Brown KH, Engle-Stone R, Kagin J, Rettig E, Vosti SA: Use of optimization modeling for selecting national micronutrient intervention strategies: an example based on potential programs for control of vitamin A deficiency in Cameroon. Food Nutr Bull 2015;36(3 suppl):S141–S148.

21 Gorstein J, Sullivan K, Parvanta I, Begin F: Indicators and Methods for Cross-Sectional Surveys of Vitamin and Mineral Status of Populations. Ottawa, The Micronutrient Initiative, and Atlanta, The Centers for Disease Control and Prevention, 2007.

22 Righetti AA, Wegmüller R, Glinz D, Ouattara M, Adiossan LG, N'Goran EK, Utzinger J, Hurrell RF: Effects of inflammation and Plasmodium falciparum infection on soluble transferrin receptor and plasma ferritin concentration in different age groups: a prospective longitudinal study in Cote d'Ivoire. Am J Clin Nutr 2013;97:1364–1374.

23 Fedosov SN, Brito A, Miller JW, Green R, Allen LH: Combined indicator of vitamin B12 status: modification for missing biomarkers and folate status and recommendations for revised cut-points. Clin Chem Lab Med 2015;53:1215–1225.

24 Brito A, Verdugo R, Hertrampf E, Miller J, Green R, Fedosov S, Shahab-Ferdows S, Sanchez H, Albala C, Castillo J, et al: Vitamin B-12 treatment of asymptomatic, deficient, elderly Chileans improves conductivity in myelinated peripheral nerves, but high serum folate impairs vitamin B-12 status response assessed by the combined indicator of vitamin B-12 status. Am J Clin Nutr 2016;103:250–257.

25 Zimmermann MB, de Benoist B, Corigliano S, Jooste PL, Molinari L, Moosa K, Pretell EA, Al-Dallal ZS, Wei Y, Zu-Pei C, et al: Assessment of iodine status using dried blood spot thyroglobulin: development of reference material and establishment of an international reference range in iodine-sufficient children. J Clin Endocrinol Metab 2006;91:4881–4887.

26 Raiten DJ, Sakr Ashour FA, Ross AC, Meydani SN, Dawson HD, Stephensen CB, Brabin BJ, Suchdev PS, van Ommen B; INSPIRE Consultative Group: Inflammation and Nutritional Science for Programs/Policies and Interpretation of Research Evidence (INSPIRE). J Nutr 2015;145:1039S–1108S.

27 Giorgi MG, Howland K, Martin C, Bonner AB: A novel HPLC method for the concurrent analysis and quantitation of seven water-soluble vitamins in biological fluids (plasma and urine): a validation study and application. ScientificWorldJournal 2012;2012: 359721.

28 Hampel D, York ER, Allen LH: Ultra-performance liquid chromatography tandem mass-spectrometry (UPLC-MS/MS) for the rapid, simultaneous analysis of thiamin, riboflavin, flavin adenine dinucleotide, nicotinamide and pyridoxal in human milk. J Chromatogr B Analyt Technol Biomed Life Sci 2012;903: 7–13.

29 Hampel D, Shahab-Ferdows S, Domek JM, Siddiqua T, Raqib R, Allen LH: Competitive chemiluminescent enzyme immunoassay for vitamin B12 analysis in human milk. Food Chem 2014;153:60–65.

30 Allen L, Hampel D, Shahab-Ferdows S, York E, Adair L, Flax V, Tegha G, Chasela C, Kamwendo D, Jamieson D, et al: Antiretroviral therapy provided to HIV-infected Malawian women in a randomized trial diminishes the positive effects of lipid-based nutrient supplements on breast milk B-vitamins. Am J Clin Nutr 2015;102:1468–1474.

31 Monahan M, Boelaert K, Jolly K, Chan S, Barton P, Roberts TE: Costs and benefits of iodine supplementation for pregnant women in a mildly to moderately iodine-deficient population: a modelling analysis. Lancet Diabetes Endocrinol 2015;3:715–722.

32 Siddiqua TJ, Ahmad SM, Ahsan KB, Rashid M, Roy A, Rahman SM, Shahab-Ferdows S, Hampel D, Ahmed T, Allen LH, et al: Vitamin B12 supplementation during pregnancy and postpartum improves B12 status of both mothers and infants but vaccine response in mothers only: a randomized clinical trial in Bangladesh. Eur J Nutr 2015, Epub ahead of print.

Dr. Lindsay H. Allen
USDA, ARS Western Human Nutrition Research Center, University of California
430, W. Health Sciences Drive
Davis, CA 95616 (USA)
E-Mail Lindsay.allen@ars.usda.gov

Biesalski HK, Black RE (eds): Hidden Hunger. Malnutrition and the First 1,000 Days of Life: Causes, Consequences and Solutions. World Rev Nutr Diet. Basel, Karger, 2016, vol 115, pp 118–124
DOI: 10.1159/000442078

The Importance of Adequate Iodine during Pregnancy and Infancy

Michael B. Zimmermann

Laboratory for Human Nutrition, Institute of Food, Nutrition and Health, Swiss Federal Institute of Technology (ETH) Zurich, Zurich, Switzerland

Abstract

Iodine requirements are increased ≥50% during pregnancy. Iodine deficiency during pregnancy can cause maternal and fetal hypothyroidism and impair neurological development of the fetus. The consequences depend upon the timing and severity of the hypothyroidism; the most severe manifestation is cretinism. In iodine-deficient areas, controlled studies have demonstrated that iodine supplementation before or during early pregnancy eliminates new cases of cretinism, increases birth weight, reduces rates of perinatal and infant mortality and generally increases developmental scores in young children by 10–20%. Mild-to-moderate maternal iodine deficiency can cause thyroid dysfunction, but whether it impairs cognitive and/or neurological function in the offspring remains uncertain. In nearly all regions affected by iodine deficiency, salt iodization is the most cost-effective way of delivering iodine and improving maternal and infant health.

Introduction

Iodine is an essential nutrient in human diets because it is a component of thyroid hormone. In healthy adults, the absorption of iodide from the diet is >90% [1, 2]. The body of a healthy adult contains 15–20 mg iodine, of which 70–80% is in the thyroid. In chronic iodine deficiency, the iodine content of the thyroid may fall to <20 μg, and

Table 1. Recommendations for iodine intake (μg/day) for pregnant and lactating women and for infants

Age or population group[a]	US Institute of Medicine [4]	Age or population group[c]	World Health Organization [2]
Infants 0–12 months[b]	110–130	Children 0–5 years	90
Pregnancy	220	Pregnancy	250
Lactation	290	Lactation	250

[a] Recommended daily allowance. [b] Adequate intake. [c] Recommended nutrient intake.

Table 2. Epidemiological criteria from the World Health Organization for the assessment of iodine nutrition in pregnant and lactating women and in infants, based on the median or a range of urinary iodine concentrations

	Iodine intake
Pregnant women	
<150 μg/l	Insufficient
150–249 μg/l	Adequate
250–499 μg/l	More than adequate
≥500 μg/l[a]	Excessive
Lactating women	
<100 μg/l	Insufficient
≥100 μg/l	Adequate
Children <2 years of age	
<100 μg/l	Insufficient
≥100 μg/l	Adequate

this limits thyroid hormone synthesis, leading to hypothyroidism and its sequelae (discussed below) [1]. The iodine requirement during pregnancy is sharply increased due to (1) an increase in maternal thyroxine production to maintain maternal euthyroidism and to transfer thyroid hormone to the fetus early in the first trimester, before the fetal thyroid is functioning; (2) iodine transfer to the fetus, particularly in later gestation, and (3) an increase in renal iodine clearance [3]. Iodine requirements from the US Institute of Medicine [4] and the World Health Organization [2] for pregnancy, lactation and infancy are shown in table 1. The recommended method to assess iodine nutrition in pregnant women is assessment of the urinary iodine (UI) concentration [2]. Because >90% of dietary iodine eventually appears in the urine, UI is an excellent indicator of recent iodine intake [1, 2]. Recommendations for using the median UI to classify the iodine status of pregnant and lactating women and that of infants are shown in table 2 [2].

Effects of Iodine Deficiency during Pregnancy on Maternal Thyroid Function and Mental Development of the Offspring

Iodine deficiency has multiple adverse effects on growth and development in animals and humans. These effects are collectively termed the iodine deficiency disorders and are one of the most important and common human diseases [1]. They result from inadequate thyroid hormone production due to a lack of sufficient iodine. Iodine deficiency during pregnancy impairs the neurological development of the fetus. In areas of severe chronic iodine deficiency, maternal and fetal hypothyroxinemia can occur from early gestation onward [3, 5]. Thyroid hormone is required for normal neuronal migration and myelination of the brain during fetal and early postnatal life, and hypothyroxinemia during these critical periods causes irreversible brain damage, with mental retardation and neurological abnormalities [3, 5]. The consequences depend upon the timing and severity of the hypothyroxinemia. The most severe manifestation of in utero iodine deficiency is cretinism. Two classic forms of cretinism, or neurological and myxedematous, have been described [1].

In landmark trials of iodine repletion during pregnancy using iodized oil in areas of severe iodine deficiency in Papua New Guinea [6] and Zaire [7], iodine supplementation was associated with a significant reduction in the prevalence of endemic cretinism and with higher psychomotor development scores in the offspring of iodine-treated mothers. In a study in western China, an area of severe iodine deficiency and endemic cretinism, participants consisted of groups of children from birth to 3 years and women at each trimester of pregnancy [8]. The intervention was oral iodized oil, and the treated children as well as babies born to the treated women were followed for 2 years. The prevalence of moderate or severe neurological abnormalities among the infants whose mothers received iodine in the first or second trimester was 2%, compared with 9% among the infants who received iodine during the third trimester (through the treatment of their mothers) or after birth. The prevalence of microcephaly was 27% in the untreated children, compared with 11% in the treated children, and the mean developmental quotient at 2 years of age was higher in the treated than in the untreated children [8]. Controlled studies in Peru [9] and Ecuador [10] also demonstrated benefits in the rates of cretinism and development when iodine deficiency during pregnancy was corrected using iodized oil.

Endemic cretinism is the extreme expression of the abnormalities in physical and intellectual development caused by iodine deficiency, but the cognitive deficits associated with iodine deficiency may not be limited to remote, severely iodine-deficient areas. Many authors have argued that even mild-to-moderate iodine deficiency in pregnancy, still present in many countries in Europe, may affect the cognitive function of the offspring. Two prospective case-control studies in iodine-sufficient women have reported that even mild thyroid dysfunction during pregnancy may impair the cognitive development of the offspring [11, 12]. There have been six controlled studies of iodine supplementation in pregnant women in Europe [13–18]. In these studies, the baseline median UI (the severity of prevailing iodine deficiency), the doses of iodine given and the duration of supplementation all varied, making comparisons between the studies difficult. However, the findings of these trials suggest that in areas of mild-to-moderate iodine deficiency, the maternal thyroid is able to adapt to meet the increased thyroid hormone requirements of pregnancy. Although supplementation was generally effective in minimizing an increase in thyroid size during pregnancy, only two of the six studies reported that the maternal thyroid-stimulating hormone level was lower (within the normal reference range) with supplementation, and none of the studies showed a clear impact of supplementation on maternal and newborn total or free thyroid hormone concentrations. Thyroid hormone concentrations may be the best surrogate biochemical marker for healthy fetal development. Thus, the results of these trials are reassuring. However, because none of the trials measured long-term clinical outcomes, such as maternal goiter or infant development, the potential adverse effects of mild-to-moderate iodine deficiency during pregnancy remain unclear. However, a recent observational study in the UK suggested that even mild-to-moderate iodine deficiency during pregnancy may have long-term adverse effects on child cognition [19].

Effects of Iodine Repletion during Pregnancy on Birth Weight

In Zaire, treatment with iodized oil during pregnancy resulted in 3.7% higher birth weights compared with the birth weights of offspring of untreated mothers [7]. In a region of endemic goiter in Algeria, treatment of pregnant women with oral iodized oil just before conception or during the first trimester significantly increased birth weights (+6.25%) compared with no treatment [20]. Household use of iodized salt correlated with increased weight for age and an increased mid-upper-arm circumference during infancy in a large Asian study [21].

Effects of Iodine Repletion during Pregnancy and Infancy on Infant Mortality

Infant survival is improved in infants born to women whose iodine deficiency is corrected before or during pregnancy. DeLong et al. [22] added potassium iodate to irrigation water over a 2- to 4-week period in three areas of severe iodine deficiency in China and found a large reduction in both neonatal and infant mortality over the following 2–3 years compared with areas that did not receive iodine. Iodized oil given intramuscularly to iodine-deficient pregnant women in Zaire at ≈28 weeks of gestation also decreased infant mortality [7]. Infant survival may also be improved by iodine supplementation in the newborn period. A randomized, placebo-controlled trial of oral iodized oil (100 mg iodine) was conducted in an area of presumed iodine deficiency in Indonesia to evaluate the effect on mortality [23]. The iodine or placebo was given in conjunction with oral poliovirus vaccine to infants (n = 617), who were treated at ≈6 weeks of age and followed to 6 months of age. There was a significant (72%) decrease in the risk of infant death during the first 2 months of follow-up. In a large cross-sectional study in Indonesia, use of adequately iodized salt was associated with a significantly lower prevalence of child malnutrition and mortality in neonates, infants, and children aged <5 years [24].

Systematic Review of the Effects of Iodine Repletion during the First 1,000 Days

A recent systematic review [25] examined the effects of iodine supplementation and/or status on the mental development of children ≤5 years. Organized by study design, the average effect sizes were (a) 0.68 (2 randomized controlled trials with iodine supplementation of mothers), (b) 0.46 (8 nonrandomized trials with iodine supplementation of mothers and/or infants), (c) 0.52 (9 prospective cohort studies stratified by mothers' iodine status), and (d) 0.54 (4 cohort stratified by infants' iodine status). Overall, this translated into 6.9–10.2 fewer IQ points in iodine-deficient children compared with iodine-replete children [25]. Thus, the available data, although limited, suggest that iodine deficiency of mild-to-moderate severity in infancy and young children has adverse effects on cognitive/motor performance and likely prevents children from attaining their full intellectual potential.

Methods to Ensure Adequate Iodine Intake in Pregnancy and Infancy

In nearly all regions affected by iodine deficiency, salt iodization is the most cost-effective way of delivering iodine to women of reproductive age, pregnant women and young children [2]. From 1990 to 2014, global population coverage by iodized salt increased from about 20 to 75%, respectively [26]. In regions where iodized salt is not available, iodine supplementation can be used to increase iodine intake in women. Iodine can be given as daily oral supplements containing 100–250 μg. Alternatively, iodized oil can be given orally to women of childbearing age, pregnant women and lactating women; usual doses are 200–400 mg iodine/year [2, 27].

Future Research

Priorities for future research should include (a) the development of new biomarkers of individual iodine status and (b) controlled trials in mildly to moderately iodine-deficient pregnant women, with the primary outcomes being long-term clinical outcomes, such as maternal goiter, postpartum thyroid dysfunction and/or infant development. Considering the potentially irreversible adverse impact of iodine deficiency during early life on neurodevelopment, regional and national public health programs should focus on effective and sustained iodine prophylaxis for pregnant women and infants.

References

1 Zimmermann MB, Jooste PL, Pandav C: Iodine deficiency disorders. Lancet 2008;372:1251–1262.
2 World Health Organization: Assessment of Iodine Deficiency Disorders and Monitoring Their Elimination, ed 2. Geneva, WHO, 2007.
3 Glinoer D: The regulation of thyroid function during normal pregnancy: importance of the iodine nutrition status. Best Pract Res Clin Endocrinol Metab 2004;18:133–152.
4 Institute of Medicine, Academy of Sciences: Dietary Reference Intakes for Vitamin A, Vitamin K, Arsenic, Boron, Chromium, Copper, Iodine, Iron, Manganese, Molybdenum, Nickel, Silicon, Vanadium and Zinc. Washington, National Academy Press, 2001.
5 Morreale de Escobar G, Obregon MJ, et al: Role of thyroid hormone during early brain development. Eur J Endocrinol 2004;151(suppl 3):U25–U37.
6 Pharoah PO, Buttfield IH, Hetzel BS: Neurological damage to fetus resulting from severe iodine deficiency during pregnancy. Lancet 1971;1:308–310.
7 Thilly CH, Delange F, Lagasse R, et al: Fetal hypothyroidism and maternal thyroid status in severe endemic goiter. J Clin Endocrinol Metab 1978;47:354–360.
8 Cao XY, Jiang XM, Dou ZH, et al: Timing of vulnerability of the brain to iodine deficiency in endemic cretinism. N Engl J Med 1994;331:1739–1744.
9 Pretell EA, Palacios P, Tello L, et al: Iodine deficiency and the maternal/fetal relationship; in Stanbury JB (ed): Endemic Goiter and Cretinism: Continuing Threats to World Health. Washington, PAHO Sci. Pub.292, 1974, pp 143–155.
10 Fierrobenitez R, Cazar R, Stanbury JB, et al: Effects on school-children of prophylaxis of mothers with iodized oil in an area of iodine deficiency. J Endocrinol Invest 1988;11:327–335.
11 Haddow JE, Palomaki GE, Allan WC, et al: Maternal thyroid deficiency during pregnancy and subsequent neuropsychological development of the child. N Engl J Med 1999;341:549–555.
12 Pop VJ, Kuijpens JL, van Baar AL, et al: Low maternal free thyroxine concentrations during early pregnancy are associated with impaired psychomotor development in infancy. Clin Endocrinol (Oxf) 1999; 50:149–155.
13 Romano R, Jannini EA, Pepe M, et al: The effects of iodoprophylaxis on thyroid size during pregnancy. Am J Obstet Gynecol 1991;164:482–485.
14 Pedersen KM, Laurberg P, Iversen E, et al: Amelioration of some pregnancy-associated variations in thyroid function by iodine supplementation. J Clin Endocrinol Metab 1993;77:1078–1083.
15 Glinoer D, De Nayer P, Delange F, et al: A randomized trial for the treatment of mild iodine deficiency during pregnancy: maternal and neonatal effects. J Clin Endocrinol Metab 1995;80:258–269.
16 Liesenkötter KP, Göpel W, Bogner U, et al: Earliest prevention of endemic goiter by iodine supplementation during pregnancy. Eur J Endocrinol 1996;134: 443–448.
17 Nøhr SB, Jørgensen A, Pedersen KM, et al: Postpartum thyroid dysfunction in pregnant thyroid peroxidase antibody-positive women living in an area with mild to moderate iodine deficiency: is iodine supplementation safe? J Clin Endocrinol Metab 2000;85: 3191–3198.
18 Antonangeli L, Maccherini D, Cavaliere R, et al: Comparison of two different doses of iodide in the prevention of gestational goiter in marginal iodine deficiency: a longitudinal study. Eur J Endocrinol 2002;147:29–34.
19 Bath SC, Steer CD, Golding J, et al: Effect of inadequate iodine status in UK pregnant women on cognitive outcomes in their children: results from the Avon Longitudinal Study of Parents and Children (ALSPAC). Lancet 2013;382:331–337.
20 Chaouki ML, Benmiloud M: Prevention of iodine deficiency disorders by oral administration of lipiodol during pregnancy. Eur J Endocrinol 1994;130: 547–551.
21 Mason JB, Deitchler M, Gilmann A, et al: Iodine fortification is related to increased weight-for-age and birthweight in children in Asia. Food Nutr Bull 2002; 23:292–308.

22 DeLong GR, Leslie PW, Wang SH, et al: Effect on infant mortality of iodination of irrigation water in a severely iodine-deficient area of China. Lancet 1997; 350:771–773.
23 Cobra C, Muhilal, Rusmil K, et al: Infant survival is improved by oral iodine supplementation. J Nutr 1997;127:574–578.
24 Semba RD, de Pee S, Hess SY, et al: Child malnutrition and mortality among families not utilizing adequately iodized salt in Indonesia. Am J Clin Nutr 2008;87:438–444.
25 Bougma K, Aboud FE, Harding KB, et al: Iodine and mental development of children 5 years old and under: a systematic review and meta-analysis. Nutrients 2013;5:1384–1416.
26 Zimmermann MB, Boelaert K: Iodine deficiency and thyroid disorders. Lancet Diabetes Endocrinol 2015; 3:286–295.
27 Bouhouch RR, Bouhouch S, Cherkaoui M, et al: Direct iodine supplementation of infants versus supplementation of their breastfeeding mothers: a double-blind, randomised, placebo-controlled trial. Lancet Diabetes Endocrinol 2014;2:197–209.

Prof. Michael B. Zimmermann, MD
Laboratory for Human Nutrition, Institute of Food, Nutrition and Health
Swiss Federal Institute of Technology (ETH) Zurich
Schmelzbergstrasse 7, LFV E19
CH–8092 Zurich (Switzerland)
E-Mail michael.zimmermann@ilw.agrl.ethz.ch

Biesalski HK, Black RE (eds): Hidden Hunger. Malnutrition and the First 1,000 Days of Life:
Causes, Consequences and Solutions. World Rev Nutr Diet. Basel, Karger, 2016, vol 115, pp 125–133
DOI: 10.1159/000442079

Zinc Deficiency in Childhood and Pregnancy: Evidence for Intervention Effects and Program Responses

Laura M. Lamberti · Christa L. Fischer Walker · Robert E. Black

Department of International Health, Johns Hopkins Bloomberg School of Public Health, Baltimore, MD, USA

Abstract

Zinc is a key micronutrient of particular importance during childhood and pregnancy. Zinc deficiency has been linked to increased infection and stunting among children and is a risk factor for adverse pregnancy outcomes and preterm delivery. Targeted interventions have the potential to alleviate the adverse effects of zinc deficiency via therapeutic and preventive supplementation, fortification and biofortification, but implementation is challenging. A growing number of low- and middle-income countries have introduced national policies for zinc treatment of diarrhea among children under 5 years in response to mounting evidence of reduced episode duration and severity as well as reduced incidence in the ensuing months, but coverage remains low in the absence of effective scale-up efforts. Implementation of preventive zinc supplementation in young children has also been slow, despite evidence linking routine daily supplementation and treatment regimens with reductions in stunting and the incidence of diarrhea and pneumonia. Acceptance of other zinc interventions, including traditional fortification, fortification with micronutrient powders and biofortification, is hindered by unclear evidence on efficacy. Additional research is therefore warranted to ascertain the efficacy of delivering zinc through fortified and biofortified foods and in combination with other micronutrients in supplements or powders. Operations research is also necessary to establish best practices for scale-up of therapeutic zinc supplementation for diarrhea.

Introduction

Zinc is an essential micronutrient with a well-established role in human health and immunity [1–3]. Deficiency in zinc, which is required for cell division and differentiation, protein synthesis and nucleic acid metabolism [1–3], is associated with growth retardation and an elevated risk of infectious disease among children and adolescents [4–6].

Acrodermatitis enteropathica is a rare genetic condition in which hindered zinc uptake causes skin lesions, persistent diarrhea, and, if untreated, subsequent death [7, 8]. More commonly, zinc deficiency results from dietary insufficiency in low- and middle-income countries and is exacerbated by the loss of endogenous zinc during diarrhea, which frequently recurs among young children in such settings [9–12]. There is a vicious cycle of zinc deficiency and diarrheal infection since zinc-deficient children are more susceptible to contracting diarrheal pathogens and since diarrhea causes the poor nutrient absorption that contributes to deficiency [13].

In this chapter, we present an overview of the global prevalence and effects of zinc deficiency in early childhood and pregnancy. We also describe the existing evidence on zinc interventions, including therapeutic supplementation, preventive supplementation, food fortification with micronutrient powders (MNPs), and biofortification. Finally, we discuss the barriers to delivering zinc interventions at scale.

Measuring Zinc Deficiency Globally

The gold-standard method of diagnosis of zinc deficiency in populations is measurement of the zinc concentration in serum or plasma. However, data on the population distribution of serum/plasma zinc concentrations are scarce. Regional estimates of the risk of zinc deficiency have instead been derived from assessments of national food availability, which indicate that 17% of the global population may have inadequate zinc intake [9]. These estimates vary greatly by region, ranging from 5.7% in Oceania to 7.6% in Europe, 9.6% in the Americas and Caribbean, 19.6% in Asia and 23.9% in Africa [9].

Though possible dietary zinc intake provides insight into the degree of population-level zinc deficiency, the serum/plasma zinc concentration remains the best biomarker. Of the 12 national surveys that have assessed the plasma zinc concentration among young children living in low- and middle-income countries, 11 indicated that the proportion of the population with low plasma zinc concentrations exceeded the proportion of the national population at risk of inadequate zinc consumption based on food availability data [14]. This finding suggests that assessment of national food availability for zinc consumption may underestimate the prevalence of zinc deficiency in young children. Furthermore, the successful completion of these studies in low- and middle-income countries indicates that the blood collection necessary for assessment of the plasma zinc concentration is feasible even in challenging settings.

The Effects of Zinc Deficiency in Childhood

The earliest study on human zinc deficiency noted growth anomalies and delayed maturation [4], and the literature has since established an increased need for zinc during periods of growth and an association between zinc deficiency and stunting in children [15–17].

There is also extensive evidence documenting the association between zinc deficiency in children and infectious disease, and specifically diarrhea and acute lower respiratory tract infection (ALRI) [1]. In a study in urban India, the prevalence rates of diarrhea and ALRI were respectively 4 and 3.5 times higher among children with low plasma zinc compared to those with normal levels [6]. However, the strongest evidence for a causal association between zinc status and diarrheal and ALRI outcomes has been derived from therapeutic and preventive zinc supplementation trials. In addition to morbidity, meta-analyses of data from randomized controlled trials (RCTs) have indicated a trend toward an elevated risk of mortality from diarrhea and pneumonia among zinc-deficient compared to nondeficient children [18].

The Effects of Zinc Deficiency in Pregnancy

Few studies have been conducted on zinc deficiency in pregnancy. The existing evidence suggests that a low plasma zinc concentration is a risk factor for maternal complications, such as hypertension, preeclampsia, intrapartum hemorrhage, infection, prolonged labor and preterm delivery, as well as congenital anomalies and low birth weight among surviving offspring [19].

Zinc Interventions: Therapeutic Supplementation

The earliest therapeutic zinc supplementation trials were conducted on young children in low-resource settings in the late 1980s and the 1990s [20–23]. These studies demonstrated the efficacy of zinc treatment for diarrhea and thus laid the groundwork for the more than one hundred additional zinc treatment RCTs to be carried out in the ensuing two decades and for the global recommendation issued by the World Health Organization (WHO) and the United Nations Children's Fund in 2004 [24]. Overall, the data pooled from this body of evidence show a reduction of approximately 25% in the relative risk of diarrheal episode duration beyond 3 days among zinc-treated children under 5 years of age [25]. Meta-analyses have also indicated statistically significant reductions in hospitalizations for diarrhea [1, 25], and one RCT reported a reduction in noninjury deaths [26]. There is less definitive evidence on the efficacy of zinc treatment in improving ALRI outcomes among children, as studies have reported variable results [1]. Similarly, zinc therapy provided no benefit to school-aged children with acute, uncomplicated falciparum malaria in a large multicenter trial [27].

Zinc Interventions: Preventive Supplementation

Studies have assessed the impact of preventive zinc supplementation on diarrhea via two intervention designs. Primary prevention includes strategies in which daily zinc supplements are administered to children with no apparent illness in an effort to prevent disease. Secondary prevention interventions are initiated in response to disease, with the goals of reducing the severity of that illness as well as illness in the subsequent months.

In a recent meta-analysis of 18 RCTs, primary preventive zinc supplementation resulted in a nonsignificant, 9% reduction in all-cause mortality as well as a 13% (95% CI: 6–19) decrease in diarrhea and a 19% (95% CI: 10–27) decrease in pneumonia among children under 5 years of age [28]. Evidence suggests that for ALRI, the effect of primary preventive zinc supplementation is stronger for cases meeting specific diagnostic criteria, as opposed to caregiver-reported ALRI [29]. A meta-analysis of RCTs assessing the effect of primary preventive supplementation with zinc reported a gain in linear growth of 0.37 cm in children receiving zinc compared to those receiving placebo [30].

Secondary preventive zinc supplementation trials have reported reductions in the incidence and prevalence of diarrhea and ALRI during the period following therapy [26, 31]. A trial in Bangladesh observed a 15% (95% CI: 4–24) reduction in diarrhea incidence and a 7% (95% CI: –10 to 22) decrease in ALRI incidence during the 2–3 months following 14 days of zinc treatment [26]. The 24-hour prevalence of diarrhea and ALRI decreased by 25% (95% CI: 9–38) and 72% (95% CI: 58–81), respectively, during the 6-month follow-up period in a cluster randomized trial in Haryana, India [31].

Zinc Interventions: Supplementation in Pregnancy

A systematic review of zinc supplementation earlier than 27 weeks of gestation reported a statistically significant, 14% decrease in the risk of preterm birth among supplemented women in low-income countries [32]. However, there was no effect on low birth weight or other maternal, fetal, neonatal or infant outcomes. There is no established benefit of prenatal zinc supplementation for postnatal linear growth [33], but studies have shown an association with reductions in diarrhea during infancy [34, 35].

Zinc Interventions: Traditional Fortification and Fortification with Micronutrient Powders

Micronutrient fortification is a method by which essential vitamins and minerals are added to commonly consumed food staples in order to improve the quality of diet in a given population. Despite the inclusion of zinc as a recommended fortificant in the WHO policy on industrial fortification of wheat and maize flour [36], the majority of governments have resisted adding zinc to national food fortification programs due to a lack of evidence of benefits. Studies have demonstrated that zinc fortification successfully increases daily zinc absorption and the serum zinc concentration among children [37, 38], but the impact of zinc fortification on health and growth outcomes has not yet been established. Further research is therefore warranted.

MNPs are single-dose packets of powdered vitamins and minerals that can be sprinkled on any semi-solid food, thus enabling home fortification [39]. A systematic review of eight trials assessing the effect of MNPs containing iron, vitamin A and zinc on children aged 6–23 months found that MNP recipients experienced reductions in anemia and iron deficiency [40]. On the basis of this result, the current WHO recommendation for children under 2 years in regions with high anemia prevalence includes daily home fortification with one MNP sachet containing 12.5 mg elemental iron, 300 μg retinol (vitamin A) and 5 mg elemental zinc [39]. However, it is important to note that studies have not found that consumption of MNPs containing zinc results in an increase in serum zinc, as has almost uniformly been observed with oral zinc supplements, and that studies have not demonstrated the reduction in infectious diseases that is associated with zinc supplements.

Zinc Interventions: Biofortification

Biofortification is a process by which the micronutrient content of crops is enhanced through biological agriculture. Examples of zinc biofortification have included biofortification of wheat, rice, beans, sweet potato and maize [41, 42]; however, further research on zinc biofortification is necessary, as the existing evidence is limited and the potential benefits, if any, are unclear.

Incorporating Zinc Interventions into National Programs

The translation of evidence on the efficacy of zinc therapy into effective programs has been fraught with challenges. There are currently at least 82 countries with national policies supporting the use of low-osmolarity oral rehydration salts (ORS) and zinc for the management of diarrhea among children under 5 years (fig. 1). Despite growing acceptance of ORS and zinc policy, regional and national scale-up has proven

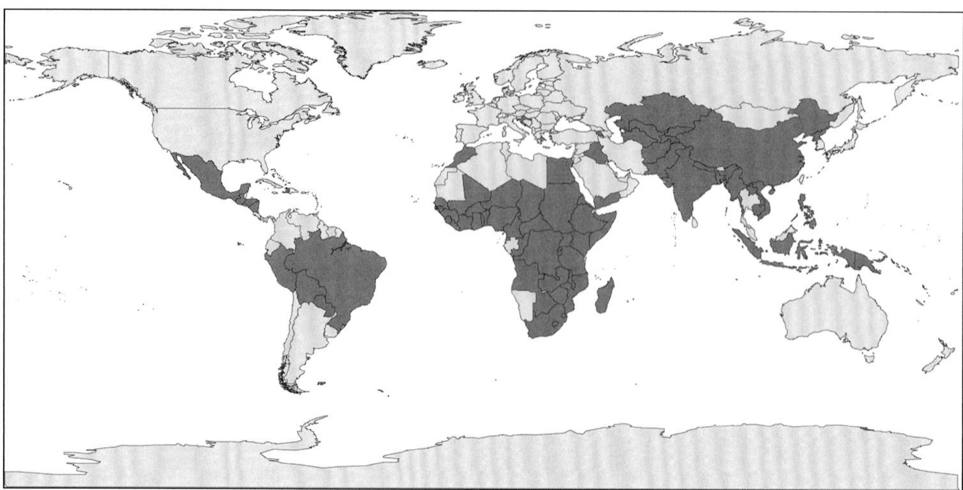

Fig. 1. Eighty-two countries with policies on the use of low-osmolarity ORS and zinc for diarrhea treatment in children under 5 years of age, 2015. The map was originally designed in 2011 using United Nations Children's Fund data on national zinc treatment policies for diarrhea among children under 5 years; the data were collected for all United Nations Children's Fund priority countries and additional countries with formative zinc research or pilot interventions. The data on the 75 countries included in the *Countdown to 2015* report were updated in August 2015 [44].

problematic in many countries due to issues with product procurement and delivery. In addition, gaining buy-in from public- and private-sector providers and generating caregiver demand are essential for maximizing coverage but are not easily achieved without political commitment and programmatic emphasis on improving diarrhea treatment practices at the community level. The first step in addressing these challenges is to ensure that the treatment of diarrhea in young children remains a focal point of national health agendas in low- and middle-income countries. Effective program implementation leading to high coverage for ORS and zinc will only be achieved through prioritized investments in product procurement, targeted training of front-line health workers and behavioral change communication to increase product demand. Continued investments in operations research and program evaluations are also critical for ascertaining lessons learned and reassessing context-specific scale-up strategies moving forward.

Barriers also exist to scale-up of primary preventive zinc supplementation. Though the benefits of zinc supplements have been established, governments are reluctant to commit to micronutrient supplementation programs that focus on zinc alone. The dearth of convincing evidence on the health effects of zinc through fortification, MNP use and biofortification presents a significant challenge that must be addressed before programmatic implementation can be considered. It is therefore important that studies assessing these preventive zinc interventions remain on the global research agenda.

For young children, studies are needed to develop a primary prevention approach in which zinc is efficacious when provided along with other micronutrients in supplements or powders. More studies are also needed to quantify the secondary prevention benefits of the use of zinc for the treatment of diarrhea. The effects of zinc supplements in pregnancy may be achieved through provision of multiple micronutrient supplements that have been shown to reduce the occurrence of both small-for-gestational-age and preterm births [43].

Conclusions

Zinc is a critical micronutrient for health and development, and deficiency has been linked to an increased risk of infectious disease and stunting. Provision of zinc for the treatment of diarrhea is efficacious in reducing episode duration and severity and has secondary prevention benefits. Nearly all low- and middle-income countries now have a policy of treating diarrhea in children under 5 years of age with zinc, but resources have been limited for implementation of this policy, and coverage for zinc treatment of diarrhea remains low. Supplementation of young children with either routine daily dosing for primary prevention or a short treatment course for secondary prevention decreases the incidence of diarrhea and pneumonia and reduces stunting. Despite the known associations between zinc deficiency and poor health outcomes and the evidence demonstrating the efficacy and acceptability of supplementation for the treatment of diarrhea and the prevention of diarrhea and severe pneumonia, implementation of zinc interventions is limited.

Improvement of dietary quality to meet the needs for zinc and other essential nutrients is the ultimate goal. Even in countries where dietary sources of zinc are not scarce, women and young children do not consume enough of these foods to ensure optimal growth and development. Reduction in poverty and inequities in low- and middle-income countries can help to accomplish this goal, but technologic advances in traditional fortification or biofortification may be advantageous. Research can improve understanding of the biological effects associated with zinc deficiency as well as the benefits of correcting for deficiency via supplementation or fortification. Program planners can build from extensive research experience to design targeted, evidence-based programs to decrease the burden of infectious diseases, poor birth outcomes and stunted growth.

References

1 Fischer-Walker C, Lamberti L, Roth D, Black R: Zinc and infectious diseases; in Rink L (ed): Zinc in Human Health. Amsterdam, IOS Press, 2011, pp 234–253.

2 Sandstead HH: Zinc deficiency. A public health problem? Am J Dis Child 1991;145:853–859.

3 World Health Organization: Trace elements in human nutrition and health. Geneva, World Health Organization, 1996.

4 Prasad AS, Miale A, Farid Z, Sanstead HH, Schulert AR, Darby WJ: Biochemical studies on dwarfism, hypogonadism and anemia. Arch Internal Med 1963;111:407–428.

5 Bondestam M, Foucard T, Gebre-Medhin M: Subclinical trace element deficiency in children with undue susceptibility to infections. Acta Paediatr Scand 1985;74:515–520.

6 Bahl R, Bhandari N, Hambidge KM, Bhan MK: Plasma zinc as a predictor of diarrheal and respiratory morbidity in children in an urban slum setting. Am J Clin Nutr 1998;68(suppl):414S–417S.

7 Barnes PM, Moynahan EJ: Zinc deficiency in acrodermatitis enteropathica: multiple dietary intolerance treated with synthetic diet. Proc R Soc Med 1973;66:327–329.

8 Walling A, Householder M, Walling A: Acrodermatitis enteropathica. Am Fam Physician 1989;39:151–154.

9 Black RE, Victora CG, Walker SP, Bhutta ZA, Christian P, de Onis M, et al: Maternal and child undernutrition and overweight in low-income and middle-income countries. Lancet 2013;382:427–451.

10 Castillo-Duran C, Vial P, Uauy R: Trace mineral balance during acute diarrhea in infants. J Pediatr 1988;113:452–457.

11 Rothbaum RJ, Maur PR, Farrell MK: Serum alkaline phosphatase and zinc undernutrition in infants with chronic diarrhea. Am J Clin Nutr 1982;35:595–598.

12 Naveh Y, Lightman A, Zinder O: Effect of diarrhea on serum zinc concentrations in infants and children. J Pediatr 1982;101:730–732.

13 Tomkins A: Recent developments in the nutritional management of diarrhoea. 1. Nutritional strategies to prevent diarrhoea among children in developing countries. Trans R Soc Trop Med Hyg 1991;85:4–7.

14 Hess SY: Overview of nationally representative zinc surveys and other zinc assessment strategies [Personal Communication] 2015.

15 Gibson RS: Zinc: the missing link in combating micronutrient malnutrition in developing countries. Proc Nutr Soc 2006;65:51–60.

16 Gibson RS, Heywood A, Yaman C, Sohlström A, Thompson LU, Heywood P: Growth in children from the Wosera subdistrict, Papua New Guinea, in relation to energy and protein intakes and zinc status. Am J Clin Nutr 1991;53:782–789.

17 Stammers AL, Lowe NM, Medina MW, Patel S, Dykes F, Perez-Rodrigo C, et al: The relationship between zinc intake and growth in children aged 1–8 years: a systematic review and meta-analysis. Eur J Clin Nutr 2015;69:147–153.

18 Fischer Walker CL, Rudan I, Liu L, Nair H, Theodoratou E, Bhutta ZA, et al: Global burden of childhood pneumonia and diarrhoea. Lancet 2013;381:1405–1416.

19 King JC: Determinants of maternal zinc status during pregnancy. Am J Clin Nutr 2000;71(5 suppl):1334S–1343S.

20 Sachdev HP, Mittal NK, Mittal SK, Yadav HS: A controlled trial on utility of oral zinc supplementation in acute dehydrating diarrhea in infants. J Pediatr Gastroenterol Nutr 1988;7:877–881.

21 Sazawal S, Black RE, Bhan MK, Bhandari N, Sinha A, Jalla S: Zinc supplementation in young children with acute diarrhea in India. N Engl J Med 1995;333:839–844.

22 Fuchs GJ: Possibilities for zinc in the treatment of acute diarrhea. Am J Clin Nutr 1998;68(2 suppl):480S–483S.

23 Black RE: Therapeutic and preventive effects of zinc on serious childhood infectious diseases in developing countries. Am J Clin Nutr 1998;68(2 suppl):476S–479S.

24 WHO/UNICEF: Joint statement on the clinical management of acute diarrhea. Geneva, World Health Assembly, 2004.

25 Lamberti LM, Walker CL, Chan KY, Jian WY, Black RE: Oral zinc supplementation for the treatment of acute diarrhea in children: a systematic review and meta-analysis. Nutrients 2013;5:4715–4740.

26 Baqui AH, Black RE, El Arifeen S, Yunus M, Chakraborty J, Ahmed S, et al: Effect of zinc supplementation started during diarrhoea on morbidity and mortality in Bangladeshi children: community randomised trial. BMJ 2002;325:1059.

27 Zinc against Plasmodium Study Group: Effect of zinc on the treatment of *Plasmodium falciparum* malaria in children: a randomized controlled trial. Am J Clin Nutr 2002;76:805–812.

28 Yakoob MY, Theodoratou E, Jabeen A, Imdad A, Eisele TP, Ferguson J, et al: Preventive zinc supplementation in developing countries: impact on mortality and morbidity due to diarrhea, pneumonia and malaria. BMC Public Health 2011;11(suppl 3):S23.

29 Roth DE, Richard SA, Black RE: Zinc supplementation for the prevention of acute lower respiratory infection in children in developing countries: meta-analysis and meta-regression of randomized trials. Int J Epidemiol 2010;39:795–808.

30 Imdad A, Bhutta ZA: Effect of preventive zinc supplementation on linear growth in children under 5 years of age in developing countries: a meta-analysis of studies for input to the lives saved tool. BMC Public Health 2011;11(suppl 3):S22.
31 Bhandari N, Mazumder S, Taneja S, Dube B, Agarwal RC, Mahalanabis D, et al: Effectiveness of zinc supplementation plus oral rehydration salts compared with oral rehydration salts alone as a treatment for acute diarrhea in a primary care setting: a cluster randomized trial. Pediatrics 2008;121:e1279–e1285.
32 Mori R, Ota E, Middleton P, Tobe-Gai R, Mahomed K, Bhutta ZA: Zinc supplementation for improving pregnancy and infant outcome. Cochrane Database Syst Rev 2012;7:CD000230.
33 Gebreselassie SG, Gashe FE: A systematic review of effect of prenatal zinc supplementation on birthweight: meta-analysis of 17 randomized controlled trials. J Health Popul Nutr 2011;29:134–140.
34 Iannotti LL, Zavaleta N, León Z, Huasquiche C, Shankar AH, Caulfield LE: Maternal zinc supplementation reduces diarrheal morbidity in Peruvian infants. J Pediatr 2010;156:960–964, 964.e1–e2.
35 Wieringa FT, Dijkhuizen MA, Muhilal, Van der Meer JW: Maternal micronutrient supplementation with zinc and beta-carotene affects morbidity and immune function of infants during the first 6 months of life. Eur J Clin Nutr 2010;64:1072–1079.
36 World Health Organization: Recommendations on wheat and maize flour fortification. Meeting Report: Interim Consensus Statement. Geneva, World Health Organization, 2009.
37 Brown KH, Wessells KR, Hess SY: Zinc bioavailability from zinc-fortified foods. Int J Vitam Nutr Res 2007;77:174–181.
38 Winichagoon P, McKenzie JE, Chavasit V, Pongcharoen T, Gowachirapant S, Boonpraderm A, et al: A multimicronutrient-fortified seasoning powder enhances the hemoglobin, zinc, and iodine status of primary school children in North East Thailand: a randomized controlled trial of efficacy. J Nutr 2006;136:1617–1623.
39 World Health Organization: Guideline: use of multiple micronutrient powders for home fortification of foods consumed by infants and children 6–23 months of age. Geneva, World Health Organization, 2011.
40 De-Regil LM, Suchdev PS, Vist GE, Walleser S, Pena-Rosas JP: Home fortification of foods with multiple micronutrient powders for health and nutrition in children under two years of age. Cochrane Database Syst Rev 2011;CD008959.
41 World Health Organization: Biofortification of staple crops 2015. http://www.who.int/elena/titles/biofortification/en/ (accessed August 28, 2015).
42 Bouis HE, Hotz C, McClafferty B, Meenakshi JV, Pfeiffer WH: Biofortification: a new tool to reduce micronutrient malnutrition. Food Nutr Bull 2011;32(1 suppl):S31–S40.
43 Christian P: Evidence of Multiple Micronutrient Supplementation (MMS) in pregnancy. Sight Life 2015;29:28–34.
44 Victora CG, Requejo JH, Barros AJ, Berman P, Bhutta Z, Boerma T, et al: Countdown to 2015: a decade of tracking progress for maternal, newborn and child survival. Lancet 2015, Epub ahead of print.

Dr. Robert E. Black
Department of International Health
Johns Hopkins Bloomberg School of Public Health
615 N Wolfe St., Baltimore, MD 21205 (USA)
E-Mail rblack1@jhu.edu

Biesalski HK, Black RE (eds): Hidden Hunger. Malnutrition and the First 1,000 Days of Life: Causes, Consequences and Solutions. World Rev Nutr Diet. Basel, Karger, 2016, vol 115, pp 134–141
DOI: 10.1159/000442080

The Second International Conference on Nutrition, as Seen by a Member State

Hanns-Christoph Eiden • Simone Welte

Federal Office for Agriculture and Food, Bonn, Germany

Abstract

For years now, providing people with food and balanced diets has been a problem unsolved by the world community. Despite numerous initiatives, the great breakthrough has still not happened, not least because the issue is so complex. Hunger and undernourishment must be fought as much as hidden hunger, overweight and obesity. Increasingly, several forms of malnutrition have been occurring simultaneously. The so-called double burden of malnutrition has become the new normal. The follow-up process of the Second International Conference on Nutrition assumes a vital role in that context. The *Rome Declaration* and the *Framework for Action* commit the international community, international organizations and civil society to undertake joint efforts across and beyond sectorial policies. Both documents also indicate numerous starting points for actions that consider individual national examples. Germany has been actively engaged at both the national and the international levels. Since its inception in 2008, the National Action Plan 'IN FORM' has taken up a number of suggestions made by the Second International Conference on Nutrition. While IN FORM is further developed, the ideas given in the *Framework for Action* shall provide a fresh impetus. Within its development cooperation, Germany is increasingly focusing on improving the nutritional situation, such as through its One World, No Hunger initiative. In the follow-up process, all stakeholders, including the Food and Agriculture Organization and the World Health Organization, will have to offer platforms to promote exchange among all parties involved and to initiate coherent actions that also reach beyond national borders. Only then can the improvement of the nutritional situation really be seen as a truly global challenge. Given the issue's complexity, it is equally important to establish priorities in each case in order for progress not to be thwarted by lengthy decision-making processes. Improving the situation of particularly vulnerable groups, such as young women and small children, shall be as prominent as the support and promotion of diversified agriculture. Building networks among partners is of equal importance for joint action and exchange between stakeholders at the national and international levels to generate added value on the way toward solving the nutrition problem. Science will also have to be more closely involved for that matter and purpose. Research is required to supply scientific evidence for certain measures to be taken, and it assumes a prominent role where political consultation, knowledge management and the implementation of measures are concerned.

The Second International Conference on Nutrition, as Seen by a Member State

The Second International Conference on Nutrition (ICN2), organized by the Food and Agriculture Organization (FAO) and the World Health Organization (WHO) on 19–21 November 2014 in Rome, was the first global intergovernmental conference toward solving food- and nutrition-related issues in the 21st century. It underlined the subject's importance and explosive nature. The issues of hunger and malnutrition remain unsolved by the world community. Progress registered in recent years is still too slow. New challenges have emerged and are increasing: overweight and obesity. Furthermore, anemia in women of reproductive age is stagnant, and stunting levels are declining slowly and are uneven.

Both the conference and the statements presented by high-ranking political and social stakeholders emphasized the will to act. The final documents, or the *Rome Declaration on Nutrition* and the *Framework for Action*, are milestones on the way toward tackling the challenges in the framework of the follow-up process, jointly directed by the FAO and the WHO, even in a decade focusing on food and nutrition [1].

Background

For many years now, the consequences of malnutrition have been discussed intensely. Irrespective of both numerous declarations of intent and general recognition of the importance of the issues of hunger and malnutrition and despite ambitious goals, such as halving the number of people who suffer from hunger by 2015 [2], progress is limited. Were recent years mainly marked by rhetorical declarations of intent? Has the world community mainly talked instead of taking action? Such across-the-board criticism would not be justified, given that the issue is complex and that success depends on many factors. Seen in this light and against the backdrop of rapid world population growth, the fact that the number of people who suffer from hunger has been reduced [3] is a big success!

However, as the focus was put on fighting hunger, the phenomenon of hidden hunger, which 2 billion people are affected by, has been given less attention for a long time. Hidden hunger often affects people who take in sufficient, or at times even excess, amounts of calories while their food lacks quality. A lack of vitamin D, iodine, zinc and iron and other vitamin and mineral deficiencies have grave and often irreversible effects on a person's development.

Hidden hunger often also occurs in countries where large parts of the population are challenged by overweight. This double burden has become the 'new normal' [4]. Overweight and obesity spread quickly; across the globe, 1.9 billion people are overweight, and 600 million of them are considered obese [5]. Margaret Chan, WHO Director-General, and the Organization for Economic Cooperation and Development are talking about a global obesity epidemic that no country has been able to curb yet [6, 7]. Overweight does not concern rich countries only. On the contrary, the global community and people living under different social and economic conditions are affected [8], but excess weight and obesity do particularly present a challenge in poorer regions around the world. Problems often start when parts of a population become wealthier and increasingly give up their traditional diets in favor of high-energy, highly processed foods with high fat and sugar contents (nutrition transition). As incomes increase, so does the share of foods of animal origin in people's diets [8].

To date, why has no one been able to realize the decisive step of providing balanced diets and sufficient food, with calorie supplies neither too low nor too high, for the majority of people? During the past 30 years, a number of efforts were undertaken to solve the food and nutrition problem: the green revolution, strengthening of both the roles of women and rural areas, involvement in international trade, etc.

The reason lies in the fact that nutrition is a very complex issue that depends on and is influenced by a number of factors; access to water, health services, climate, soils, agricultural technology, education, and the value of agricultural goods in the national and international markets are only a few of the aspects that determine the nutrition situation.

In the individual states concerned, a good political framework is indispensable to providing people with optimal food and nutrition. Additionally, priorities must be clearly established, and respective policies must involve all areas and all stakeholders affected. For the longest time, countless initiatives at the state and international levels have managed neither to translate the manifold issues into coherent and target-oriented actions nor to firmly place the fight against hunger and malnutrition on the world community's agenda as a vital field of action.

For some years, however, this picture has been changing! Initiated by the Food Price Crisis [9] and the Lancet Series in 2008 [10], which supplied a scientifically sound and concentrated presentation of the grave consequences of maternal and child undernutrition in particular, the Scaling Up Nutrition (SUN) movement has, since 2010, motivated a growing number of countries to make the improvement of their populations' nutrition a central and cross-sectoral issue at the government level.

Within the movement, donor countries, civil society, international organizations and economic partners are joining efforts toward the success of these individual state initiatives. A report that evaluated the work done by the SUN movement between 2010 and 2015 [11] illustrated various achievements and also made important suggestions on how to further develop and permanently establish the initiative's work, in which more than 50 states are currently participating.

In addition to intensifying the dynamics of this process, the ICN2 final documents also spread the conference's contents to every state within the world community. Both the *Rome Declaration* and the *Framework for Action* also suggest pursuing approaches that involve various policy areas and all stakeholders concerned. However, while SUN currently focuses on fighting undernutrition due to insufficient food supplies, the *Declaration* and the *Framework* include all forms of malnutrition, i.e. overweight and obesity in particular, and address all governments.

The ICN2 conclusions underline the need to enshrine the fight against hunger and malnutrition as a prominent goal of global sustainable development [12]. The conference asked for a multisectoral and multistakeholder approach, including, inter alia, the improvement of water, sanitation and hygiene, and access to health services and education, which is already at the center of all SUN activities.

The General Assembly of the United Nations (UN) acknowledges the need for action and welcomes the fact that the FAO and the WHO are offering to provide the platform for states and governments to exchange experiences and form alliances to benefit from each other and to achieve more by joining efforts [13].

Against this background, the question as to the steps to be taken by the FAO and WHO member states in the wake of the ICN2 arises with particular emphasis.

Germany's Answer to the Challenges regarding the Nutritional Situation in the 21st Century: 'IN FORM'

The German government took action several years ago already. The National Action Plan 'IN FORM', Germany's initiative for healthy diets and more physical activity [14], was started in 2008. IN FORM was initiated in response to the growing numbers of Germans who are malnourished. More than half of all women and 67% of all men in Germany are overweight, and every 1 in 5 Germans is considered obese [15].

IN FORM is a joint initiative undertaken by the Federal Ministry of Food and Agriculture and the Federal Ministry of Health. It intends to sustainably improve people's habits regarding their diets and their physical activity. IN FORM identifies, develops and implements measures to prevent malnutrition, lack of physical activity, overweight and related diseases.

IN FORM's aims are as follows:

- Adults should live healthier lives
- Children should grow up healthier
- The entire population should benefit from a higher quality of life and increased activity

As a long-term action plan, IN FORM runs until 2020. By then, it intends to achieve both a significant decrease in noncommunicable diseases and a reduction of costs arising in the public health sector. For these purposes, IN FORM counts on

- people's personal initiative;
- information;
- sustainable structures;
- stakeholders and projects forming networks to interact with each other.

Germany has agreed to the ICN2 final documents. The contents and aims of the IN FORM action plan already cover a large part of the recommendations for action given in the *Framework for Action*. The *Rome Declaration* and the *Framework for Action* confirm, simultaneously, that the National Action Plan presents an appropriate framework for tackling nutrition-related problems in Germany.

This, however, does not mean that Germany has already done its homework and can sit back and relax, because despite all progress and all our efforts within IN FORM, the fact remains that the number of overweight citizens in Germany is just stagnating at a high level [15]. In addition, the 2012 Food and Nutrition Report states that regarding the prevalence of obesity in Germany between 1999 and 2009, neither it nor its increase stagnated, and that there is no trend reversal in sight [16].

As social realities in Germany are changing, new challenges arise. Hence, new target groups need to be addressed in the future, measures and actions taken must have a much broader impact, and networking structures need further improvement. Against the background of the *Framework for Action*, we will have to check to what extent the National Action Plan IN FORM sufficiently considers social developments such as the trend toward external catering for day care centers, schools, canteens and cafeterias, hospitals and retirement homes; whether sections of society with low levels of academic achievement are reached; whether a sufficient number of multipliers are included, and whether a sound basis of data is provided in order to initiate the necessary steps. Both the *Rome Declaration* and the *Framework for Action* support this action plan's further development and adaptation to new conditions on the ground, and decisions adopted by the ICN2 enter into the IN FORM process.

Additionally, the new German Prevention Act will put a particular emphasis on strengthening public health promotion in Germany. Food and nutrition will play an important role in that context, as they can sustainably contribute to preventing certain noncommunicable diseases from arising [17].

International Food and Nutritional Policy: Germany Is Involved

At the international level, the German Federal Ministry of Food and Agriculture defines the agriculture and nutrition policy. Moreover, it promotes bilateral cooperation between application-oriented pilot projects on food security and nutrition. Within the framework of the Bilateral Trust Fund, the ministry supports FAO projects to improve the food and nutrition situation based on the human right to adequate food. Examples are projects with a focus on nutrition education and highly efficient, sustainable agriculture and food systems that prevent negative effects on health, the environment and society along the entire value chain [18].

Where development cooperation is concerned, Germany is also increasingly focusing on nutrition and food security. The initiative One World, No Hunger, started by the German Federal Ministry for Economic Cooperation and Development, emphasizes inclusive approaches to fight undernutrition. This ministry is also providing the financial means for the Global Nutrition Report 2015 to be drafted [19].

Breaking the Cycle of Malnutrition

Malnutrition in all its forms prevents people from developing and realizing their full potential in life. Malnourished children do less well in school and will later face challenges in their professional life. Malnourished adults are less able to work, will face limitations when they exercise their professions and will thus have fewer opportunities to gain sufficient income for themselves and their families. Malnourished mothers give birth to malnourished babies and lack the capacity to adequately care for them. The cycle of poverty, malnutrition and economic stagnation closes only to restart over and over again [20].

Establish Priorities
Cross-sectoral cooperation is key to the termination of hunger and malnutrition. However, working comprehensively toward a holistic approach to food and nutrition and across the various sectors involved is not an easy task. Nonetheless, the process that led up to the ICN2 has shown that it is indeed possible to cooperate internationally with many stakeholders and thee two large UN organizations involved, despite time-consuming coordination processes among the member states. This success should now be utilized, and this process has triggered dynamics that should encourage us to take further action.

In order for the ICN2 not to turn into a mere rhetorical declaration of intentions, the following aspects are particularly relevant:

- The political decision makers must quickly become aware of what is important in a country's concrete situation. This purpose requires an in-depth analysis of available data.
  Generally speaking, the targeted evaluation of available information already leads further [4]. Other countries' experiences or the expertise of countries with similar problems are also helpful. Case studies already conducted by other countries and regions always provide guidelines as to the proper placement of interventions.
- In many cases, arriving at a clear conclusion will be difficult because of a lack of sufficient scientific evidence that would point out the necessary steps to be taken. In such cases, further data will have to be collected in order to allow more accurate decisions on particular situations. Lacking data indicate that scientific expertise and networking activities among scientific institutions as well as their dialog with policy makers need to be more strongly promoted in the country concerned.
- A decision goes along with the establishment of priorities. Given that the challenge of improving the nutrition situation is complex and manifold, people might run the risk of debating for too long about the proper way to reach the aim instead of taking action. Priorities must be established in each country concerned. However, no matter how complex the issue, as a group particularly at risk, small children and young women will always deserve special attention. Only well-nourished women can give

birth to healthy children, who in turn will only then have a chance for a healthy start in life and the opportunity to develop their full potential as they grow up.

- The same applies to the promotion of a sustainable and varied agriculture and food systems. Farmers have the task of feeding people and steadily providing them with varied, healthy and affordable food. The sustainable improvement of the food situation, which considers climatic and environmental aspects and contributes to crisis prevention, is only possible if we develop nutrition-sensitive agriculture and food systems and improve the capacities of farmers.
- In all this, the UN and its organizations must assume a decisive role as promoters and monitors of the process. They must make networking come alive for the multitude of individual activities to become a global movement that spurs stakeholders on and that supports and encourages everyone involved. Jointly, the UN and its member states have a mandate to improve the food and nutrition situation and to incorporate food security and nutrition, a major goal on the international agenda, prominently in the *Sustainable Development Goals*. Networks such as SUN, which, during the past 5 years, has decisively contributed to the fact that the issue of balanced diets figures prominently on the international agenda, do deserve support. By involving all the stakeholders concerned, the movement has initiated, in the SUN countries, the process toward change that it needs to make progress. The UN's role and SUN complement each other. Both are part of the process: the UN by way of its comprehensive activity, and SUN by way of its bottom-up approach.

Conclusive Remarks

Malnutrition, in its various degrees and forms, affects the entire globe. The double burden of malnutrition, with too much and too little unbalanced and occurring simultaneously, is the new normal.

Although every country must come to its own conclusions in the sense of the ICN2, not every country must solve its problems alone! Even though situations vary from country to country, the necessary approaches toward solutions are similar. We must learn from one another, and we must build networks and exchange information and experiences!

In that sense, now is the time to pick up where the ICN2 and its spirit left off and to implement its conclusions. Everybody is called upon to join in the effort: the UN member states, civil society, the private sector, and the UN organizations themselves.

References

1 Food and Agriculture Organization, World Health Organization: Rome Declaration on Nutrition and Framework for Action. November 19, 2014. http://www.fao.org/about/meetings/icn2/documents/en/ (accessed July 3, 2015).

2 United Nations Organization: Millenium development goals. http://www.un.org/milleniumgoals/ (accessed June 11, 2015).

3 von Grebmer K, Saltzman A, Birol E, Wiesmann D, Prasai N, Yin S, Yohannes Y, Menon P, Thompson J, Sonntag A: Global hunger index: the challenge of hidden hunger. 2014. http://dx.doi.org/10.2499/9780896299580 (accessed June 11, 2015).

4 International Food Policy Reasearch Institute: Global nutrition report: actions and accountability to accelerate the world's progress on nutrition. 2014. http://dx.doi.org/10.2499/9780896295643 (accessed June 3, 2015).

5 World Health Organization: Overweight and obesity facts. January 2015. http://www.who.int/mediacentre/factsheets/fs311/en/ (accessed July 2, 2015).

6 Sassi F: Obesity and the Economics of Prevention. Fit Not Fat. Paris, OECD, 2010.

7 Chan M: World Health Organization Director-General addresses health promotion conference. Opening address at the 8th Global Conference on Health Promotion. Helsinki, June 10, 2013.

8 Welthungerhilfe, Weingärtner L, Trentmann C: Handbuch Welternährung. Frankfurt am Main, Campus, 2011.

9 SUN in Outline: An introduction to the SUN movement. February 2014. http://scalingupnutrition.org/about (accessed July 30, 2015).

10 Lancet: Series on maternal and child undernutrition. January 16, 2008. http://www.thelancet.com/series/maternal-and-child-undernutrition (accessed June 9, 2015).

11 Mokoro: Independent Comprehensive Evaluation of the Scaling Up Nutrition Movement: Final Report – Main Report and Annexes. Oxford, Mokoro Ltd, 2015.

12 United Nations Organization: Sustainable development goals. https://sustainabledevelopment.un.org/post2015/transformingourworld (accessed June 11, 2015).

13 UN General Assembly: A-RES-69-310: follow-up to the Second International Conference on Nutrition. Resolution adopted by the General Assembly. New York, United Nations Organization, 2015.

14 Federal Ministry of Food and Agriculture: IN FORM: the National Action Plan for the prevention of poor dietary habits, lack of physical activity, overweight and related diseases. Bonn, Federal Ministry of Food and Agriculture, 2008.

15 Kurth MB: Erste Ergebnisse aus der Studie zur Gesundheit Erwachsener in Deutschland (DEGS). Bundesgesundheitsbl 2012;55:980–990.

16 German Nutrition Society eV 12: Ernährungsbericht 2012. Bonn, German Nutrition Society eV, 2012.

17 Federal Ministry of Health: Gesetz zur Stärkung der Gesundheitsförderung und der Prävention (Präventionsgesetz – PrävG). Federal Gazette 2015;31:1368–1379.

18 Federal Ministry of Agriculture and Food: Konzept Welternährung. 2015. http://www.bmel.de/SharedDocs/Downloads/Broschueren/Konzept-Welternaehrung.html (accessed July 3, 2015).

19 Federal Ministry for Economic Cooperation and Development: One World – No Hunger. 2015. http://www.bmz.de/de/was_wir_machen/themen/les/ernaehrung/basiswissen/sonderinitiative_einewelt_ohne_hunger/index.html (accessed June 3, 2015).

20 Biesalski HK: Der verborgene Hunger – Satt sein ist nicht genug. Berlin, Springer Spektrum, 2012.

Dr. Hanns-Christoph Eiden
Federal Office for Agriculture and Food
Deichmanns Aue 29
DE–53179 Bonn (Germany)
E-Mail hanns-christoph.eiden@ble.de

Biesalski HK, Black RE (eds): Hidden Hunger. Malnutrition and the First 1,000 Days of Life: Causes, Consequences and Solutions. World Rev Nutr Diet. Basel, Karger, 2016, vol 115, pp 142–152
DOI: 10.1159/000442100

The Second International Conference on Nutrition: Implications for Hidden Hunger

Leslie Amoroso

Nutrition and Food Systems Division, Food and Agriculture Organization of the United Nations (FAO), Rome, Italy

Abstract

The Second International Conference on Nutrition (ICN2) was jointly organized by the Food and Agriculture Organization of the United Nations (FAO) and the World Health Organization (WHO) and was held at the FAO Headquarters in Rome, Italy, from 19 to 21 November 2014. The ICN2 was a high-level intergovernmental meeting that focused global attention on addressing malnutrition in all its forms: undernutrition, including micronutrient deficiencies, overweight, and obesity. The ICN2 was held to specifically address the persistent and unacceptably high levels of malnutrition. Despite much progress in reducing hunger globally, 795 million people remain undernourished, over 2 billion people suffer from various micronutrient deficiencies, and an estimated 161 million children under 5 years of age are stunted, 99 million underweight, and 51 million wasted. Meanwhile, more than 600 million adults are obese. Global problems require global solutions. The ICN2 brought together national policy-makers from food, agriculture, health, education, social protection and other relevant sectors to address the complex problem of malnutrition through a multi-sectoral approach. Two outcome documents – the *Rome Declaration on Nutrition* and the *Framework for Action* – were endorsed by participating governments at the Conference, committing world leaders to establishing national policies aimed at eradicating malnutrition in all its forms and transforming food systems to make nutritious diets available to all. The *Rome Declaration on Nutrition* is a political statement of 10 commitments for more effective and coordinated action to improve nutrition, while the *Framework for Action* is a voluntary technical guide of 60 recommendations for the implementation of the political commitments. This chapter provides information on the ICN2 and its outcomes as well as follow-up activities. Emphasis is placed on the *Rome Declaration on Nutrition* and the *Framework for Action*, with special focus on hidden hunger problems that have to be addressed through different interventions and a multi-sectoral approach.

Introduction

The Second International Conference on Nutrition (ICN2), co-organized by the Food and Agriculture Organization of the United Nations (FAO) and the World Health Organization (WHO), was successfully held at the FAO Headquarters in Rome, Italy, from 19 to 21 November 2014. The ICN2 was a high-level intergovernmental conference that focused global attention on malnutrition in all its forms: undernutrition, including micronutrient deficiencies, overweight, and obesity. Over 2,200 people participated in the Conference. Besides eminent special guests, the ICN2 brought together a total of 164 members of FAO and WHO, including senior national policy-makers from agriculture, health and other relevant ministries and agencies; leaders of the United Nations (UN) and other intergovernmental organizations as well as civil society and private sector organizations; parliamentarians; opinion leaders; researchers, and development experts [1].

The Conference was convened to (i) review progress made since the 1992 International Conference on Nutrition (ICN), respond to new challenges and opportunities, and identify policy options for improving nutrition; (ii) bring food, agriculture, health and other sectors together and align their sectoral policies to improve nutrition in a sustainable manner; (iii) propose adaptable policy options and institutional frameworks that can adequately address major nutrition challenges in the foreseeable future; (iv) encourage greater political and policy coherence, alignment, coordination and cooperation among food, agriculture, health and other sectors; (v) mobilize the political will and resources to improve nutrition, and (vi) identify priorities for international cooperation on nutrition in the near and medium terms.

Two outcome documents – the *Rome Declaration on Nutrition* [2] and the *Framework for Action* [3, 4] for its implementation – were endorsed at the ICN2. The Conference addressed the persistent and unacceptably high levels of malnutrition, which are having serious consequences for individuals and families, societies and nations. While the global food system has succeeded in increasing the quantity of food produced to feed a growing population in terms of providing enough dietary energy, ensuring the availability, accessibility and affordability of a variety of food products that contribute to healthy diets for all remains a challenge.

Second International Conference on Nutrition: Background and Rationale

The first ICN, held in 1992 and jointly convened by the FAO and WHO, unanimously adopted a World Declaration and Plan of Action for Nutrition [5]. Delegates from 159 countries and the European Community pledged to eliminate or substantially reduce starvation and famine; widespread chronic hunger; undernutrition, especially among children, women and the aged; micronutrient deficiencies, and especially mineral and vitamin deficiencies; diet-related communicable and noncommunicable diseases (NCDs); impediments to optimal breastfeeding, and inadequate sanitation, poor hygiene and unsafe drinking water. Following the 1992 ICN, countries committed to prepare and implement National Plans of Action for Nutrition reflecting country priorities and strategies for alleviating hunger and malnutrition. Nevertheless, implementation and progress have been patchy and often unsatisfactory due to inadequate commitment and leadership, a lack of financial investments, weak human and institutional capacities and a lack of appropriate accountability mechanisms [4].

In the two decades following the first ICN, notwithstanding great improvements in a number of individual countries, progress in reducing hunger and malnutrition has been uneven and unacceptably slow. The latest available estimates indicate that 795 million people globally – just over 1 in 9 people – were or will be undernourished in 2014–2016 (i.e. unable to meet their dietary energy requirements), which is down by 167 million relative to the last decade and 216 million fewer than in 1990–1992 [6]. Over 2 billion people (about 30% of the world's population) suffer from one or more micronutrient deficiencies or hidden hunger [7], with serious public health consequences. An estimated 161 million children under 5 years of age are stunted or chronically malnourished; 99 million underweight for their age, and 51 million wasted or acutely malnourished [8]. At the same time, more than 1.9 billion adults are overweight, of which over 600 million are obese [9], increasingly in low- and middle-income countries, with consequences ranging from an increased risk of premature death to serious chronic health conditions, including an increased prevalence of diet-related NCDs. Changes in diets in recent decades, associated with changing lifestyles, rising incomes and increased consumption of convenience foods together with reductions in physical activity levels, are believed to be associated with this transition.

Many developing countries now face multiple burdens of malnutrition, with people living in the same communities – sometimes even the same households – suffering from undernutrition, micronutrient deficiencies or obesity. The most nutritionally vulnerable communities often include low-income, resource-poor, socially excluded and economically marginalized food-insecure households. Unacceptably high levels of malnutrition will likely persist unless these communities have access to health care, water and sanitation, agricultural inputs and technical support, education, employment and social protection, services that are essential for good nutrition [10].

In the meantime, the food system has continued to evolve, with a greater proportion of food now processed and traded internationally. The availability of highly processed commercial food products high in fat, sugars and salt/sodium has increased, often replacing healthy local diets and foods with the needed micronutrients and also resulting in excessive consumption of energy, fats, sugars and salt. The important challenge today is to sustainably improve nutrition through implementation of coherent policies and better-coordinated actions across all concerned sectors, strengthening, preserving and recovering healthy and sustainable food systems.

Global problems require global solutions. Malnutrition is a global problem requiring coordinated multi-sectoral actions and solutions. Only an intergovernmental conference can commit stakeholders to address all forms of malnutrition. The ICN2 was held to specifically address the persistent and unacceptably high levels of malnutrition and to unite countries as well as parliamentarians, civil society and the private sector in the common goal of improving diets and raising levels of nutrition and keeping nutrition high up on the development agenda [10].

Why Invest in Nutrition?

Malnutrition in all its forms is an intolerable burden, not only on national health systems but also on the entire cultural, social and economic fabric of nations, and is a major impediment to development and the full realization of human potential. People who are undernourished have a weakened immune system, become ill easily and more frequently and are less able to recover quickly and fully from disease. Malnourished children are limited in reaching their full potential in school, affecting their future job and income opportunities and thus perpetuating a cycle of poverty [11, 12]. Globally, the prevalence of overweight and obesity continues to rise, increasing the risk of NCDs such as cardiovascular diseases, diabetes, some cancers and osteoarthritis, which poses a significant threat to public health.

While the cost of dealing with the effects of malnutrition – whether in fiscal, economic or human terms – is high, the cost of prevention is much less. Malnutrition in all its forms costs USD 2.8–3.5 trillion, equivalent to 4–5% of the global gross domestic product, or USD 400–500 per person [7]. Investing in nutrition therefore not only is a moral imperative but also makes economic sense, as it improves productivity and economic growth, reduces health care costs, and promotes education, intellectual capacity and social development.

The most nutritionally vulnerable households tend to consume diets that are monotonous and nutrient-poor, often carbohydrate-rich staples with little diversity. In line with the ICN2 slogan 'Better nutrition, better lives', the lives of all people around the world will improve if we can improve their diets.

Second International Conference on Nutrition Outcome Documents: The *Rome Declaration on Nutrition* and the *Framework for Action*

Two outcome documents – the *Rome Declaration on Nutrition* and the *Framework for Action* – were endorsed by participating governments at the ICN2, committing world leaders to establishing national policies aimed at eradicating malnutrition in all its forms and transforming food systems to make nutritious diets available to all. The *Rome Declaration on Nutrition* is a political statement of 10 commitments for more

Table 1. Summary of the 10 commitments to action in the *Rome Declaration on Nutrition*

1	Eradicate hunger and prevent all forms of malnutrition worldwide
2	Increase investments for effective interventions and actions to improve people's diets and nutrition
3	Enhance sustainable food systems by developing coherent public policies from production to consumption and across relevant sectors
4	Raise the profile of nutrition within relevant national strategies, policies, action plans and programmes and align national resources accordingly
5	Improve nutrition by strengthening human and institutional capacities through relevant research and development, innovation and appropriate technology transfer
6	Strengthen and facilitate contributions and action by all stakeholders and promote collaboration within and across countries
7	Develop policies, programmes and initiatives for ensuring healthy diets throughout the life course
8	Empower people and create an enabling environment for making informed choices about food products for healthy dietary practices and appropriate infant and young child feeding practices through improved health and nutrition information and education
9	Implement the commitments of the *Rome Declaration on Nutrition* through the *Framework for Action*
10	Give due consideration to integrating the vision and commitments of the *Rome Declaration on Nutrition* into the post-2015 development agenda process, including a possible related global goal

Source: Joint FAO-WHO ICN2 Secretariat, Information Note on the *Framework for Action*, November 2014.

effective and coordinated action to improve nutrition, while the *Framework for Action* is a voluntary technical guide of 60 recommendations for the implementation of the political commitments.

The ICN2 outcome documents recognize that food systems have a fundamental role to play in promoting healthy diets and improving nutrition. Food systems comprise the resources, environment, people, institutions and processes with, in and for which food is produced, processed, stored, distributed, prepared and consumed [7]. The food system influences the availability and accessibility of diverse nutritious foods and thus the ability of consumers to choose healthy diets. The food system – in terms of how food is produced, processed, distributed and marketed – as well as the culture of food influences consumer choices, diets and nutrition. In turn, the demand generated through consumer preferences affects the food supply. Food systems are changing rapidly, generally becoming more industrial, commercial and global, with profound implications for diets and nutrition as well as for small-scale farmers. Governments have a role in shaping food systems to ensure food safety and balanced diets for all.

The *Rome Declaration on Nutrition* is a milestone in global efforts to advance food security and eliminate hunger and malnutrition. The 10 commitments of the *Rome Declaration* (table 1) set out a common vision and provide a mandate, as well as out-

Table 2. *Framework for Action*: thematic areas

– Creating an enabling environment for effective action (Recommendations 1–7)
– Increasing actions for sustainable food systems promoting healthy diets (Recommendations 8–16)
– Achieving global food and nutrition targets through trade and investment policies (Recommendations 17–18)
– Enhancing social protection, nutrition education and information to build capacities (Recommendations 19–24)
– Creating strong and resilient health systems to address all forms of malnutrition (Recommendations 25–57)
– Improving accountability mechanisms for nutrition (Recommendations 58–60)

lining obligations, for governments to address nutrition in the coming decades. It aims to do this by increasing investments in sustainable food systems and ensuring access to balanced and healthy diets and nutrition for all [2].

Everyone has the right to adequate food and the highest attainable standard of physical and mental health. The *Rome Declaration on Nutrition* emphasizes the importance of all individuals having a diversified, balanced and healthy diet at all stages of life. In particular, it calls for special attention to be given to the first 1,000 days from the start of pregnancy to 2 years of age and to pregnant and lactating women, women of reproductive age, and adolescent girls by promoting and supporting adequate care and feeding practices, including exclusive breastfeeding for 6 months and continued breastfeeding until 2 years of age and beyond with appropriate complementary feeding. Other groups that will receive priority attention are the most vulnerable, neglected, socially excluded and economically marginalized parts of the population, including those affected by humanitarian crises. These groups must be included in the development process and provided with decent employment as well as essential water, sanitation, hygiene and education services.

The *Framework for Action* provides a set of voluntary options and strategies – in the form of 60 recommended actions – that governments, acting in dialog with a wide range of stakeholders, may incorporate, as appropriate, into their national nutrition, health, agriculture, development and investment plans [3, 4].

The *Framework for Action* sets out how to create an enabling environment for effective action and calls for strengthening of sustainable food systems, including through investments in pro-poor agriculture and smallholder agriculture to improve diets and raise levels of nutrition. It also refers to actions in other related sectors and thematic areas (i.e. trade and investment, education, social protection, health) in order to improve nutrition (table 2). The *Framework* is underpinned by recommendations for ensuring accountability.

Table 3. Summary of key messages from the *Framework for Action*

– For effective implementation of policies to improve nutrition, an *enabling policy environment* is essential. This means explicit political commitment, greater investment and cross-government policies and plans, along with multi-stakeholder governance mechanisms
– *Sustainable food systems* are key to promoting healthy diets, and innovative food system solutions are needed
– Information and education concerning healthy dietary practices are vital, but consumers must also be empowered through enabling *food environments* that provide safe, diverse and healthy diets
– While a food systems approach is important, *coherent action* is also needed in other sectors. These include international trade and investment, nutrition education and information, social protection, health system delivery of direct nutrition interventions and other health services to promote nutrition, water, sanitation and hygiene, and food safety
– For the purpose of *accountability*, the *Framework for Action* adopts existing global targets for improving maternal, infant and young child nutrition and for noncommunicable disease risk factor reduction

Source: Joint FAO-WHO ICN2 Secretariat, Information Note on the *Framework for Action*, November 2014.

As governments have primary responsibility for taking action at the country level, in dialog with a wide range of stakeholders, including affected communities, the recommendations are principally addressed to government leaders. These leaders will consider the appropriateness of the recommended policies and actions in relation to national and local needs and conditions as well as national and regional priorities, including in legal frameworks (table 3).

The *Rome Declaration on Nutrition* called upon the UN General Assembly (UNGA) to endorse the *Rome Declaration on Nutrition* and the *Framework for Action* and to consider declaring a Decade of Action on Nutrition from 2016 to 2025 (paragraph 17) [2]. The purpose of the Decade of Action on Nutrition is to translate the agreed-upon commitments of the ICN2 outcome documents into sustained and coherent action by governments and the UN system, with overall international coordination provided by the FAO and WHO. The Decade of Action on Nutrition would provide the opportunity for effective action with a period of 10 years to support countries to make significant progress in addressing malnutrition, with clearly set goals and objectives to be achieved.

Second International Conference on Nutrition: Implications for Hidden Hunger

Although the most severe problems of micronutrient malnutrition are found in developing countries, people of all population groups in all regions of the world can be affected by micronutrient deficiencies. This is one of the most serious impediments to socio-economic development, contributing to the vicious cycle of malnutrition, underdevelopment and poverty. Micronutrient malnutrition has long-ranging effects

Table 4. *Rome Declaration on Nutrition:* implications for hidden hunger

We Ministers and Representatives of the Members of the Food and Agriculture Organization of the United Nations (FAO) and the World Health Organization (WHO)...

Multiple challenges of malnutrition to inclusive and sustainable development and to health:

- Para 4: ... acknowledge that malnutrition, in all its forms, including undernutrition, micronutrient deficiencies, overweight and obesity, not only affects people's health and wellbeing by impacting negatively on human physical and cognitive development ... but also poses a high burden in the form of negative social and economic consequences to individuals, families, communities and States
- Para 12: ... note with profound concern that:
  d over two billion people suffer from micronutrient deficiencies, in particular vitamin A, iodine, iron and zinc, among others

A common vision for global action to end all forms of malnutrition:

- Para 13: We reaffirm that:
  a the elimination of malnutrition in all its forms is an imperative for health, ethical, political, social and economic reasons, paying particular attention to the special needs of children, women ... other vulnerable groups as well as people in humanitarian emergencies
- Para 14: We recognize that:
  h responsible investment in agriculture[1], including small holders and family farming and in food systems, is essential for overcoming malnutrition

Commitment to action:

- Para 15: We commit to:
  a eradicate hunger and prevent all forms of malnutrition worldwide ... and anaemia in women and children among other micronutrient deficiencies...
  c enhance sustainable food systems by developing coherent public policies from production to consumption and across relevant sectors to provide year-round access to food that meets people's nutrition needs and promote safe and diversified healthy diets
  e improve nutrition by strengthening human and institutional capacities to address all forms of malnutrition through, inter alia, relevant scientific and socio-economic research and development, innovation and transfer of appropriate technologies...
  g develop policies, programmes and initiatives for ensuring healthy diets throughout the life course, starting from the early stages of life to adulthood, including of people with special nutritional needs...

[1] The term 'agriculture' includes crops, livestock, forestry and fisheries.

on health, learning ability and productivity, leading to high social and public costs, reduced work capacity in populations due to high rates of illness and disability and loss of human potential. Therefore, overcoming micronutrient deficiencies is a precondition for ensuring rapid and appropriate development [11, 12].

The ICN2 *Rome Declaration on Nutrition* and *Framework for Action* set out, inter alia, commitments and recommendations to prevent and control micronutrient deficiencies. Tables 4 and 5 show a detailed analysis of the ICN2 outcome documents, with special focus on hidden hunger.

Table 5. *Framework for Action:* implications for hidden hunger

Sustainable food systems promoting healthy diets

- Rec. 10: Promote the diversification of crops including underutilized traditional crops, more production of fruits and vegetables, and appropriate production of animal-source products as needed, applying sustainable food production and natural resource management practices
- Rec. 13: Develop, adopt and adapt, where appropriate, international guidelines on healthy diets
- Rec. 15: Explore regulatory and voluntary instruments ... to promote healthy diets

Nutrition education and information

- Rec. 21: Conduct appropriate social marketing campaigns and lifestyle change communication programmes to promote physical activity, dietary diversification, consumption of micronutrient-rich foods such as fruits and vegetables...

Social protection

- Rec. 23: Use cash and food transfers, including school feeding programmes and other forms of social protection for vulnerable populations to improve diets through better access to food ... and which is nutritionally adequate for healthy diets

Strong and resilient health systems

- Rec. 25: Strengthen health systems ... to enable national health systems to address malnutrition in all its forms

Anaemia in women of reproductive age

- Rec. 42: Improve intake of micronutrients through consumption of nutrient-dense foods, especially foods rich in iron, where necessary, through fortification and supplementation strategies, and promote healthy and diversified diets
- Rec. 43: Provide daily iron and folic acid and other micronutrient supplementation to pregnant women as part of antenatal care; and intermittent iron and folic acid supplementation to menstruating women where the prevalence of anaemia is 20% or higher...

Health services to improve nutrition

- Rec. 47: Provide zinc supplementation to reduce the duration and severity of diarrhoea, and to prevent subsequent episodes in children
- Rec. 48: Provide iron and, among others, vitamin A supplementation for pre-school children to reduce the risk of anaemia

Hidden hunger problems have to be addressed through a multi-sectoral approach and different interventions. Food systems are important to promote healthy diets, improve nutrition and combat micronutrient deficiencies, but complementary actions have to be adopted in health, education and other related sectors. On the one hand, in order to prevent and control micronutrient deficiencies in the medium and long term, food-based strategies are key, e.g. not only through the production of foods that are naturally rich in micronutrients but also through the promotion of healthy and diversified diets. On the other hand, in order to combat hidden hunger in the short term, especially among groups at high risk and in emergencies, supplementation is necessary, as it can save many lives and prevent much suffering. Other complementary strategies to address hidden hunger include fortification (the addition of micronutrients to staple foods and also the addition micronutrient-enriched paste to home foods) and, more recently, biofortification.

Second International Conference on Nutrition Follow-Up Activities

The 39th session of the FAO Conference (6–13 June 2015) endorsed the ICN2 outcome documents and urged FAO Members to implement the commitments set out in the *Rome Declaration on Nutrition* and the recommendations in the *Framework for Action*. Specific FAO follow-up activities include (i) mainstreaming nutrition as a cross-cutting theme under the FAO's reviewed Strategic Framework; (ii) identifying priority activities in support of member countries, covering different areas of the *Framework for Action*; (iii) strengthening the FAO's capacity to enhance its role in nutrition; (iv) establishing the Action for Nutrition Trust Fund, with the aim of supporting governments in transforming the ICN2 commitments, recommendations and strategies into concrete actions, and (v) establishing initiatives to ensure monitoring of and reporting on the ICN2 follow-up to the FAO Governing Bodies [13].

Follow-up activities being undertaken by the FAO in collaboration with other partners, and particularly the WHO, include (i) steps taken to enable the UNGA to endorse the *Rome Declaration on Nutrition* and the *Framework for Action* as well as to consider declaring a Decade of Action on Nutrition (2016–2025); (ii) efforts to improve interagency coordination and collaboration on nutrition through existing mechanisms (e.g. with the Committee on World Food Security serving as the appropriate intergovernmental and multi-stakeholder forum on nutrition), including to set up monitoring and reporting mechanisms, and (iii) promotion of ICN2-related messages and outcomes via Expo Milano 2015 'Feeding the Planet, Energy for Life' to focus attention on food security and nutrition [13].

On 6 July 2015 in New York, the UNGA adopted a resolution on 'Follow-Up to the Second International Conference on Nutrition (ICN2)' [14]. The resolution welcomes the ICN2 outcome documents and invites governments, UN agencies, funds and programs as well as other stakeholders to implement the *Framework for Action* in a coordinated manner so as to achieve better nutrition for all.

On 25 September 2015, the UNGA adopted the 2030 Agenda for Sustainable Development, a global plan of action for people, planet and prosperity, with 17 Sustainable Development Goals (SDGs) and 169 targets [15]. Nutrition is explicitly addressed in SDG 2 'End hunger, achieve food security and improved nutrition and promote sustainable agriculture'. However, nutrition has also a role to play in achieving other goals of the 2030 Agenda, including, inter alia, goals related to poverty, health, education, gender, work, growth, inequality and climate change. Together, the ICN2 and the 2030 Agenda have placed nutrition firmly at the heart of the development agenda.

With reference to the proposed Decade of Action on Nutrition, a discussion was called for in the 70th session of the UNGA. To this end, a second resolution on ICN2 follow-up is expected to be introduced for consideration by the UNGA. Once the Decade of Action on Nutrition is approved, it will provide an umbrella within which to coordinate nutrition actions across sectors and disciplines for impact.

Conclusions

The ICN2 is not an end but part of a wider process. The Conference clearly recognized the problem of hidden hunger and the slow progress in addressing it. The *Rome Declaration on Nutrition* and the *Framework for Action* set out commitments and recommendations to address micronutrient deficiencies. These commitments and recommendations now need to be translated into firm national actions. Furthermore, there is a need for sustained and coordinated international support and cooperation, including, inter alia, through the proposed Decade of Action on Nutrition.

References

1 FAO, WHO: Second International Conference on Nutrition: report of the Joint FAO/WHO Secretariat on the Conference. 2014. http://www.fao.org/3/a-mm531e.pdf (accessed July 20, 2015).
2 FAO, WHO: Second International Conference on Nutrition (ICN2). Rome Declaration on Nutrition. 2014. http://www.fao.org/3/a-ml542e.pdf (accessed July 20, 2015).
3 FAO, WHO: Second International Conference on Nutrition (ICN2). Framework for Action. 2014. http://www.fao.org/3/a-ml542e.pdf (accessed July 20, 2015).
4 FAO, WHO: Joint FAO-WHO ICN2 Secretariat. Information note on the Framework for Action. 2014. http://www.fao.org/fileadmin/user_upload/faoweb/ICN2/documents/InfoNote-e.pdf (accessed July 20, 2015).
5 FAO, WHO: International Conference on Nutrition. World Declaration and Plan of Action on Nutrition. Rome, FAO/WHO, 1992. http://www.fao.org/docrep/015/u9260e/u9260e00.pdf (accessed July 20, 2015).
6 FAO, IFAD, WFP: The State of Food Insecurity in the World 2015. Meeting the 2015 International Hunger Targets: Taking Stock of Uneven Progress. Rome, FAO, 2015. http://www.fao.org/3/a-i4646e.pdf (accessed July 20, 2015).
7 FAO: The State of Food and Agriculture 2013. Food Systems for Better Nutrition. Rome, FAO, 2013. http://www.fao.org/docrep/018/i3300e/i3300e.pdf (accessed July 20, 2015).
8 UNICEF, WHO, World Bank: Levels and trends in child malnutrition (summary). 2013. http://www.who.int/nutgrowthdb/summary_jme_2013.pdf (accessed July 20, 2015).
9 WHO: Obesity and overweight, factsheet No 311. 2015. http://www.who.int/mediacentre/factsheets/fs311/en/ (accessed July 20, 2015).
10 FAO: Second International Conference on Nutrition (ICN2). 2014. www.fao.org/ICN2 (accessed July 20, 2015).
11 Thompson B, Amoroso L (eds): Combating Micronutrient Deficiencies: Food-based Approaches. Rome, FAO, and Wallingford, CAB International, 2011. http://www.fao.org/docrep/013/am027e/am027e.pdf (accessed July 20, 2015).
12 Thompson B, Amoroso L (eds): Improving Diets and Nutrition: Food-based Approaches. Rome, FAO, and Wallingford, CAB International, 2014. http://www.fao.org/3/a-i3030e.pdf (accessed July 20, 2015).
13 FAO: 39th session FAO Conference – C 2015/30, Joint FAO/WHO Second International Conference on Nutrition (ICN2) (19–21 November 2014). 2015. http://www.fao.org/3/a-mn236e.pdf (accessed July 20, 2015).
14 United Nations General Assembly Resolution 69/310. Follow-Up to the Second International Conference on Nutrition. http://www.un.org/en/ga/search/view_doc.asp?symbol=A/RES/69/310 (accessed March 14, 2016).
15 United Nations General Assembly Resolution 70/1. Transforming Our World: The 2030 Agenda for Sustainable Development. http://www.un.org/ga/search/view_doc.asp?symbol=A/RES/70/1&Lang=E (accessed March 14, 2016).

Leslie Amoroso
Nutrition and Food Systems Division
Food and Agriculture Organization of the United Nations (FAO)
Viale delle Terme di Caracalla
IT–00153 Rome (Italy)
E-Mail leslie.amoroso@fao.org

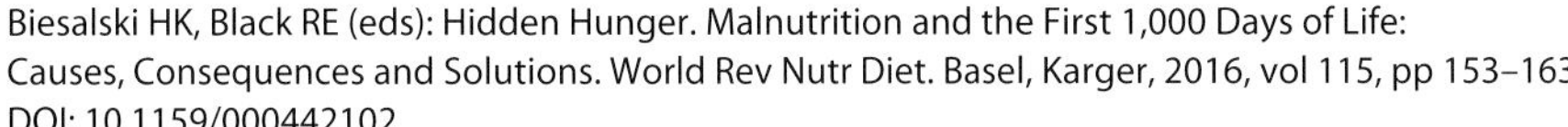

Biesalski HK, Black RE (eds): Hidden Hunger. Malnutrition and the First 1,000 Days of Life: Causes, Consequences and Solutions. World Rev Nutr Diet. Basel, Karger, 2016, vol 115, pp 153–163
DOI: 10.1159/000442102

Genetically Modified Organisms and the Future Global Nutrient Supply: Part of the Solution or a New Problem?

Peter W.B. Phillips

Johnson-Shoyama Graduate School of Public Policy, University of Saskatchewan, Saskatoon, SK, Canada

Abstract

For almost a generation now, scientists and policy makers have enthusiastically advanced genetically modified (GM) crops as a solution to both global food security and, specifically, the micronutrient needs of the hidden hungry. While genetic modification offers the prospect of overcoming technological barriers to food security, the gap between the vision and reality remains large. This chapter examines the impact of GM crops at three levels. Undoubtedly, at the micro level, bio-fortification offers a real opportunity to enhance the availability of micronutrients. However, the inexorable 'research sieve' ruthlessly culls most technical candidates in the agri-food system. GM bio-fortified foods, such as Golden Rice™, remain only a promise. At the meso level, GM crops have generated benefits for both producers and consumers who have adopted GM crops, but given that the technology has been differentially applied to maize, the average diet for the food insecure has become somewhat less balanced. Finally, while GM crops have increased yields and the global food supply, these have come at the cost of more complex and costly trade and market systems, which impair access and availability. In essence, while biotechnology offers some tantalizing technological prospects, the difficulties of getting the corresponding benefits to the most needy have dampened some of the enthusiasm.

Introduction

Hunger is a pervasive 21st-century problem. While the proportion of the global population that goes hungry episodically or regularly has gone down over the past 2 decades, about 842 million people in 2011–2013, or around 1 in 8 people around the world, were estimated to be suffering from chronic hunger due to not regularly getting enough food to conduct an active life. Chronic hunger leads to physical and mental stunting, which decreases the length and quality of life for individuals and undercuts the development objectives of many governments around the world.

In response to climate variability, volatile prices and episodic famines around the world, food security has moved to the top of the international policy agenda in the past decade. The Food and Agriculture Organization (FAO) [1, 2], the Organization for Economic Cooperation and Development (OECD) [3], and the heads of government of the 'Group of 20' leading economies [4] have each issued statements and directives about the need to accelerate food productivity and to ensure more effective distribution of food. The FAO defines security as a complex condition involving 'availability, access, utilization and stability' [2]. Interestingly, the focus is disproportionately on macro-level global production and distribution. Largely missing from the debate is any consideration of the meso level – specifically, the capacity of self-sufficient, small landholders in vulnerable parts of the world to either earn adequate incomes or access the market – and the micro level – where restricted dietary choices limit access to the full array of micronutrients.

This chapter reframes the hunger challenge at the micro, meso and macro levels and assesses the potential for genetically modified (GM) organisms (GMOs) to address and respond effectively to the challenges at each level.

The Biotechnological Response to Hidden Hunger

GMOs are proposed by policy makers, scientists and seed companies as solutions to the three-level problem. At the micro level, there has been significant effort and discussion about the potential to bio-fortify crops through genetic modification; Golden Rice™ is the iconic example, but there is a wide range of other efforts to change specific crops in ways that will improve nutrition. Meanwhile, economists and seed companies note that, somewhat counterintuitively, hidden hunger tends to be concentrated in subsistence farming communities, in effect at the meso level. Realized and potential farm-level adaptation and adoption of the existing and prospective arrays of GM commodity crops (especially maize, soybeans, canola, rice, wheat and potatoes) actually support farm families by generating higher incomes that allow families to purchase a greater variety of foods, which goes a long way towards realizing community-based food security. Finally, at the macro level, GM crops, where they have been adopted, have unambiguously boosted yields and created a greater global supply, albeit with some perverse impacts due to uneven acceptance and the serious challenges of segmenting and differentiating supplies between markets with different regulations and preferences.

The Micro Level

At the micro level, the unit of analysis is the individual. Individuals suffering from hidden hunger have diets that are deficient in micronutrients, including iodine, vitamin A, calcium, folic acid (vitamin B_9), iron and zinc [5]. The International Food Policy Research Institute (IFPR) [6] estimates that about 1.8 billion people suffer from iodine deficiency, 1.6 billion from iron deficiency, and 1.2 billion from inadequate zinc, and that 190 million preschool-age children suffer from vitamin A deficiency. The effects include anaemia; impaired motor, visual and cognitive development; weakened immune systems; increased maternal mortality, and premature death [6].

In most societies, individuals with access to a greater variety of foods, such as fruits, vegetables, animal and fish products and eggs, are able to gain the appropriate range and amounts of micronutrients to sustain their health. Many people, however, are simply too poor to be able to afford foods that are rich in micronutrients or otherwise lack access to these foods.

Biotechnology offers one solution. With the capacity to identify, isolate and move or selectively turn on or off specific genes, scientists and plant breeders now can biofortify staple crops so that people may access and consume appropriate levels of the essential micronutrients for health, without any fundamental change in their other circumstances. Phillips [7] undertook a review of the nutritional value of wheat, rice and maize using the US Department of Agriculture nutrient database and concluded that while none of the crops by itself would provide an adequate mix of protein, fibre and micronutrients for health, wheat was unambiguously a more balanced source of nutrition. One hundred grams of maize and rice, for instance, provides less than 15% of the recommended daily allowance of the B complex of vitamins for adult health and less 10% of the recommended dietary allowance for iron, magnesium or zinc.

A range of foods and micronutrients have been targeted, including higher levels of phytosterols for reduced cholesterol in rapeseed and soybeans; higher levels of carotenoids for increased vitamin A in rice (Golden Rice™), sorghum, tomatoes and bananas; higher levels of antioxidants in potatoes; higher levels of essential fatty acids in a range of oilseeds, including low-linolenic soybeans and canola, and higher lysine and tryptophan levels in maize [8].

While all technologically feasible, there is a long way between the scientific breakthroughs and an accessible and available variety of food. Graff et al. [9] showed the scale of the challenge. Their analysis showed that what they call the 'research sieve' culls up to 99% of innovations before they reach markets and end users. They undertook a survey of the US system to identify 560 biotechnology-derived traits that had achieved 'proof of concept' and then traced these technologies to their terminal use. An estimated 383 of these inventions were put into early trials, 47 made it to advanced trials, 14 were prepared and presented to regulators for review, 5 were approved by regulators and introduced to the market, and only 2 (or less than 1%) achieved any sustained market success. It is worth noting that this extreme culling happens in the USA, which many would argue is the most accommodating and responsive marketplace in the world. The culling is the result of decisions by a wide range of actors. Researchers often subject an invention to a trial simply to see if it works, withdrawing it from further scrutiny once they have achieved the evidence that they need for their scientific purposes. The process of assembling the regulatory dockets and the review process sometimes reveals flaws or weaknesses in a construct. While there are few identifiable examples of regulators rejecting new products over identified health and safety concerns, proponents routinely abandon candidates when they can see that the decision is likely to be unfavourable. Moreover, proponents need to see prospects for commercial success. The processes of reducing to practice and scaling up provide greater clarity about commercial prospects; many proponents find that the benefit-cost calculus does not justify a push to full commercialization. A recent industry-supported study by the consultancy Phillips McDougall [10] reported that the cost of taking a new commercial GM variety through the full discovery, development, review and global market introduction stages is USD 136 million and takes 283 months (27% of that in regulatory review). The challenge is that because of the nature of the global marketplace, the leading biotechnology firms assume that they need approval in at least two major producing countries and the top five importing countries. Costs, duration and uncertainty have risen in the past decade in almost all key markets. In short, the hurdle for regulatory and commercial success has risen, so that new traits with niche, often concessionary markets are less likely to be realized.

The iconic example of this is Golden Rice™, a variety developed by two public-sector scientists in Switzerland that expresses genes that produce and accumulate β-carotene in the rice endosperm (the edible part of the plant) [11, 12]. When the rice is consumed, β-carotene is either stored in the fatty tissues of the body or converted into vitamin A. Given that rice provides up to 80% of the daily caloric intake of 3 billion people, the expression of β-carotene offers the potential to directly combat vitamin A deficiency, which can lead to childhood blindness and early mortality. An estimated 250,000–500,000 children go blind annually around the world [13]. Golden Rice™ was a technological breakthrough in 2000; 15 years later, it remains only a promise. In the first instance, the inventors discovered that they did not have the freedom to operate; Kryder et al. [14] identified that the new rice variety had used 70 proprietary technologies that would require up to 40 licenses from up to 20 entities, depending on the country of use. While this barrier was resolved by an innovative licensing agreement [15], the development and review of the regulatory docket have stalled development. Efforts to undertake confined regulatory field trials in the Philippines were jeopardized in 2013 when protestors destroyed the crops. In spite of funding from the Rockefeller Foundation, the Bill and Melinda Gates Foundation, the Syngenta Foundation, the International Rice Research Institute, the US Agency for International Development, the European Union and the Philippine government and support from the FAO, the Pope and many scientific foundations, Golden Rice™ remains tantalizingly out of reach; as of late 2015, there was no firm date for the first release of Golden Rice™. The other bio-fortified targets, lacking supporters with such deep pockets and influence, are less likely to navigate the research sieve.

At the other end of the supply chain, it remains unclear if or how farmers and producers will respond if offered the chance to use bio-fortified products. The regulatory processes and systems in many of the targeted food-insecure countries are underdeveloped or dysfunctional, presenting real barriers to diffusion to the most needy markets. Moreover, farmer adoption is not clear; many of the bio-fortified traits have been expressed in less competitive varieties, which will make them relatively, if not absolutely, less competitive with other cropping opportunities for farmers. Most are currently designed to be single-trait options, while the rest of the seed business is moving to stacked-trait crops, which are significantly more competitive in most growing areas. Finally, the scientific and development community has so far assumed that the public and consuming populations in the target markets will accept these new traits. Right now, the best that we can say is that acceptance is indeterminate. While GM varieties have gained significant market shares in those developing countries accepting them (e.g. South Africa, Burkina Faso and the Sudan), much of these are cotton or maize for animal feed. Nutritionally altered crops are not generally available. In a few instances, governments have rejected trade and aid flows because of 'fears' of contamination with GM traits [16].

The best that we can conclude at this point is that transgenically modified bio-fortified crops offer a 'promise' of more nutritious foods, but realizing that promise remains uncertain.

The Meso Level

At the meso level, the unit of analysis is the family or community. While the availability of a sufficient array and supply of foodstuffs may be a necessary condition for addressing hidden hunger, it is not sufficient. Somewhat counterintuitively, the highest incidence of hidden hunger is in and among farm families and farming communities. Subsistence farming in many marginal growing areas of the world, such as Sub-Saharan Africa, simply is unable to generate either adequate food supplies or adequate farm incomes to allow families and, in many cases, whole communities to achieve a balanced diet. Many small landholders face gaps in availability, access, utilization and stability, none of which is directly fixed by nutritionally enhanced crops.

GM technology generally makes modified crops more resilient, efficient, robust and profitable. Although the first commercial GM crop was planted in 1994 (tomatoes), 1996 was the first year in which a significant area of crops containing GM traits were planted (1.66 million hectares) [17]. Since then, there has been a dramatic increase in plantings; by 2014, the global planted area reached 181 million hectares [18]. While 130 events have been commercialized in more than a dozen crops, GM traits have had their greatest impact on four main crops – canola, corn, cotton and soybeans – although small areas of GM crops of sugar beets (adopted in the USA and Canada since 2008), papaya (in the USA since 1999 and in China since 2008) and squash (in the USA since 2004) have also been planted. In 2014, 28 countries planted GM crops. More than half the countries are developing nations, and more than half the crop area is in those countries. Two traits – herbicide tolerance and insect resistance – dominate. GM seeds account for 70% of the global acreage for soybeans, 52% for cotton, 26% for corn, and 20% for canola. In those countries adopting GM varieties, GM seed market share has risen above 80%. GM crops have also been pro-trade, in that adoption and production are concentrated in leading export nations. Brookes and Barfoot [17] estimated that biotechnology producers account for between 72% of cotton and 95% of soybean global trade. James [18] estimated that in 2014, approximately 18 million farmers grew biotechnological crops; remarkably, about 90%, or 16.5 million, were risk-averse small and poor farmers in developing countries, most cultivating fewer than 3 hectares in their operations.

Economists have invested a great deal of time and energy trying to quantify the scale and distribution of the impacts of GM crops. Smyth et al. [19] presented a range of summative reports on the impacts of specific crops in specific markets, while Klümper and Qaim [20] performed a meta-analysis on 147 studies conducted over the preceding 20 years that used primary data from farm surveys or field trials. Their meta-analysis concluded that, on average, GM crop adoption reduced chemical pesticide use by 37%, increased crop yields by 22%, and increased farm profits by 68%. Yield and pesticide reductions were estimated to be larger for insect-resistant crops than for herbicide-tolerant crops. Most importantly for the issue of hidden hunger, yield and profit gains were estimated to be 'higher in developing countries than in developed countries'.

Economic studies have gone on to show that the diffusion of GM technologies can have a dark side. Those producers unable or unwilling to adapt to and adopt the more competitive crop varieties have the potential to lose, as the market prices for their crops will be depressed by greater competition from advanced varietals. This is where regulatory, commercial, technological, economic and social barriers can make or break a farmer.

The Macro Level

Much of the effort and debate about GMOs revolves around the notion that bioscience innovation will accelerate crop yields, which, through trade, will fulfil the FAO's four-fold goals of availability, access, utilization and stability. Clearly, this goes well beyond the technical and into the economic, social and political systems that are part of supporting research, development, commercialization and trade.

The global agri-food research system was estimated to encompass investments totalling about USD 40 billion (in purchasing power parity) in 2008 [21]. About 80% of this (USD 31.7 billion) was contributed by the public sector, distributed across a wide array of institutions, programs and crop and livestock areas. Meanwhile, just over 20% (USD 8.3 billion) came from private sources, most directed to downstream research in support of commercialization of new traits for a few large-area commercial crops.

The GM traits flowing from this global effort, while concentrated in a few crops, have generated an estimated USD 100 billion of net benefit, shared among producers, consumers and innovators [22].

A recent partial analysis of the impacts related to soybeans illustrates the profound effects of technological change. Alston et al. [22] estimated that Roundup Ready™ technology, developed and owned by Monsanto Company, has generated global benefits exceeding USD 40 billion over 1996–2009, with 55% accruing to producers, 31% to consumers, and 14% to the innovator. They estimated that this technology not only reduced the price of soybeans by an average of 2% over the period but also, through competitive forces, pushed down prices for sunflower, canola, and palm oil by an average of 0.7%, causing a cascading set of winners (consumers) and losers (producers). Meanwhile, the increasing competitiveness of soybeans has caused farmers to shift land from other less profitable crops, such as corn and wheat, which causes the prices of those crops to be relatively higher than they would otherwise be (with the effect that producers gain and consumers lose). In short, any new technology has a cascading set of effects, depending on whether one is an adopter, competitor or consumer; in the analysis, a full 10% of the net gain from the technological change flows beyond the adopting regions.

While those benefits flowing to producers and consumers contribute at the meso level to addressing hidden hunger, the narrow focus and uneven uptake and use of GM technology create a real downside to this positive story at the micro and macro levels.

In the first instance, the focus on a narrow range of traits and crops is having a significant effect on global crop production and nutritional availability. For all the reasons discussed above, both public and private research and development (R&D) are increasingly focused on three food crops: maize, rapeseed and soybeans. Meanwhile, cotton is increasingly competing for cropping area due to new GM traits. The net effect of the differential investments in these crops is that they have become relatively more competitive. Yields for maize, rapeseed and soybeans rose only slowly in 1985–1995, immediately before the introduction of GM technologies. Since then, average annual yields have surged for the three main crops to above almost all other staple crops (table 1).

With changing yields comes changing production. Maize, rapeseed and soybeans made up about 41% of the global primary crop area in 1995–2013, up significantly from the 1985–1995 period (table 2). Rapeseed and soybeans, in particular, increased their acreage by more than one third since GM traits were introduced. In contrast, most other large-area staple crops lost acreage, with wheat's share of crop area dropping by 12% between the two periods.

Keeping in mind the discussion earlier about the relative nutritional characteristics of maize, rice and wheat, this shift in production undoubtedly contributes to hidden hunger, as maize, the least balanced of the crops, is relatively less expensive and more available, while wheat, the most balanced, is absolutely more expensive and less available.

Table 1. Average annual percent change in yield

	1985–1995	1995–2013	Difference in rate of change after 1995
GM crops			
Maize	0.2	2.5	943%
Rapeseed	1.0	2.2	115%
Soybeans	0.7	1.2	90%
Non-GM crops			
Lentils	1.8	1.8	1%
Peas, dry	1.7	0.4	–76%
Plantains	1.1	–5.6	–614%
Potatoes	0.2	1.2	506%
Rice, paddy	1.2	1.3	7%
Wheat	1.6	1.7	7%
Yams	5.1	0.9	–83%

Source: FAO Stat 25-2-2015; Author's calculations.

Table 2. Harvested area by major primary crop

	Average share of primary crop area 1995–2013	Change in area between 1985 and 1995 and after 1995
GM crops		
Maize	22.4%	3%
Rapeseed	4.1%	36%
Soybeans	12.9%	39%
Non-GM crops		
Lentils	0.6%	7%
Peas, dry	0.9%	–33%
Plantains	0.8%	6%
Potatoes	2.8%	–5%
Rice, paddy	22.9%	–4%
Wheat	32.1%	–12%
Yams	0.7%	66%

Source: FAO Stat 25-2-2015; Author's calculations.

The difficulties arising from unbalanced productivity growth and production are compounded by the uneven availability of GMOs. In a perfectly competitive world, one would not care where production arises, as comparative advantages and competitive markets would both drive production to the lowest-cost markets and trade would even out supplies and prices, so that the gains from these innovations would be spread widely and contribute to balanced nutrition globally. In reality, however, markets are not operating efficiently, and real or imagined barriers to technological transfers, international trade and exchange all work to isolate many of the most food insecure and malnourished from the benefits of these technologies.

Table 3. Regulatory decisions related to GM events in 19 key markets, 1995–2011

	Recorded decisions, n			% of maximum possible decisions		
	species	enviro. approval	food approval	species	enviro. approval	food approval
Average	4.6	12.0	26.5	29%	12%	24%
Max	16	102	97	–	–	–

Source: Author's calculation of tabulations from GM Crops Database (http://cera-gmc.org/index.php?action=gm_crop_database). Adapted from Phillips [24].

Asynchronous approval truncates diffusion and adoption of the technology, complicating an already challenging global trading system. A 50-year effort to create a more open, transparent and competitive international trading regime culminated in 1995 with the World Trade Organization, an agreement that bound the vast majority of nations to opening food markets and permitting competitive markets to determine production, trade and prices. Coincident with that development, the emergence of GM crops has diverted attention as farmers, consumers, environmental groups, agro-chemical biotechnology companies and governments have disputed if, how, where, when and by whom these new technologies should be used. Instead of agri-food trade being liberalized, governments around the world have renationalized much of the regulation of agri-food technologies, with the end result being that we have a patchwork of differentiated markets. Some countries approve all traits for production and consumption, some countries only approve them for import and consumption, some only approve some traits, and a few reject all traits; even among those approving and accepting GM crops, they approve these traits on their own schedules and sometimes under different conditions. The end result is that asynchronous regulatory decisions have fragmented the regulatory landscape, causing the global commodity market to segment (table 3).

There is significant evidence that supply chains that receive and handle GM crops are struggling to adapt. In the largest sense, there are 340 million metric tonnes of grains and oilseeds in the international trading system flowing between 195 countries. Each major crop has upwards of 20 different grades or differentiations (in some cases, more than 100), each with their own specifications. The underlying R&D system turns over the seed stock in some crops every 3–5 years, with new varieties, new traits and new attributes. In Canada, for instance, there are more than a dozen centres of public-private research effort involving hundreds of actors, more than 3,000 seed growers who multiply the foundation seed for commercial sale and about 250,000 farmers who plant an array of crops and varieties in sophisticated rotations on more than 50 million acres. The grains and oilseeds are then harvested and largely stored on farm and called forward by public and private market aggregators through about 1,000 delivery points. The average commodity shipments then involve a minimum of three domestic transfers, in unit sizes ranging from 300 bushels to 6,000 tonnes, ultimately being aggregated in unit trains for shipment to the USA or free on board at export position in cargo holds of over 20,000 tonnes in ocean-going ships. Beyond our borders, shipments usually involve at least a further two transfers before they reach the specific buyer who contracted for that product.

GM crops and differentiated markets complicate this system. In theory, it should be possible to match differentiable supplies with differentiated demands. In practice, that is getting much harder. GM crop production is highly concentrated in a few countries that, at least for maize, soybeans and rapeseed/canola, are major producers and correspondingly large net exporters. Almost all of the exportable supplies of soybeans come from countries that have approved GM crops, while about 70% and more than half of the maize and rapeseed trade originate in GM-producing countries. Exporters then need to sort through the large number of buyers (up to 200) to match buyer specifications. One report suggests comingling mitigation costs in excess of USD 1 billion as of 2012 due to trade disputes, trade disruptions and litigation [23].

In short, GMOs offer significant benefits at the meso level but at the expense of increased macro uncertainties. Ultimately, all these uncertainties cause governments and firms either to slow down their R&D investments or to redirect their efforts to a narrow set of research interests with lower uncertainties, which, on the face of it, simply exacerbates food insecurity for many at-risk consumers and markets [24]. The net effect is undoubtedly lost opportunity and maybe some pockets of absolute damage.

Conclusions

Bioscience innovation can undoubtedly improve the nutritional profile of foods, but fixing diets requires more. Micro strategies may be necessary but are unlikely to be sufficient; they are probably too narrow and uncertain given uneven regulatory and market systems. Meso strategies are working but are limited by uneven social and political acceptance. Macro policies are generating large gains, but at the cost of fragmenting markets and unintended effects on trade and R&D. All in all, biotechnology and genetic modification present a conundrum: an exciting tool that may be ahead of its time.

References

1 FAO: How to feed the world 2050: issues brief. High-Level Expert Forum, Rome, 2009, pp 12–13. http://www.fao.org/wsfs/forum2050/wsfs-background-documents/issues-briefs/en/ (accessed October 29, 2014).

2 FAO: The state of food insecurity in the world 2013: the multiple dimensions of food security. Rome, FAO, 2013. http://www.fao.org/docrep/018/i3434e/i3434e.pdf (accessed July 13, 2015).

3 OECD: Communiqué from the Ministers Meeting of the Committee for Agriculture at ministerial level. Paris, OECD. 2010. http://www.oecd.org/agriculture/communiquefromtheministers-meetingofthecommitteeforagricultureatministeriallevel.htm (accessed July 13, 2015).

4 Group of 20: Ministerial Declaration: action plan on food price volatility and agriculture. Paris, G20, June 22 and 23, 2011. www.oecd.org/site/agrfcn/48479226.pdf (accessed July 13, 2015).

5 Micronutrient Initiative. http://www.micronutrient.org/ (accessed February 24, 2016).
6 International Food Policy Research Institute (IFPRI): Global Hunger Index 2014: The Challenge of Hidden Hunger. Washington, IFPRI, 2014. http://www.ifpri.org/sites/default/files/ghi/2014/contents.html (accessed August 22, 2015).
7 Phillips P: Give us this day our daily bread: the iconic role of wheat in the modern world; in Culver K, O'Doherty K (eds): Fishing and Farming Iconic Species: Cod and Salmon and Social Issues in Genomics Science. Concord, Captus Press, 2014, pp 261–277.
8 International Service for the Acquisition of Agribiotech Applications: Pocket K No 29: Functional Foods and Biotechnology. http://www.isaaa.org/resources/publications/pocketk/29/default.asp (accessed February 24, 2016).
9 Graff GD, Zilberman D, Bennett AB: The contraction of agbiotech product quality innovation. Nat Biotechnol 2009;27:702–704.
10 Phillips McDougall: The cost and time involved in the discovery, development and authorization of a new plant biotechnology derived trait: a consultancy study for CropLife International. Midlothian, Phillips McDougal, 2011.
11 Ye X, Al-Babili S, Klöti A, Zhang J, Lucca P, Beyer P, Potrykus I: Engineering the provitamin A (β-carotene) biosynthetic pathway into (carotenoid-free) rice endosperm. Science 2000;287:303–305.
12 Dubock A: The present status of Golden Rice. J Huazhong Agricult Univ 2014;33:69–84.
13 Golden Rice Project. Frequently asked questions. http://www.goldenrice.org (accessed February 24, 2016).
14 Kryder RD, Kowalski SP, Krattiger AF: 2000. The intellectual and technical property components of provitamin A rice (GoldenRice™): a preliminary freedom-to-operate review. ISAAA Briefs No 20. http://www.isaaa.org/Briefs/20/ (accessed August 22, 2015).
15 Golden Rice Project. Golden rice and intellectual property. http://www.goldenrice.org (accessed February 24, 2016).
16 Paarlberg R: Starved for Science: How Biotechnology Is Being Kept Out of Africa. Cambridge, Harvard University Press, 2009.
17 Brookes G, Barfoot P: GM Crops: Global Socio-Economic and Environmental Impacts 1996–2008. Dorchester, PG Economics Ltd, 2010. http://www.pgeconomics.co.uk/pdf/2010-global-gm-crop-impact-study-final-April-2010.pdf (accessed August 22, 2015).
18 James C: Brief 49: global status of commercialized biotech/GM crops: 2014. ISAAA. 2015. http://www.isaaa.org/resources/publications/briefs/49/default.asp (accessed August 22, 2015.)
19 Smyth S, Castle D, Phillips P (eds): Handbook on Agriculture, Biotechnology and Development. Cheltenham, Edward Elgar, 2014.
20 Klümper W, Qaim M: A meta-analysis of the impacts of genetically modified crops. PLoS One 2014;9:e111629.
21 Beintema N, Stads G-J, Fuglie K, Heisey P: ASTI global assessment of agricultural R&D spending: developing countries accelerate investment. Washington, IFPRI, 2012. http://www.asti.cgiar.org/global-overview (accessed August 22, 2015).
22 Alston J, Kalaitzandonakes N, Kruse J: The size and distribution of the benefits from the adoption of biotech soybean varieties; in Smyth S, Castle D, Phillips P (eds): Handbook on Agriculture, Biotechnology and Development. Cheltenham, Edward Elgar, 2014, pp 728–751.
23 Phillips P: Forthcoming LLP impacts on agricultural innovation; in Kalaitzandonakes N, Phillips P, Smyth S, Wesseler J (eds): The Co-Existence of Genetically Modified, Organic and Conventional Foods: Government Policies and Market Practices. Dordrecht, Springer, in press.
24 Smyth SJ, Kerr WA, Phillips PWB: Managing trade in products of biotechnology – which alternative to choose: science or politics? Ag Bio Forum 2013;16:126–139.

Prof. Peter W.B. Phillips
Johnson-Shoyama Graduate School of Public Policy
University of Saskatchewan
101 Diefenbaker Place, Saskatoon, SK S7N 5B5 (Canada)
E-Mail Peter.phillips@usask.ca

Biesalski HK, Black RE (eds): Hidden Hunger. Malnutrition and the First 1,000 Days of Life: Causes, Consequences and Solutions. World Rev Nutr Diet. Basel, Karger, 2016, vol 115, pp 164–174
DOI: 10.1159/000442594

SAFO: A Systematic Partnership to Reduce Vitamin A Deficiency in Tanzania

Christina Tewes-Gradl[a, b] · Andreas Bluethner[c, d]

[a]CSR Initiative, Harvard Kennedy School, Cambridge, MA, USA; [b]Endeva, Berlin, [c]Food-Fortification and Partnerships, BASF SE, Lampertheim, and [d]International Economic Law, University of Mannheim, Mannheim, Germany

There is a need to work in partnership with the private sector. The local milling industry needs support with better quality processing to add valuable micronutrients. We need to work with other development partners and with civil society to educate the public on the value of fortified foods. Food fortification is a whole industry, but a legislative and regulatory framework is crucial to impose discipline and standards.

Ronald Sibanda, Resident Representative of the World Food Programme in Tanzania [1]

Background

Vitamin A deficiency is a serious problem in most developing and emerging countries, including Tanzania. Fortification of oil with vitamin A is an effective approach to reduce vitamin A deficiency across the population, especially when fortification is made mandatory. The Strategic Alliance for the Fortification of Oil and other Staple Foods (SAFO) was created by the chemical company BASF and the development agency Gesellschaft für Internationale Zusammenarbeit GmbH (GIZ) to advance fortification of oil in selected target countries. Tanzania was selected as one country of intervention due to its high burden of vitamin A deficiency and conductive local structures.

Vitamin A Deficiency

Vitamin A deficiency is a serious problem in more than 70 countries around the world. People affected by this form of malnutrition can go blind and more easily contract infections like measles or diarrhea because of their weakened immune systems. The World Health Organization estimates that 140–250 million children under 5 years of age are suffering from vitamin A deficiency worldwide. Additionally, women with vitamin A deficiency are at a much greater risk of dying during pregnancy or childbirth [2].

The human body cannot produce vitamin A itself, and this vitamin may only be absorbed when eaten with food. In developing and emerging countries, many people often cannot afford expensive foods like high-fat fish and meat or even dairy products and vegetables, which contain natural supplies of vitamin A. They mainly eat cheap staple foods with less nutritional value, such as corn, rice, flour and oil.

Tanzania has a severe vitamin A deficiency problem. A national health survey in 2010 found that 33% of children had low serum retinol levels and that 37% of women had low breast milk retinol levels [3]. According to the 2005 Demographic Health Survey, the data used when SAFO started, only 52% of children in rural areas consumed fruits and vegetables rich in vitamin A on the previous day. In urban areas, the rate was 61%. A national supplementation program had helped to reduce infant mortality rates since 1987. Through that program, all children between 5 and 59 months old receive a vitamin A supplement twice a year. Although the program has achieved great coverage, it does not reach the rest of the population. Furthermore, supplements should not be the only source of vitamin A in a child's diet [1].

Food Fortification

Food fortification is a simple and inexpensive solution to combat micronutrient deficiency. With this method, food is enriched with vitamins and minerals that it does not naturally contain at all or only in small amounts. For example, edible oil is a good carrier for vitamin A because the micronutrient itself is oily and dissolves easily in oil and because people need fat to digest and take up vitamin A. The process of fortifying oil is rather simple: the micronutrient is simply added to cooking oil at the end of the production process. When properly packaged, it remains stable during the whole shelf-life of oil (12–18 months old) (fig. 1).

While the technical process to fortify food is simple, particularly in the case of oil, the governance process is much more complicated. Products for the upper market segment, such as bottled oil or snacks, are often fortified by producers on a voluntary basis in order to achieve a unique selling proposition vis-a-vis their customers. The poorer the target group, the harder it is to market such additional benefits sustainably. Consumers at the base of the economic pyramid (BoP) typically buy oil in small quan-

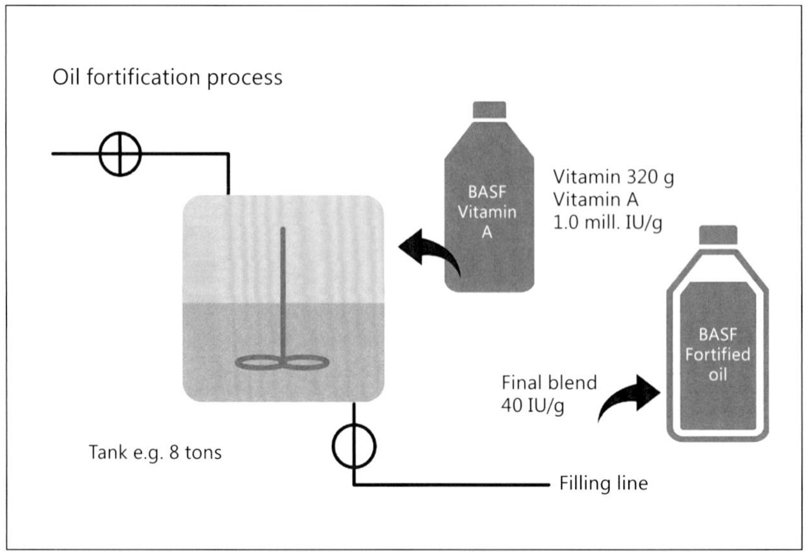

Fig. 1. Oil fortification process. Source: BASF.

tities from barrels and care much more about price than about branding or nutrition (fig. 2).

To reach these BoP consumers, regulation that makes fortification mandatory is usually the most effective approach. Fortification increases the production cost only minimally, thus fortified staple foods can be affordable for low-income consumers. For maximum impact, regulation should be paired with a targeted public awareness campaign.

The SAFO Initiative

SAFO is a project-based alliance to fight malnutrition [4]. The German development agency GIZ and the German chemical company BASF have teamed up to strengthen market-based approaches for affordable fortified food in developing countries. BASF invests into the technical aspects, providing technical support to companies and helping them to develop a sustainable business model, including corporate social responsibility thinking. GIZ mainly advises the public sector and facilitates multi-stakeholder dialogue at the national level. The initiative was launched in 2008 and improved nutrition for more than 140 million people at risk of vitamin A deficiency in several developing countries by 2012.

BASF has been working in the area of food fortification for many years. The cost-effectiveness of its nutrients is acknowledged by a number of scientific studies. BASF helps staple food producers install the right equipment and implement the best pro-

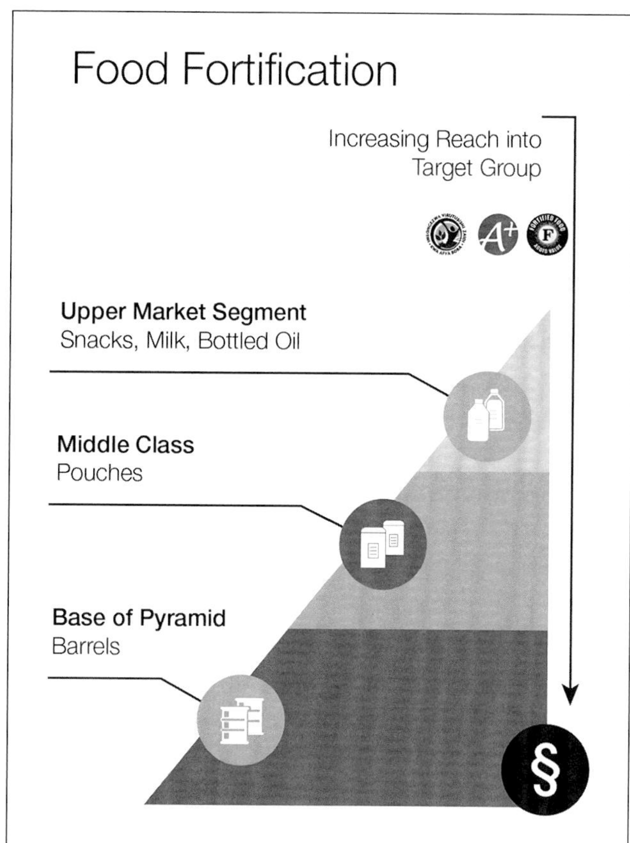

Fig. 2. Food fortification along the income pyramid. Source: BASF 2010.

cesses to produce affordable nutritious foods based on BASF's nutrients. BASF's efforts to combat micronutrient deficiency are part of its strategic goal of sustainability.

BASF joined forces with the German development agency GIZ in a project-based alliance called SAFO. This alliance was set up under develoPPP.de, a public-private partnership scheme in which GIZ offers financial and technical support to companies that invest in projects in developing countries.

SAFO supported several countries chosen based on multiple factors, including the prevalence of micronutrient deficiency, the existence of local GIZ structures, the political demand for food fortification and the domestic presence of a significant edible oil production sector. The specific interventions for each country were informed by an overarching framework, including advocacy targeting local stakeholders, technical trials, voluntary fortification and development of a standard, and, finally, the development of laws for mandatory fortification and related compliance processes [5].

The United Republic of Tanzania met all the requirements for SAFO's support: micronutrient deficiency remained widespread; GIZ had an extensive, long-established health program, and a National Food Fortification Alliance (NFFA) had been estab-

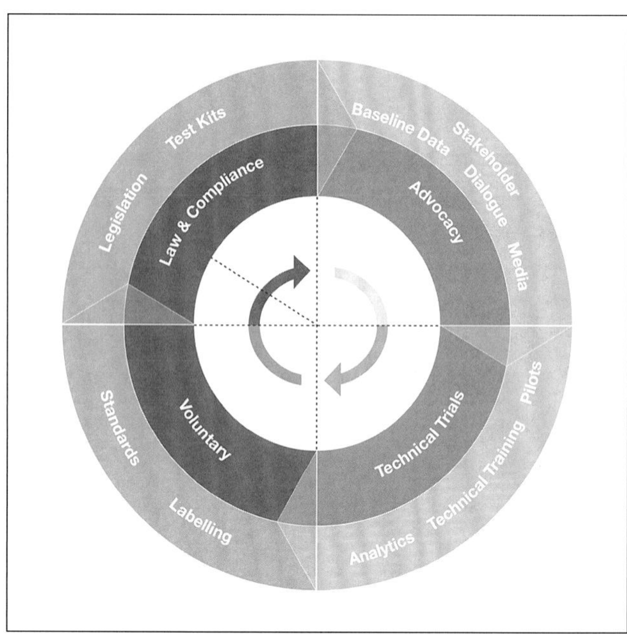

Fig. 3. Clock model by Bluethner and Vierck [5].

lished and aimed to scale up food fortification programs. Finally, Tanzania is a significant country, with approximately 40 million citizens, and BASF was already in business there via local distribution partners. Two large companies, East Coast Oils and Fats Ltd. and Murzah Oil Mills Ltd., make up the majority of the edible oil market. Edible oils are affordable, locally processed and widely consumed among BoP consumers (fig. 3).

Achieving Mandatory Oil Fortification in Tanzania

Local producers rely on certain framework conditions in order to sustainably supply fortified foods [6]:

- First, fortification needs to be transparent for consumers so that they understand what they buy. This requires a label that consumers can easily recognize. It also requires education of consumers regarding the need for micronutrients and healthier diets in general.
- Second, a standard defining at what level certain vitamins and minerals are to be added must be in place. Because nutritious food is essential for people's health, the selling of food is typically heavily regulated. In Tanzania, the Tanzania Food, Drugs and Cosmetics Act requires that fortified food be registered based on national or international standards on fortification.
- Third, to reach the lower-income groups in society, fortification often needs to be made mandatory through national regulation; otherwise, only higher-value products, for which a premium price can be charged, will be fortified.

Table 1. Timeline of establishing food fortification in Tanzania

Date	Event
2002	Tanzania participates in the 36th Regional Health Ministers conference, passing a resolution on enhanced public-private collaboration for food fortification
2003	The National Food Fortification Alliance (NFFA) is established
2004–2009	East, Central and Southern Africa Health Community (ECSA) conducts regional meetings, training workshops for laboratory personnel, and technical workshops to develop regional standards
March 2007	The ECSA workshop 'Harmonization of Regional Regulations and Standards of Fortified Foods' (Arusha, Tanzania) is held
December 2007	World Bank assesses status of nutrition in Tanzania and provides recommendations [7]
February 2008	The Strategic Alliance for the Fortification of Oil and Other Staple Foods (SAFO) is set up between GIZ and BASF
September 2008	SAFO undertakes an exploratory mission to Tanzania
November 2008	At the International Food Fortification workshop in Arusha, Tanzania, participants commit to accelerate action
February 2009	A SAFO stakeholder workshop and expert workshop in Dar es Salaam, co-hosted by the NFFA, defines the contribution of SAFO
February 2009	Two consultants financed by the World Bank begin drafting the National Action Plan together with stakeholders
March 2009	SAFO presents its support program to the NFFA
September 2009	The High Level Forum, under the auspices of the Prime Minister's office, is assembled to agree with and adopt the Food Fortification Action Plan
January 2010	World Bank board approves USD 2 million to support the implementation of the Food Fortification Action Plan
February 2010	The label for fortified oil is finalized, with support from SAFO/GIZ
March 2010	The Government of Japan approves a USD 2.69 million grant to support sustainable approaches to rural food fortification
October 2010	East Coast Oils and World Bank host a meeting to celebrate progress in food fortification; BASF provides test kits
October 2010	Standards for the fortification of oil are finalized
December 2010	The Global Alliance for Improved Nutrition (GAIN) approves USD 650,000 to be implemented by Helen Keller International (HKI) to maintain the momentum in food fortification
March 2011	Regulation for fortification of oil with vitamin A and wheat and maize flour with iron, zinc, vitamin B_{12} and folic acid is gazetted
August 2011	Regulation for fortification is passed
October 2011	The Department for International Development (UK) provides a grant for social marketing and other activities (also managed by HKI)

Without these framework conditions, producers will often have no incentives and limited ability to fortify food, especially for the lower-income consumers who need it most.

SAFO's Intervention in Tanzania

SAFO aimed to improve the ecosystem for the fortification of oil with vitamin A in Tanzania in 3 steps:

- research: data and stakeholder mapping to identify who plays which role;
- design: stakeholder dialogue to specify concrete deliverables for all actors, including GIZ and BASF;
- implementation: GIZ and BASF delivered their contributions locally.

Table 1 summarizes the most important milestones of the process, including activities by SAFO (highlighted) and by other players.

Research
The project started with a fact-finding mission to Tanzania in September 2008 to identify all relevant stakeholders for the fortification of oil and flour presented by SAFO during a meeting of the NFFA, a stakeholder alliance offering to fill the gaps in the existing support landscape [8]. The project hosted a workshop with the Tanzania Food and Nutrition Centre, a public body under the Ministry of Health and Social Welfare and the secretariat of the NFFA, to define the value added by SAFO in Tanzania.

Design
Based on this on-the-ground research, a workshop was co-organized with the NFFA on February 4 and 5, 2009, in Dar es Salaam [9]. The workshop aimed to re-energize the process of food fortification in Tanzania and to pitch the support that SAFO could provide. All national stakeholders were invited. International experts came to present relevant food fortification strategies, knowledge and technologies.

In March 2009, another workshop was held to present the results of the joint work. The stakeholders decided that SAFO's role was to facilitate and finance the label creation and review process, to support the establishment of monitoring procedures, and to provide technical assistance to oil producers. The other stakeholders committed to do their part to move the process along, including the drafting of standards, the development of monitoring regulations and building the corresponding technical capacity.

Implementation
In subsequent months, the SAFO partners realized their defined deliverables.

Label
GIZ was responsible for supporting label development. It requested proposals and received a number of suggestions. During an NFFA meeting, the participants chose one proposal as their favorite, and the submitting company was asked to further develop the label and to undergo pre-testing among the Tanzanian population in order to incorporate its view on the label. Via the lead of a label task force and an extensive consultation process within and beyond the NFFA, the final label was chosen by the stakeholders, including food producers. The whole process took about a year. The label was presented in November 2010. With regulation now passed, companies that fortified oil according to the Tanzania Food and Drug Authority (TFDA) standards were allowed to display the label on their products.

Technical Assistance
BASF was responsible for technical assistance. A technical workshop was hosted to facilitate technical progress with edible oil fortification and to identify further needs and next steps. Representatives from companies and public authorities learned about the food fortification process, quality control, and monitoring approaches. BASF's technical team trained the millers and demonstrated and explained the use of vitamin A test kits (fig. 4).

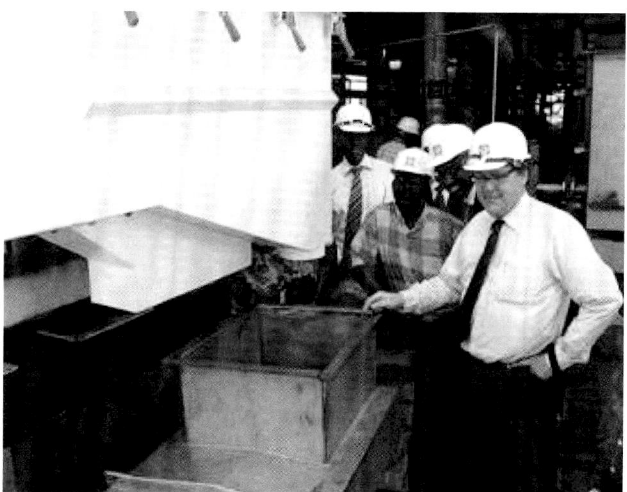

Fig. 4. Technical advice. Source: SAFO 2010.

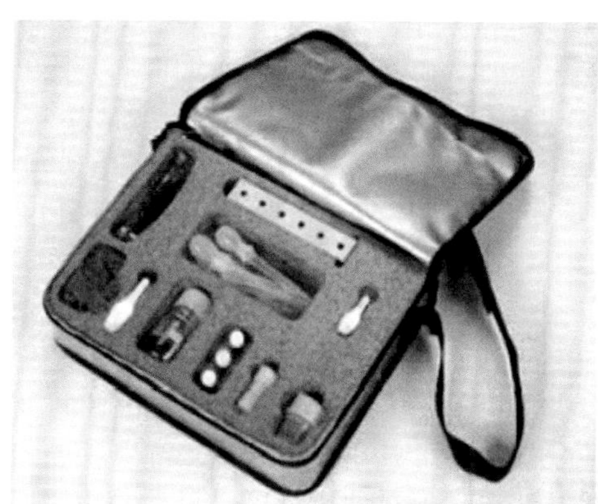

Fig. 5. Semi-quantitative test kit. Source: SAFO 2010.

Test Kits

BASF introduced a mobile testing device that had specifically been designed for its staple food fortification efforts. The device allows for a qualitative measurement of the vitamin A content in oil through a simple and quick test. While exact tests via high performance liquid chromatography cost USD 50–100 per sample, testing with the test kit costs only USD 0.02–0.05 per sample. To conduct monitoring once regulations are in place, the test kit was also supplied free of charge to smaller companies without lab equipment as to field inspectors of the TFDA (fig. 5).

In order to enable a fully quantitative measurement of the vitamin A content in oil, SAFO, via BASF, partnered with BioAnalyt, a German provider of analytical equipment, to provide a second generation test kit. The 'iCheckChroma' is as accurate as high-end laboratory equipment but comes at a tenth of the cost and is only the size of a large cell phone.

Both test kits are highly complementary in cost and use and enable companies and authorities to cost-effectively measure the quality of their oil and flour fortification programs.

Standard-Setting and Regulation

SAFO had not taken a role in technically supporting the standard setting and regulation process for food fortification, apart from providing information during the standard setting workshop. Neither GIZ nor BASF had a mandate to intervene on this political level, so while technical capacities were brought in place, these critical market frameworks still needed support.

Initially, the World Bank was assigned the mandate and the resources needed to support the Tanzania Bureau of Standards to conclude the standard-setting process with other government entities, such as the Ministry of Health. This process was complemented by a media campaign on the benefits of improved nutrition and food fortification. The standards were finalized, printed, and disseminated to relevant companies by December 2010. Along with the development of these standards, the World Bank supported the development of food fortification guidelines and manuals for food manufacturers and for the TFDA (on measurement and evaluation), as well as the training of food and laboratory inspectors.

Two oil manufacturers, East Coast Oils and Murzah Oil Mills, expressed their support for fortification once the government passed regulation that would mandate fortification and provide a 'level playing field' relative to other producers and imports.

In December 2010, a stakeholder meeting was held to comment on the draft national food fortification regulation. The TFDA incorporated the comments and sent the regulation to the Ministry of Health and Social Welfare for signature. In March 2011, the regulation was gazetted; it finally passed in August 2011 [10].

After the standards and the regulation were in place, Helen Keller International (HKI), an NGO dedicated to preventing blindness and reducing malnutrition that has been working in Tanzania since 1985, supported industry to procure fortificants through funds from the Department for International Development (UK) and the Global Alliance for Improved Nutrition (GAIN).

One critical element for the acceptance of mandatory fortification was social marketing. Many people, especially those in lower-income segments and in rural areas, were not aware of micronutrient deficiency and the benefits of oil fortified with vitamin A. To fund these activities, GAIN funded HKI to manage social marketing activities. These awareness-raising campaigns used scientific health messages combined with the logo to allow consumers to recognize fortified foods in resale stores.

All in all, it has taken almost 10 years to establish a standard and regulation for oil fortification in Tanzania. SAFO has strengthened the food fortification process with very targeted yet critical technical support for the process: a label, test kits and technical sup-

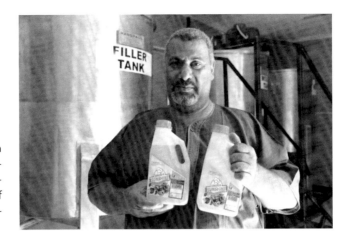

Fig. 6. Mr. Khalfan, Singida Sunshine, a small- and medium-size enterprise oil producer, with his first bottles of fortified oil (in front of the production unit). Source: BASF.

port. Yet, without the other stakeholders such as HKI, GAIN and the World Bank and a big push for standardization and regulation, this process might have taken even longer.

This case shows that it often takes several actors taking on different roles in a multi-year process to improve and strengthen an inclusive business system, especially a system in which standard setting is involved.

Results and Outlook

Since the introduction of regulation mandating the fortification of oil with vitamin A, all oil sold in Tanzania has to be fortified. Currently, 10 million Tanzanians are reached, and approximately 670,000 metric tons of edible oil have been fortified [11].

The National Action Plan for the Enrichment of Staple Food, produced by the NFFA, includes a cost-benefit assessment of food fortification in Tanzania: vitamin A deficiency causes economic losses of more than USD 32 million per year [1]. The plan conservatively estimates that vitamin A deficiency in Tanzania will be reduced by 30% [1]. Comparatively, the costs of vitamin A fortification are small. All in all, the cost per metric ton of oil is just USD 1.67 [1]. This roughly equals a just 0.17% cost increase per unit of edible oil, not even a fifth of a cent. Accordingly, a tiny cost can generate a large impact: it is estimated that every USD 1 invested in nutrition can result in benefits worth USD 60 [12].

Outlook

Today, GIZ continues to work with HKI and TFDA in strengthening the monitoring systems for fortified foods by providing technical advice and targeted resources, such as micronutrient test kits. BASF maintains the momentum with food producers by providing technical seminars and training, in particular on quality assurance.

A challenge remains to include smaller oil producers in the program, and addressing this challenge demands specific technical advice and efforts by BASF. In order to tackle these challenges, GIZ, BASF, BioAnalyt and Mühlenchemie founded a new project called Affordable Nutritious Foods for Women, which will support Tanzania's fortification program until full self-sufficiency, which is aimed to be achieved in the year 2017.

In summary, SAFO has been effective in combining the respective strengths of public and private sector actors to tackle the development challenge of vitamin A deficiency. This case study also shows that alliances like SAFO will often require the right momentum among key stakeholders as well as contributions from other key actors to be successful (fig. 6).

References

1 NFFA: Action Plan for the Provision of Vitamins and Minerals to the Tanzanian Population through Enrichment of Staple Foods. 2009.

2 BASF: Microcapsules against Malnutrition. Ludwigshafen, BASF, 2009.

3 THDS: Tanzania demographic and health survey 2010. 2010. http://www.nbs.go.tz/takwimu/references/2010TDHS.pdf (accessed September 23, 2015).

4 Gradl C, Jenkins B: Tackling Barriers to Scale: From Inclusive Business Models to Inclusive Business Ecosystems. Cambridge, CSR Initiative at the Harvard Kennedy School, 2011.

5 Bluethner A, Vierck L: Setting standards for business and development: how legal frameworks can support market-based nutrition partnerships. EFFL 2009;4: 104–118.

6 Natalicchio M, Garrett J, Mulder-Sibanda M, Ndegwa S, Voorbraak D (eds): Carrots and Sticks: The Political Economy of Nutrition Policy Reforms. Washington, World Bank, 2009.

7 World Bank: Tanzania – Advancing Nutrition for Long-Term Equitable Growth. Washington, World Bank, 2007.

8 Krawinkel M, Temu A: Vitamin A Deficiency in Tanzania and Needs for Improvement. Report for SAFO. 2009.

9 Künkel P, Wildschut G: Documentation of the SAFO Stakeholder Workshop 'Towards a Sustainable Cost-Effective Food Fortification Partnership for Tanzania'/Expert Workshop 'Standards Setting in Food Fortification in Tanzania'. Report for SAFO. 2009.

10 TBS: Finalized Tanzania Standard – Fortified Edible Fats and Oils – Specification. Dar es Salaam, TBS, 2011.

11 Assey V: Tanzania food-fortification country experience. Presentation at Food-Fortification Summit, Arusha, 2015.

12 Copenhagen Consensus: Post-2015 consensus – nutrition. 2015. http://www.copenhagenconsensus.com/post-2015-consensus/nutrition (accessed September 23, 2015).

Dr. Andreas Bluethner, Director Food Fortification and Partnerships
BASF SE, ENS/HR – F31 – Room 231
DE–68623 Lampertheim (Germany)
E-Mail andreas.bluethner@basf.com

Biesalski HK, Black RE (eds): Hidden Hunger. Malnutrition and the First 1,000 Days of Life:
Causes, Consequences and Solutions. World Rev Nutr Diet. Basel, Karger, 2016, vol 115, pp 175–183
DOI: 10.1159/000442103

Genetically Engineered Crops and Certified Organic Agriculture for Improving Nutrition Security in Africa and South Asia

Carl Pray[a] • Samuel Ledermann[b]

[a]Department of Agricultural, Food and Resource Economics, Rutgers, The State University of New Jersey, New Brunswick, NJ, USA; [b]Independent Scholar, Zurich, Switzerland

Abstract

In Africa and South Asia, where nutrition insecurity is severe, two of the most prominent production technologies are genetically modified (GM) crops and certified organic agriculture. We analyze the potential impact pathways from agricultural production to nutrition. Our review of data and the literature reveals increasing farm-level income from cash crop production as the main pathway by which organic agriculture and GM agriculture improve nutrition. Potential secondary pathways include reduced prices of important food crops like maize due to GM maize production and increased food production using organic technology. Potential tertiary pathways are improvements in health due to reduced insecticide use. Challenges to the technologies achieving their impact include the politics of GM agriculture and the certification costs of organic agriculture. Given the importance of agricultural production in addressing nutrition security, accentuated by the post-2015 sustainable development agenda, the chapter concludes by stressing the importance of private and public sector research in improving the productivity and adoption of both GM and organic crops. In addition, the chapter reminds readers that increased farm income and productivity require complementary investments in health, education, food access and women's empowerment to actually improve nutrition security.

Introduction

Genetically modified (GM) agriculture and certified organic agriculture have experienced, on average, double-digit annual growth rates (11 and 12%, respectively) since the beginning of the century. This growth took place as the agricultural sectors of emerging and developed countries underwent a significant nutritional shift, from supplying food for direct consumption to growing raw materials for the food processing industry [1]. Prices fell and consumer demand increased for empty calories, such as from refined fats and sugars [2]. It is in this context of new nutritional challenges that the these two technologies show promise not only in providing increased production and higher incomes to the adopters but also in having an impact on global diets, including through diversification of production (i.e. organic agriculture) and biofortification (i.e. GM agriculture) [3].

Africa and South Asia provide a unique perspective on studying the impact of these technologies on nutrition security. As seen in figure 1, while GM agriculture is more prominent in South Asia, certified organic agriculture in Africa is widespread and untouched by major regulatory issues. From a food security perspective, key differences exist. In South Asia, production exceeds demand, resulting in improving food access being the main area of concern. In Sub-Saharan Africa, food production per capita is declining, with family farmers constituting the largest class of Africa's hungry population [4]. Moving beyond production, however, soil health is in decline in both regions, with both macronutrient and micronutrient (i.e. zinc) deficiencies recorded [5].

Given the focus of the post-2015 development agenda on sustainable agriculture, our ensuing review of the potential impact of the two agricultural technologies on nutrition security highlights additional research avenues aligned with 'calls for more nutrition-sensitive agricultural policies with foci on increasing household income and improving access to high-quality diets' [6, p. 536].

Methods

Our research analyzes how nutrition can be improved by GM and organic agriculture production. Ruel and Alderman [6] provide an overview of potential pathways in the literature regarding how agriculture can impact nutrition, which includes not only its function as a source of food, income or lowered food prices but also its empowerment of women, reduction of their burden, and improvement of their health status. Using the most recent data on organic [7] and GM [8] agriculture available, we draw on the adapted conceptual pathways [9] between agriculture and nutrition in figure 2 to analyze the potential of these two technologies to contribute to nutrition security in Africa and South Asia.

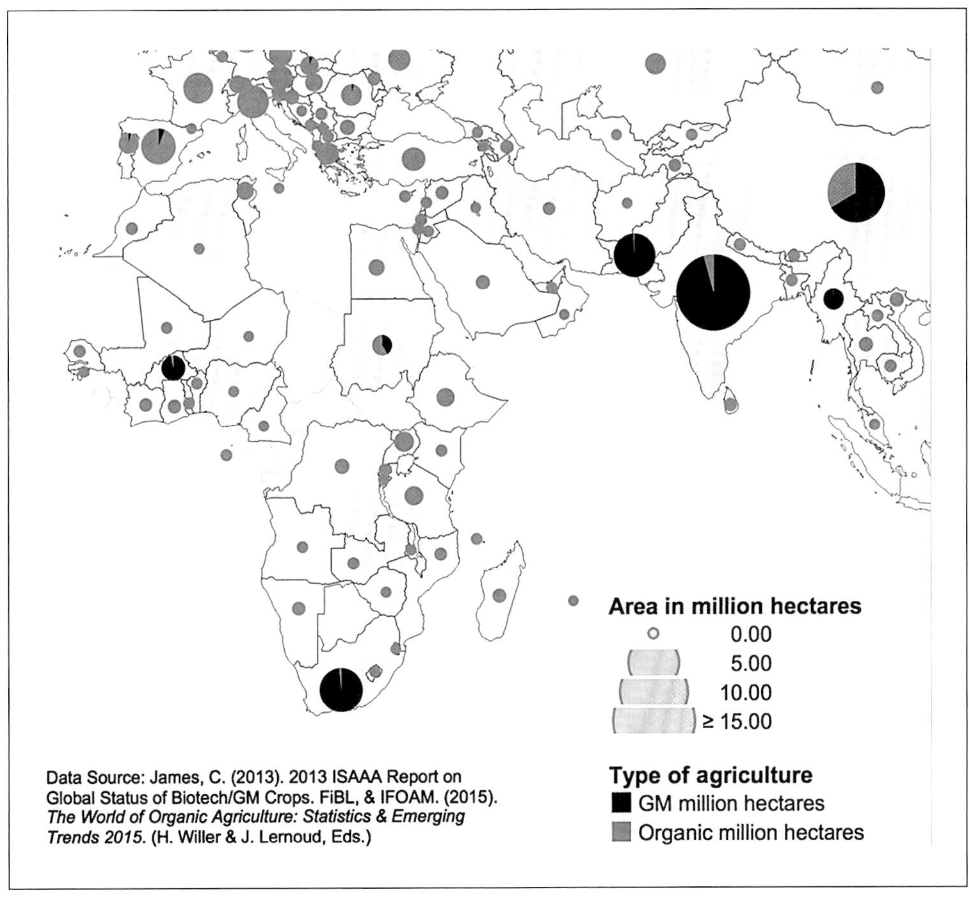

Fig. 1. Certified organic and GM agriculture areas in 2013 (in million hectares).

Impact on Nutrition by GM Crops

With more than an estimated 425 million acres under production by GM agriculture in 2013, developing countries have managed to surpass their developed counterparts [8]. Globally, however, production continues to be limited to four major field crops – soybean, cotton, maize and canola – with nutrient-rich [10] crops lacking (the main exception being papaya).

Agricultural income thus represents the primary pathway for the impact of GM crops on nutrition, mostly through the production of cash crops. Both in China and in India, Bt cotton is the only major field crop adopted and approved, grown by 7.5 million Chinese (2013) [11] and 7.7 million Indian (2014) [12] farmers. In both Africa and South Asia, the only exception is South Africa, where Bt maize for food consumption is grown mainly by large-scale farmers [13]. As a result, the main impact on nutrition is through additional income generated.

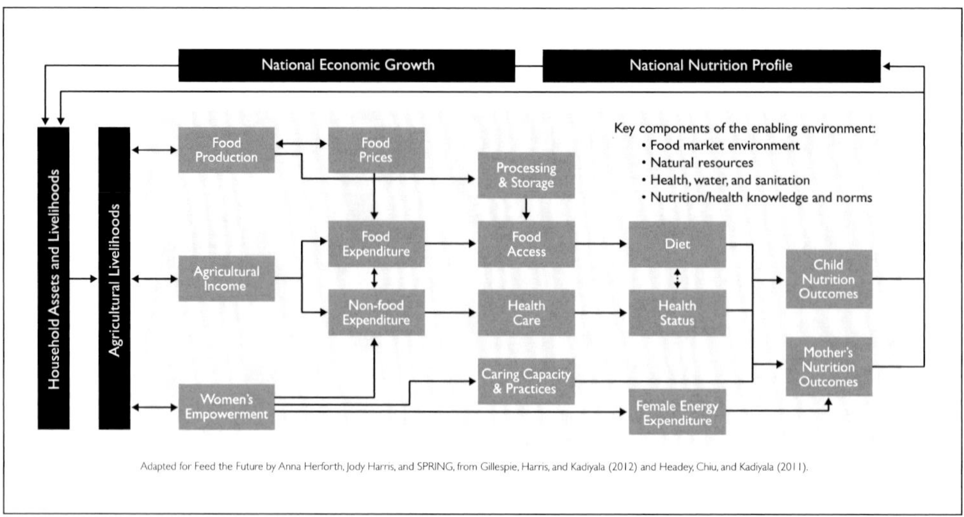

Fig. 2. Conceptual pathways between agriculture and nutrition [9, p. 3].

The secondary pathway to improving nutrition is through food prices. The global yield and production effect of adopting GM cotton, maize, and soybean is reduced prices; it is estimated that maize prices would have been 12–27% higher in the absence of GM varieties [14]. However, further studies on how changes in food prices benefit rural producers are needed, as in the case of India; the impact will depend on the extent to which the rural poor are net producers or consumers of food [15]. Their impact is furthermore compounded by changes in diets, with micronutrient malnutrition commonly arising from diets heavy on staple grains in India, thus highlighting the necessity of increasing diversification of agricultural systems, including pulse production for proteins [15].

The third pathway of positive impacts on health by GM agriculture can include biofortification. Beyond vitamin A-enriched golden rice, which still is stuck in regulatory processes, recent examples include confined field trials for biofortification of sorghum with increased levels of iron, zinc, and vitamins A and E under a research consortium led by Africa Harvest in Kenya [16]. Additional potential exists in breeding plants with better micronutrient uptake [5].

In addition to potential impacts, there are documented health impacts of GM technologies' reduced insecticide use in India and China, which has led to considerable reductions in the exposure of farmers and farm workers to pesticides, ultimately lowering sickness levels [17]. Reductions in herbicide use and replacement of herbicides containing more toxic compounds, such as atrazine, can also have a positive impact. Additionally, in South Africa, Bt maize has led to a reduction in mycotoxins, such as fumonisin, which is associated with neural tube defects [16]. Overall reduction of pesticide use can have a positive effect on the environment (i.e. improved biocontrol services in China [18]). However, increasing levels of herbicide use in some countries, changes in weed control programs due to herbicide-resistant weeds in the USA [19] and elsewhere, as well as debates about whether glyphosate is carcinogenic [20] raise some questions about how big the positive health impact will be. Finally, although higher productivity reduces the cost of energy-dense foods, their negative effect on nutrition is dampened by lower feed prices in meat production. Imported corn goes into pork in China and into poultry production in South Asia, thus contributing to more nutrient density by lowering meat prices.

Impact on Nutrition by Certified Organic Agriculture

Globally, Africa and Asia combined account for only 4% of certified organic land but make up 65% of the world's 2 million organic producers, with the 2 largest reporting countries being India, with 650,000 producers, and Uganda, with 189,610 producers [7]. In stark contrast to GM crops, which are planted in 5 countries in South Asia and Africa, 34 African and 7 South Asian countries engage in certified organic production. While the GM area (13.8 million ha) dwarfs the organic area in South Asia (0.6 million ha), in Africa, the organic acreage amounts to 1.2 million ha, compared to 3.5 million ha of GM area. In Africa, cash crops – coffee, olives, oilseeds, and textile crops – make up the largest share of the organic planted area, while in Asia, most of the organic area reported is for food crops, such as cereals, nuts, fruits, and vegetables [7].

Given the focus of certified organic agriculture on cash crops, price premiums are expected to be the main drivers increasing agricultural income [21], ultimately translating into higher food and nonfood expenditures at the household level. Long-term trials of Bt and organic cotton from 2007 to 2010 in India showed that farm incomes were higher from organic cotton, even with a 10–15% lower yield per hectare compared to Bt cotton [22]. This was attributable to a 10–15% increase in prices and 32% lower costs due to savings on seeds, a lack of use of synthetic fertilizers and pesticides, their substitution with botanicals or organic manure, and similar labor costs [22].

China is an exception, as the crops grown on 1.3 million ha out of its 2.1 million certified organic hectares are destined for the domestic market. With its reported sales of EUR 2.4 billion in 2013, China itself represents the world's fourth largest organic market [7]. The crops include nutrient-dense crops, as one sixth (50,000 ha) of the world's organic vegetables are grown in China, albeit only amounting to 0.3% of the total Chinese vegetable area [7]. China also holds 74% of the total acreage of organic cereals grown in Asia, with the three largest being organic rice (170,728 ha), wheat (162,931 ha) and maize (102,967 ha) [23]. Domestic demand is also fueled by continued food safety scares, with a lack of trust in food certificates driving innovative technologies developed by internet giants (i.e. Alibaba, Lenovo) to link wealthy urban consumers with producers [7, 24].

Producers engaging in certified organic agriculture are expected to uphold organic standards in production, which include required or recommended production strategies expected to benefit farm-level nutrition. These can be classified at two levels: diversification in production and seasonal diversification. In regard to the former, mandatory crop rotations and recommended intercropping of (edible) legumes for nitrogen fixation are the most prominent. In particular, the latter is relevant for both South Asia – in India, between 1960 and 2007, consumption of nutrient-dense pulses declined by 50% [15] – and Africa – in Malawi, households have reported more feeding of edible legumes to their children after implementation of legume-intercropping strategies [25]. Additional diversification can occur through the integration of locally adapted seeds to withstand biotic or abiotic stresses, the holding of animals for farm yard manure, and subsequent access to dairy products. Seasonal diversification is also key, as high-value crops can increase the saving of capital for the lean period. In India, the hungry season in particular has resulted in widening gender inequities in intra-household allocations to food [15]. Better organization of farmers via cooperatives can also result in improved access to storage and subsequent timing of their marketing at favorable prices. In addition, saved input costs and improved soil health can increase their resilience to shocks.

This holistic approach to organic agriculture aims to have an impact on nutrition via improved health. At the farm level in South Asia and Sub-Saharan Africa, both reduced pesticide usage at the production stage and sustainable soil fertility management can improve health. In Africa, soil nutrients are regarded as one of the major limiting factors, and not improved crop varieties [4]. The direct effects of soil degradation on food insecurity include not only lower yields but also resultant lower protein and micronutrients contents [5], as soil quality is a determinant of the nutritional value and safety of foods grown [26]. Additional indirect negative health effects of soil degradation include air, soil and water pollution [5, 27]. The potential impact on health is, however, complex, as organic products are often cash crops and as evidence on positive impact of organic consumption is disputed [28]. Ideally, a secondary impact would be expected through increased dietary diversity. Home gardening interventions – which lie outside of certified organic agriculture – enact positive changes in the diet of the beneficiary households, but due to substitution effects, the overall impact remains unclear [3].

Discussion

Clear conceptual pathways to improvement of nutrition by organic and GM agriculture exist, and their main pathways are through increasing farm-level income. The impact of specific GM or organic techniques will be context dependent. For organic agriculture, this includes the de facto organic setting of smallholder agriculture in Africa, with low use of synthetic fertilizer and pesticides, while in South Asia, synthetic fertilizers and pesticides are used extensively. Maximizing the benefits of GM agriculture will depend on proper crop management, especially to slow the development of resistant pests. Overall, though, both technologies show potential to improve health and nutritional security through lowered pesticide exposure. In GM agriculture, there is some potential to reduce mycotoxins in food. On the consumption level, diversification at the farm level and production of more nutrient-rich crops for consumers might increase nutritional health in organic agriculture. The higher prices in organic markets, however, stand in stark contrast to lower staple prices for GM agriculture and their subsequent impact pathway.

We expect that both technologies will face multiple challenges to realizing their impact potential on nutrition security. In GM agriculture, the production of genetically engineered food crops in India (eggplant), China (rice and maize) and Kenya (maize and soybean) was stopped by political decisions. Urban elites and environmental interest groups as well as a lack of domestic support from economic interest groups are likely to continue slowing down the adoption of more diverse GM crops. While governments share an interest in increasing food production and food security, they fear that approving GM food would lead to a loss of sovereignty over the seed market (i.e. China), negative environmental impacts (i.e. India), or potential negative impacts on European donors (i.e. Kenya). However, several new GM seeds might receive approval: Bt maize in China (by 2017) and India (by 2020); hybrid mustard for vegetable oil (by 2017); biofortified sorghum, banana or cassava in Africa, and outside South Asia and Africa, pinto beans in Brazil (by 2017) [16].

In certified organic agriculture, slowed growth in Africa and Asia over recent years accentuates the need to move beyond its current niche to have an impact on nutrition. From the demand side, this could take place via increased urban demand from rapidly growing affluent customer segments, such as in China. From the supply end, it includes moving beyond the niche generated by high certification costs, toward Organic 3.0 [7]. This includes cutting certification costs by 70–90% through participatory guarantee systems. Aimed at production for the regional market, these systems are growing rapidly in Africa, although Asia still leading (19,094 producers, out of which 7,234 are certified) [7]. This move could extend organic agriculture's reach to increase farmers' diversification and food security throughout the year. The challenges are in obtaining government certification of the new standard and the limited capacity of governments and nongovernmental organizations to provide support for organic extension to farmers. From the private sector, major agricultural input industries have limited incentives in performing research and development (R&D) for sustainable management technology that depends on on-farm inputs. Three potential new avenues to accelerate organic agriculture could be payments for ecosystem services, the implementation of the Sustainable Development Goals (Goal 2), and technical assistance to farmers from integrated value-chain drivers, such as supermarkets. Finally, even for the large-scale conventional input firms, incentives are growing to invest in alternative solutions, such as biopesticides and biofertilizers, which are now the focus of major investments by Monsanto, Bayer, BASF and Syngenta.

Conclusions

As we find ourselves in a dietary transition, the potential for agricultural technologies to contribute to nutrition security becomes more prominent. Our work has tried to highlight two of the most prominent development strategies and their potential impact in regions where nutrition insecurity is the most severe. Since empirical studies are limited, resulting in an overall weak evidence base [15], we strongly advocate a more systematic integration of nutrition security in impact assessments of the pathways shown. Given that each agricultural technology needs to continuously be adapted to new challenges, limited funding will have implications for the global division of R&D labor between the private and the public sectors. For maize, cotton and soybean, the R&D investment of the private sector is so strong that the government's role is to ensure competition between the companies, coupled with strategic investments to improve specific adaptations of these main crops. For wheat and rice, both the conventional public and private sectors will need to contribute. However, for the most nutrient-rich products, such as vegetables, legumes, fruits and nuts, the public sector should take the lead in sustainable development to increase productivity and reduce macro- and micronutrient deficiency [1]. Finally, solutions will need to move beyond production and include complementary improvements, as reflected in our pathways, in enhancing market access and reducing food loss and wastage in an enabling environment to reach full impact.

References

1 Pinstrup-Andersen P: Nutrition-sensitive food systems: from rhetoric to action. Lancet 2013;382:375–376.

2 Tilman D, Clark M: Global diets link environmental sustainability and human health. Nature 2014;515:518–522.

3 Masset E, Haddad L, Cornelius A, et al: Effectiveness of agricultural interventions that aim to improve nutritional status of children: systematic review. BMJ 2012;344:d8222.

4 Sanchez PA, Swaminathan MS: Hunger in Africa: the link between unhealthy people and unhealthy soils. Lancet 2005;365:442–444.

5 Lal R: Soil degradation as a reason for inadequate human nutrition. Food Secur 2009;1:45–57.

6 Ruel MT, Alderman H: Nutrition-sensitive interventions and programmes: how can they help to accelerate progress in improving maternal and child nutrition? Lancet 2013;382:536–551.

7 Willer H, Lernoud J: The World of Organic Agriculture: Statistics and Emerging Trends 2015. Frick/Bonn, FiBL/IFOAM, 2015.

8 James C: 2013 ISAAA Report on Global Status of Biotech/GM Crops. 2013. http://www.isaaa.org/resources/publications/briefs/46/pptslides/Brief-46slides.swf.

9 Herforth A, Harris J: Understanding and Applying Primary Pathways and Principles. 2014. Improving Nutrition through Agriculture Technical Brief Series. Arlington, USAID/Strengthening Partnerships, Results, and Innovations in Nutrition Globally (SPRING) Project, 2014.

10 Fulgoni VL, Keast DR, Drewnowski A: Development and validation of the nutrient-rich foods index: a tool to measure nutritional quality of foods. J Nutr 2009;139:1549–1554.

11 James C: Biotech Facts and Trends 2014: China. Ithaca, ISAAA, 2013.

12 Choudhary B, Gaur K: Biotech Cotton in India, 2002 to 2014. Ithaca, ISAAA, 2014.

13 Gouse M, Pray CE, Kirsten J, et al: A GM subsistence crop in Africa: the case of Bt white maize in South Africa. Int J Biotechnol 2005;7:84–94.

14 Barrows G, Sexton S, Zilberman D: The impact of agricultural biotechnology on supply and land-use. Environ Dev Econ 2014:1–28.
15 Gillespie S, Harris J, Kadiyala S: The Agriculture-Nutrition Disconnect in India: What Do We Know? Washington, IFPRI, 2012.
16 Chambers JA, Zambrano P, Falck-Zepeda J, et al: GM Agricultural Technologies for Africa 2014. Côte d'Ivoire, The African Development Bank, 2014.
17 Hossain F, Pray CE, Lu Y, et al: Genetically modified cotton and farmers' health in China. Int J Occup Environ Health 2001;10:296–303.
18 Lu Y, Wu K, Jiang Y, et al: Widespread adoption of Bt cotton and insecticide decrease promotes biocontrol services. Nature 2012;487:362–365.
19 Fernandez-Cornejo J, Nehring R, Osteen C, et al: Pesticide use in US Agriculture: 21 Selected Crops 1960–2008. Washington, US Department of Agriculture, Economic Research Service, 2014.
20 Guyton KZ, Loomis D, Grosse Y, et al: Carcinogenicity of tetrachlorvinphos, parathion, malathion, diazinon, and glyphosate. Lancet Oncol 2015;16:490–491.
21 Crowder DW, Reganold JP: Financial competitiveness of organic agriculture on a global scale. Proc Natl Acad Sci USA 2015;112:7611–7616.
22 Forster D, Andres C, Verma R, et al: Yield and economic performance of organic and conventional cotton-based farming systems – results from a field trial in India. PLoS One 2013;8: e81039.
23 FiBL: Survey 2015 based on national data sources. Unpublished.
24 Stevenson A, Mozur P: China's long food chain plugs in. New York Times, March 1, 2015, pp 3–6.
25 Bezner Kerr R, Snapp S, Chirwa M, et al: Participatory research on legume diversification with Malawian smallholder farmers for improved human nutrition and soil fertility. Exp Agric 2007;43:437–453.
26 Pepper IL: The soil health-human health nexus. Crit Rev Environ Sci Technol 2013;43:2617–2652.
27 Pimentel D, Cooperstein S, Randell H, et al: Ecology of increasing diseases: population growth and environmental degradation. Hum Ecol 2007;35:653–668.
28 Dangour A, Lock K, Hayter A, et al: Nutrition-related health effects of organic foods: a systematic review. Am J Clin Nutr 2010;92:203–210.

Prof. Carl Pray
Department of Agricultural, Food and Resource Economics
Rutgers, The State University of New Jersey
55 Dudley Road, New Brunswick, NJ 08901-8520 (USA)
E-Mail pray@aesop.rutgers.edu

Biesalski HK, Black RE (eds): Hidden Hunger. Malnutrition and the First 1,000 Days of Life: Causes, Consequences and Solutions. World Rev Nutr Diet. Basel, Karger, 2016, vol 115, pp 184–192
DOI: 10.1159/000442104

Behavioral Change Strategies for Improving Complementary Feeding and Breastfeeding

Saskia J.M. Osendarp • Marion L. Roche

The Micronutrient Initiative, Ottawa, ON, Canada

Abstract

Improving infant and young child feeding (IYCF) practices, including breastfeeding and complementary feeding, has been identified as one of the most effective interventions to improve child survival, stunting and wasting. Evidence from randomized controlled trials suggests that effective promotion of breastfeeding and complementary feeding, with or without food provision, has the potential to improve IYCF practices and child nutrition. However, in many countries, breastfeeding practices and complementary feeding practices are still far from optimal. The lack of implementation of available, effective, affordable interventions in scale-up programs is in part attributed to a lack of innovative, creative and effective behavioral change strategies that enable and encourage caregivers. Successful behavioral change strategies should be based on a rigorous situational analysis and formative research, and the findings and insights of formative research should be used to further design interventions that address the identified barriers and enablers, to select delivery channels, and to formulate appropriate and effective messages. In addition, successful behavioral change interventions should a priori define and investigate the program impact pathway to target behavioral change and should assess intermediary behavioral changes and indicators to learn why the expected outcome was achieved or not achieved by testing the program theory. The design of behavioral change communication must be flexible and responsive to shifts in societies and contexts. Performance of adequate IYCF also requires investments to generate community demand through social mobilization, relevant media and existing support systems. Applying these principles has been shown to be effective in improving IYCF practices in Vietnam, Bangladesh and Ethiopia and is recommended to be adopted by other programs and countries in order to accelerate progress in improving child nutrition.

Introduction

Despite improvements in recent decades, undernutrition, including fetal growth restriction, stunting, wasting and deficiencies of vitamin A and zinc combined with suboptimal breastfeeding, is estimated to cause 45% of all child deaths, resulting in 3.1 million deaths annually [1]. In recent years, there has been an increased focus of attention on interventions targeting undernutrition in the so-called first 1,000 days, from conception until the child's second birthday, because this is the time in life in which much of the growth faltering (stunting) takes place and during which good nutrition can have lasting benefits throughout life. The data show that globally, the estimated number of stunted children is decreasing, but still at least 162 million children under 5 years in 2012 suffer from stunting. This number is not on track to meet the World Health Assembly (WHA) goal of 100 million by 2025 [2]. While substantial progress has been achieved in Asia, the prevalence of stunting is still high (over 25% in 2010), with almost 60% of all stunted children globally living in Asia.

Of all proven preventive health and nutrition interventions, adequate infant and young child feeding (IYCF) promotion, consisting of promotion of exclusive breastfeeding (EBF), continued breastfeeding after 6 months of age and timely and adequate introduction of complementary foods, is one of the most important solutions to directly address the causes of childhood undernutrition [1]. The World Health Organization (WHO) and the United Nations Children's Fund recommend EBF for the first 6 months and continued breastfeeding with appropriate complementary feeding for up to 2 years and beyond as part of the IYCF strategy [3]. Infants are particularly at risk when they first receive complementary foods, which often occurs earlier than the recommended 6 months. At 6 months of age, when their nutritional needs are greatest, children are first exposed to foods which may be nutritionally inadequate and potentially contaminated with micro-organisms, causing diarrhea and other infectious diseases [4]. With the small quantities these children can consume, energy density and nutrient density of complementary foods is usually an issue in many low-income settings. Consequently, in many low-income regions, a drastic growth drop among children especially between 6 and 23 months is observed, and caused by diets that do not provide adequate nutrition and by high rates of infectious diseases due to a lack of hygiene, access to a safe water supply, and sanitation [5, 6].

In this chapter, we will first describe the recent global trends in IYCF practices and will then review the evidence from intervention studies on the impact of behavioral change strategies to improve rates of EBF and adequate complementary feeding. However, despite the fact that these intervention studies consistently demonstrate the efficacy and affordability of behavioral change interventions, there is very little experience documented describing how to successfully introduce these interventions in large-scale programs. In the last part of this chapter, we will therefore describe what is required to implement effective programs at scale.

Infant and Young Child Feeding Practices

Eight population-level indicators have been defined by the WHO in response to the need for simple, practical indicators of appropriate feeding practices in children aged 0–23 months that can be developed from large-scale survey data that describe trends

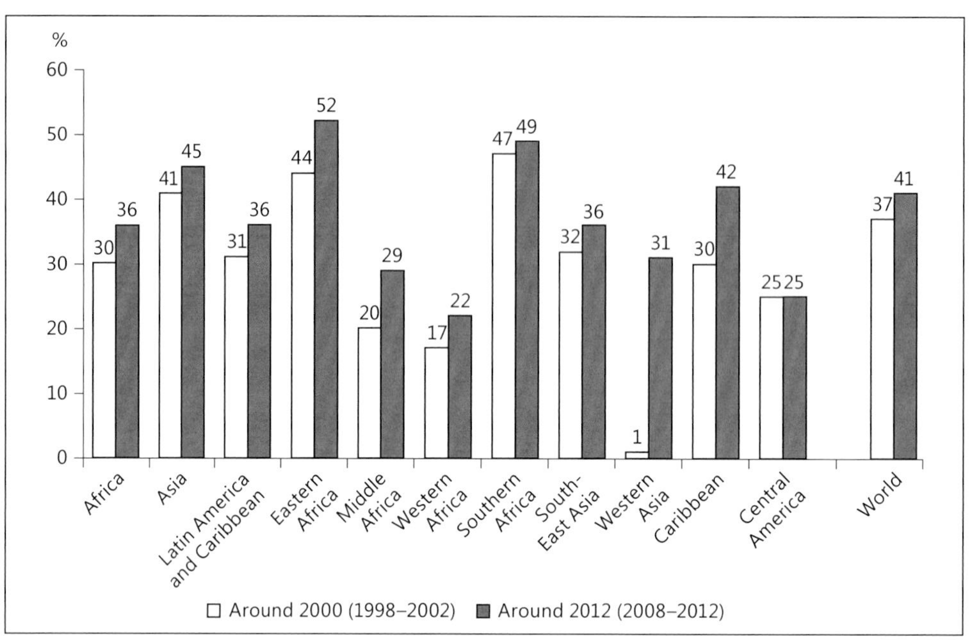

Fig. 1. Percentage of infants 0–5 months of age who are exclusively breastfed, by region, in 2002 and 2012. Source: International Food Policy Research Institute, Global Nutrition Report, 2014 [2].

over time and that compare regions and countries [7]. These eight core indicators include measures of appropriate breastfeeding practices, dietary diversity, feeding frequency, and consumption of iron-rich foods. Since the publication of these indicators, 46 countries now routinely collect data on IYCF practices as part of their Demographic and Health Survey [8].

Examination of these data revealed that breastfeeding practices and, especially, complementary feeding practices are still far from optimal, particularly in Sub-Saharan Africa and South Asia [2]. Although the rates of EBF have increased in most countries from 2002 to 2012, still less than 50% of children globally are exclusively breastfed until 6 months of age (fig. 1). Complementary feeding practices are even worse. In the 27 countries with data on complementary feeding practices, only 3–15% of children 6–23 months of age receive a minimum acceptable diet (a composite score of adequate dietary diversity and feeding frequency), and 27% receive a diet with minimum dietary diversity (received foods from a minimum of four food groups) (fig. 2) [2].

Suboptimal IYCF practices are of concern, as breastfeeding indicators and complementary feeding-related indicators of dietary diversity have been associated with child nutrition, health and survival. A systematic review modeling the effect of maternal and child nutrition interventions on lives saved suggested that adequate breastfeeding practices (early initiation of breastfeeding and EBF until 6 months of age) are associated with a 44–45% reduction in all-cause mortality [9]. In addition, increased dietary

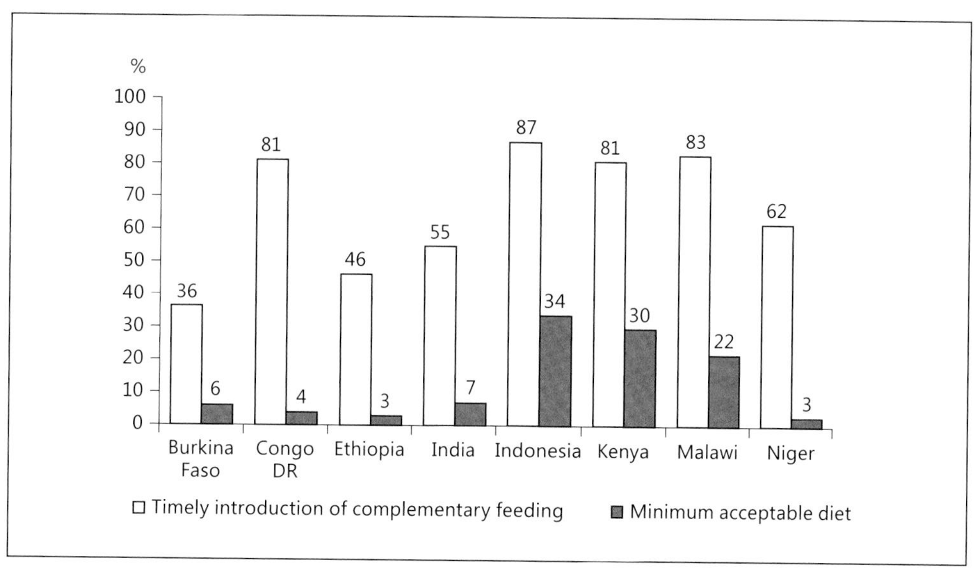

Fig. 2. Complementary feeding practices in selected countries with national data for these indicators. Source: Demographic and Health Survey data from these countries, 2010–2013.

diversity was positively associated with height-for-age Z-scores (HAZ) in nine of the 11 countries with Demographic and Health Survey data for this indicator [9]. In a recent analysis of national representative data from India, the total dietary diversity score and achieving minimum dietary diversity for children 6–23 months of age were most strongly and significantly associated with increased HAZ, weight-for-age Z-scores, stunting and underweight. In contrast, in this analysis, early initiation of breastfeeding and EBF were not associated with any of the nutrition outcomes considered [10]. Indicators of dietary diversity and overall diet quality were also found to be positively associated with HAZ in Bangladesh, Ethiopia, India and Zambia [8].

Strategies for Improving Exclusive Breastfeeding

EBF for the first 6 months clearly has benefits for protecting a child from morbidity and mortality: compared to exclusively breastfed infants, 'no breastfeeding' was associated with a significant 165% increase in diarrhea incidence in 0- to 5-month-old infants and a 32% increase in 6- to 11-month-old infants [11]. Breastfeeding also has long-term effects: the results of a meta-analysis [12] of 14 observational studies showed that breastfeeding was associated with an increase of 3.5 points (95% CI: 1.9–5.0) on intelligence tests in childhood and adolescence, and there is recent evidence from Brazil suggesting that these beneficial effects of breastfeeding might even be associated with improved performance on intelligence tests at 30 years of age [13].

There are interventions which have been proven effective in supporting and enabling women to exclusively breastfeed. In a systematic review of studies on the effect of promotion of breastfeeding, Haroon et al. [14] estimated that adequate education and counseling could increase the prevalence of EBF at 6 months in developing countries by 188% (relative risk: 2.88; 95% CI: 2.11–3.93), while the impact was nonsignificant for developed countries. Combined individual and group counseling and combined pre- and postnatal counseling were the most effective for increasing the rate of EBF at 6 months [15].

The difference in effect size between developing and developed countries could be because routine breastfeeding education in hospitals and during home visits, as well as healthy baby follow-up visits, are less common in less developed health systems than in the developed world, leading to gaps in mothers' knowledge of EBF and potentially lower self-efficacy and perceived support for managing any challenges. These mothers may benefit more from any educational intervention. In addition, breastfeeding may be more socially accepted as the norm in many cultures in developing countries, whereas mothers in developed countries may have lower EBF rates due to a wider availability of high-quality formula, work constraints and social perceptions which do not foster an enabling environment, rather than knowledge acting as the main barrier [14].

Although these interventions were successful, the achieved rates of EBF in these trials were still modest (<50%), most likely because none of these trials addressed the issue of practical barriers for mothers to change behavior, including work environments, social pressures inside or outside the home, and supportive strategies such as maternity leave provision.

Strategies for Improving Adequate Complementary Feeding

Adequate complementary feeding for infants 6–23 months of age refers to the timely introduction of safe and nutritionally adequate foods in addition to breastfeeding. In the Guiding Principles for Complementary Feeding of the Breastfed Child [16], the WHO recommends that the complementary feeding should be (1) timely, meaning that all infants should start receiving other foods in addition to breastmilk from 6 months onwards; (2) adequate, in that the nutritional value of the complementary foods in combination with breastmilk should fulfill the needs of the rapidly growing child, and (3) appropriate, meaning that the foods should be diverse, safe, appropriately textured and sufficiently abundant.

The available evidence to date indicates that there is no single universal best package of complementary feeding interventions, yet in every context, consideration of the available and culturally acceptable nutrient-dense foods is key to potential adoption. Findings from systematic reviews pooling the effects of 16 randomized and nonrandomized controlled trials and programs concluded that in a food secure context, nutrition education alone, especially when promoting animal-source foods, resulted in significant increases in height [standard mean difference (SMD): 0.35; 95% CI: 0.08–0.62) and HAZ (0.22; 0.01–0.43], whereas its effect on stunting was not significant. In food insecure populations, nutrition education alone showed significant effects on HAZ (SMD: 0.25; 95% CI: 0.09–0.42), stunting (relative risk: 0.68; 95% CI: 0.60–0.76) and weight-for-age Z-scores (SMD: 0.26; 95% CI: 0.12–0.41) [9]. Provision of appropriate (fortified) complementary foods in addition to nutritional counseling resulted in an extra gain of 0.25 kg (±0.18) in weight and 0.54 cm (±0.38) in height in children aged 6–24 months [17]. In addition, there is ample evidence from studies assessing actual intake of complementary foods, as well as studies modeling optimal intake for children 6–23 months of age based on local available foods. These studies concluded that in most developing country settings, children 6–23 months of age are not able to fulfill dietary adequacy for some micronutrients, notably iron, zinc and calcium, with local foods alone; thus, additional interventions to improve intake of these micronutrients remain required [18, 19]. Fortified complementary foods and/or the provision of home fortificants, including multiple-micronutrient powders or small-quantity lipid-based nutrient supplements, have been shown to improve micronutrient intake and to reduce anemia [20, 21] without reducing or displacing breastmilk intake in children 6–23 months of age [22].

Effective Programs at Scale

In their 2013 review of nutrition interventions, Bhutta et al. [9] estimated that combined promotion of breastfeeding and education, with or without provision of appropriate complementary feeding, would result in an estimated savings of 221,000 deaths per year among children under 5 years old if 90% coverage was achieved. Although the evidence from randomized controlled trials described above indicates that efficacious solutions exist to achieve this target, these findings have not yet been translated into successful programs with interventions that resulted in widespread adoption of these behavioral changes at scale or in improved outcomes at a national level.

In a comprehensive review documenting the experiences and lessons learned by Alive and Thrive for a rapid scale-up of programs to prevent stunting [23], the lack of scale-up implementation of breastfeeding and complementary feeding programs is attributed to a combination of reasons: a lack of scaling strategies and resources to support them, incomplete understanding of economic and cultural barriers, and incorrect assumptions about the determinants of poor feeding practices, such as assuming that food insecurity or poverty is the underlying cause of poor complementary feeding.

Other reasons include a lack of clarity on program approaches due to insufficient documentation of different ways to deliver results and an absence of creative behavioral change communication strategies, such as social marketing, that are based on successful marketing strategies employed by the private sector [23]. An absence of effective and creative behavioral change communication strategies often occurs because we do not know enough about what makes these interventions work: for whom, when, why, at what cost and for how long [24]. Successful and effective behavioral change campaigns therefore have to be evidence-informed through situational analysis, stakeholder consultations, formative research, and feasibility studies. The design of behavioral change communication must be flexible and responsive to contexts and shifts in societies. Performance of adequate IYCF also requires investments to generate community demand and support through social mobilization, relevant media and existing support systems. Both grandmothers and fathers have potentially unique roles in supporting mothers in adopting and sustaining recommended infant and young child feeding practices [25]. Insights from commercial marketing have yet to be used effectively in generating demand for adequate IYCF in public health. For instance, focusing on what consumers want or eliciting an emotional response (desire, fear, hope, etc.), instead of what they need or 'should do', is likely to result in more effective and appealing behavioral change messages, but there is limited documentation and evidence describing the successful application of these creative approaches in public health. The Alive and Thrive Viet Nam 'talking babies' campaign is an encouraging example, in which adorable babies in TV commercials and well-crafted, simple messages have been part of a strategy that has been designed to be effective and to measure improved feeding practices [26].

In a review identifying the determinants of effective complementary feeding-related behavioral change interventions in developing countries, Fabrizio et al. [24] concluded that effective interventions utilize two critical determinants. First, these interventions conducted rigorous formative research in preparation and, more importantly, used the findings and insights of that formative research to identify barriers and enablers for change, to further design the intervention and the delivery channels and to formulate appropriate and effective messages. Second, successful interventions a priori defined and investigated the program impact pathway (PIP) to target behavioral change and assessed intermediary behavioral changes and indicators to learn why the expected outcome was achieved or not [27]. We will describe each of these two requirements in a bit more detail below.

A detailed situational analysis should guide the development of effective communication strategies. Insights into the determinants of behavior, including barriers and enablers to change, and the application of exchange theory to understand the costs and benefits associated with current and proposed behaviors can help to prioritize the IYCF practices to focus on. It is recommended to focus campaigns on a small number of practical behavioral objectives that have the highest chance of success or are the biggest threat to the desired behavior. These can be selected by balancing the likelihood of the target audience to adopt the behavior (by minimizing the perceived and real costs and by increasing benefits) and the potential for a positive impact on nutrition if the behavior is adopted [28]. For instance, in its mass media campaign on EBF in Vietnam, Alive and Thrive focused on the practice that was the biggest threat to EBF: giving water before 6 months of age [26]. Interventions benefit from responding to the specific insights revealed by formative research, and formative research should be designed with the goal of influencing intervention design. For instance, formative research performed by the Micronutrient Initiative for an IYCF program in Ethiopia provided an example of incorrect assumptions about determinants of poor feeding practices [29]. In addition to poor availability of affordable foods, the barriers to adequate IYCF practices included cultural constraints, which prevented caregivers from providing certain foods to young children, thereby limiting food diversification. Additionally, some communities were traditionally reliant on food aid and therefore resistant to participate in activities that did not provide food. Moreover, barriers at the level of the health system prevented caregivers from applying adequate IYCF practices; these barriers included heavy workloads, high staff turnover at health facilities and limited capacity and skills of the health workers responsible for the delivery of IYCF services [29].

Information derived from situational analysis can help to develop a conceptual framework and PIP describing the steps through which a given intervention in a program is expected to have an impact on the desired outcomes of interest: IYCF practices and nutrition. A PIP thus provides a detailed picture of program processes and assumptions, as well as the organizational requirements to deliver the interventions [27]. A lack of knowledge about the intermediate steps and assumptions in the PIP represents a 'black box' that prevents a full understanding of why interventions are expected to work, as well as for whom, when, at what costs and for how long [24].

Applying these principles to the design and implementation of large-scale behavioral change campaigns has been shown potential to be successful. For instance, in Vietnam, a combination of mass media and interpersonal counseling increased the EBF rate from 21 to 80% within just 14 months of implementation [26]. These innovative and tested approaches are recommended to be adopted by other countries and programs [23], and promoting the adoption of best practices by implementers is expected to accelerate progress in improving infant and young child feeding and nutrition in the critical first 1,000 days.

References

1 Black RE, Victora CG, Walker SP, et al: Maternal and child undernutrition and overweight in low-income and middle-income countries. Lancet 2013;382:427–451. Erratum in Lancet 2013;382:396.

2 International Food Policy Research Institute: Global Nutrition Report 2014: Actions and Accountability to Accelerate the World's Progress on Nutrition. Washington, International Food Policy Research Institute (IFPRI), 2014.

3 World Health Organization/UNICEF: Global strategy for infant and young child feeding. 2003. http://www.who.int/nutrition/publications/infantfeeding/9241562218/en/ (accessed 17 September 2015).

4 Black RE, Allen LH, Bhutta ZA, et al: Maternal and child undernutrition: global and regional exposures and health consequences. Lancet 2008;371:243–260.

5 Victora CG, de Onis M, Hallal PC, et al: Worldwide timing of growth faltering: revisiting implications for interventions. Pediatrics 2010;125:e473–e480.

6 Prentice AM, Ward KA, Goldberg GR, et al: Critical windows for nutritional interventions against stunting. Am J Clin Nutr 2013;97:911–918.

7 WHO, UNICEF, USAID, et al: Indicators for Assessing Infant and Young Child Feeding Practices: Part 1: Definitions. Geneva, World Health Organization, 2008. http://www.who.int/nutrition/publications/infantfeeding/9789241596664/en/index.html (accessed 17 September 2015)

8 Jones AD, Ickes SB, Smith LQ, et al: World Health Organization infant and young child feeding indicators and their associations with child anthropometry: a synthesis of recent findings. Mat Child Nutr 2014;10:1–17.

9 Bhutta ZA, Das JK, Rizvi A, et al: Evidence-based interventions for improvement of maternal and child nutrition: what can be done and at what cost? Lancet 2013;382:452–477. Erratum in Lancet 2013; 382:396.

10 Menon P, Bamezai A, Subrandoro A, et al: Age-appropriate infant and young child feeding practices are associated with child nutrition in India: insights from nationally representative data. Mat Child Nutr 2015;11:73–87.

11 Lamberti LM, Fischer Walker CL, Noiman A, et al: Breastfeeding and the risk for diarrhea morbidity and mortality. BMC Public Health 2011;11(suppl 3):S15.

12 Horta BL, Victora CG: Long-term Effects of Breastfeeding: A Systematic Review. Geneva, World Health Organization, 2013.

13 Victora CG, Horta BL, Lore de Mola C, et al: Association between breastfeeding and intelligence, educational attainment, and income at 30 years of age: a prospective birth cohort study from Brazil. Lancet Global Health 2015;3:e199–e205.

14 Haroon S, Das JK, Salam RA, et al: Breastfeeding promotion interventions and breastfeeding practices: a systematic review. BMC Public Health 2013; 13(suppl 3):S20.

15 Imdad A, Yakoob MY, Bhutta ZA: Effect of breastfeeding promotion interventions on breastfeeding rates, with special focus on developing countries. BMC Public Health 2011;11(suppl 3):S24.

16 Pan American Health Organisation (PAHO)/World Health Organisation (WHO): Guiding Principles for Complementary Feeding of the Breastfed Child. Washington, PAHO, 2003. http://www.who.int/nutrition/publications/guiding_principles_compfeeding_breastfed.pdf (accessed 17 September 2015).

17 Imdad A, Yakoob MY, Bhutta ZA: Impact of maternal education about complementary feeding and provision of complementary foods on child growth in developing countries. BMC Public Health 2011; 11(suppl 3):S25.

18 Osendarp SJM, Broersen BC, van Liere MJ, et al: Complementary feeding diets made of local foods can be optimized, but additional interventions will be needed to meet iron and zinc requirements in 6–23 month old children in low and middle income countries (submitted).

19 Allen LH: Adequacy of family foods for complementary feeding. Am J Clin Nutr 2012;95:785–786.

20 De-Regil LM, Suchdev PS, Vist GE, et al: Home fortification of foods with multiple micronutrient powders for health and nutrition in children under two years of age. Cochrane Database Syst Rev 2011;CD008959.

21 Dewey KG, Yang Z, Boy E: Systematic review and meta-analysis of home fortification of complementary foods. Matern Child Nutr 2009;5:283–321.

22 Kumwenda C, Dewey KG, Hemsworth J, et al: Lipid-based nutrient supplements do not decrease breast milk intake in Malawian infants. Am J Clin Nutr 2014;99:617–623.

23 Piwoz E, Baker J, Frongillo EA: Documenting large-scale programs to improve infant and young child feeding is key to facilitating progress in child nutrition. Food Nutr Bull 2013;34:S143–S145.

24 Fabrizio CS, van Liere M, Pelto G: Identifying determinants of effective complementary feeding behavior change interventions in developing countries. Mat Child Nutr 2014;10:575–592.

25 Aubel J: The role and influence of grandmothers on child nutrition: culturally designated advisors and caregivers. Mat Child Nutr 2012;8:19–35.

26 Shangvi T, Jimerson A, Hajeebhoy N, et al: Tailoring communication strategies to improve infant and young child feeding practices in different countries. Food Nutr Bull 2013;34:S169–S180.

27 Rawat R, Nguyen PH, Ali D, et al: Learning how programs achieve their impact: embedding theory-driven process evaluation and other program learning mechanisms in Alive & Thrive. Food Nutr Bull 2013;34:S212–S225.

28 Lee NR, Kotler P: Social Marketing: Influencing Behaviors for Good. Thousand Oaks, Sage, 2011.

29 Roche ML, Sako B, Osendarp SJ, et al: Community-based grain banks using local foods for improved infant and young child feeding in Ethiopia. Mat Child Nutr 2015, Epub ahead of print.

Saskia J.M. Osendarp
The Micronutrient Initiative
180 Elgin Street, Suite 1000
Ottawa, ON K2P 2K3 (Canada)
E-Mail sosendarp@micronutrient.org

Biesalski HK, Black RE (eds): Hidden Hunger. Malnutrition and the First 1,000 Days of Life: Causes, Consequences and Solutions. World Rev Nutr Diet. Basel, Karger, 2016, vol 115, pp 193–202
DOI: 10.1159/000442105

Rights-Based Approaches to Ensure Sustainable Nutrition Security

Sweta Banerjee

Welthungerhilfe, South Extension Phase II, New Delhi, India

Abstract

In India, a rights-based approach has been used to address large-scale malnutrition, including both micro- and macro-level nutrition deficiencies. Stunting, which is an intergenerational chronic consequence of malnutrition, is especially widespread in India (38% among children under 5 years old). To tackle this problem, the government of India has designed interventions for the first 1,000 days, a critical period of the life cycle, through a number of community-based programs to fulfill the rights to food and life. However, the entitlements providing these rights have not yet produced the necessary changes in the malnutrition status of people, especially women and children. The government of India has already implemented laws and drafted a constitution that covers the needs of its citizens, but corruption, bureaucracy, lack of awareness of rights and entitlements and social discrimination limit people's access to basic rights and services. To address this crisis, Welthungerhilfe India, working in remote villages of the most backward states in India, has shifted from a welfare-based approach to a rights-based approach. The Fight Hunger First Initiative, started by Welthungerhilfe in 2011, is designed on the premise that in the long term, poor people can only leave poverty behind if adequate welfare systems are in place and if basic rights are fulfilled; these rights include access to proper education, sufficient access to adequate food and income, suitable health services and equal rights. Only then can the next generation of disadvantaged populations look forward to a new and better future and can growth benefit the *entire* society. The project, co-funded by the Federal Ministry for Economic Cooperation and Development, is a long-term multi-sectoral program that involves institution-building and empowerment.

Introduction

Parmila Hembram, a 22-year-old resident of Siri village in the Deoghar district, Jharkhand, used to dish out the same old fare every meal: rice, potatoes and, sometimes, dal (pulses). Despite the fact that wild greens and pumpkins grew in the vicinity of her home, they were never generally cooked because, traditionally, food in the family was all about rice and potatoes. Thousands of kilometers away, in the tribal village of Mundipadar in the Rayagada district in Odisha, Runi, 20 years old, delivered a low-weight baby boy at home. Weighing just 1.2 kg, the newborn was in a critical state, and the couple could not afford the necessary transportation and treatment costs.

Pramila and Runi are only two of the thousands of women living in India, one of the largest democracies in the world. Even after 68 years of independence, the people of India experience extreme malnutrition due to ignorance, poverty and food insecurity and are denied their basic right to survival. The government of India can boast a well-developed constitution and a strong legal system that protect the rights of its citizens, but corruption, bureaucracy, lack of awareness of rights and entitlements and social discrimination limit people's access to basic rights and services, and poor communities – especially women and children – become inevitable victims of this vicious cycle of poverty and malnutrition.

Background

In spite of the significant progress India has achieved in food production and sufficiency over the last 68 years, the majority of the rural population has had to deal with food insecurity on a daily basis year after year, generation after generation. As a result, over one fifth of India's population suffers from chronic hunger. Even though the percentage of malnourished people has dropped by 1 percentage point between 2002 and 2005 [according to the National Family Health Survey (NFHS-3) implemented by the government of India], their number has increased in absolute terms. The Indian figures for stunting, the main indicator of chronic malnutrition, are the highest among all countries globally. The epidemic nature of food insecurity in India coupled with a rapid opening of the agricultural sector to foreign competition has led to a rise in rural poverty and a reduction in food security. The distribution of vastly subsidized imported food grains from developed countries (as well as internally produced food grains) has adversely affected local varieties of produce and has led to a serious change in consumption patterns. Farmers have shifted to cash crops at the expense of their own food security. At the same time, in the last decade, this collapse in rural livelihood and income has occurred simultaneously with a higher overall rate of GDP growth.

The lack of accurate data, another major problem in India, considerably hinders appropriate planning. The last NFHS was conducted 10 years ago. A recent Rapid

Survey on Children (RSOC), which was conducted by UNICEF and the Indian government in 2013–2014, showed a reduction in the proportion of underweight children from 42.5 to 30%; unfortunately, the full study has not yet been published.

In India, malnutrition, hunger and poverty are not so much a problem of availability but rather of governance, in terms of inequality in access to food, rights and services. Even though the Indian government has set up 28 programs for poverty reduction, undernutrition rates are still very high due to poor governance, corruption and illiteracy, with Dalits (lowest caste), ethnic minorities and women being the most severely affected. Based on the above situation, Public Interest Litigations were filed by activists and 2 very pertinent movements on the rights to information and food gathered momentum in India in the early 20th century, giving rise to the Right to Information Act (2005) and the Right to Food Act (2013). These events transformed these programs to rights and shifted the situation from a welfare-based system to a rights-based system [1].

The Rights-Based Approach: Why Is It the Best Approach for India?

In India's functioning democracy, malnutrition and hunger have never been given the proper consideration on the electoral agenda. As elections are one of the few mechanisms that allow the state to connect with its citizens, a multitude of issues are addressed through them – this tends to work against single big issues like hunger, which are often neglected.

Based on the Indian constitution, the government of India initiated 'safety net' programs in India to provide special benefits for below-poverty-line [2] households; these programs include the Public Distribution System (PDS) for subsidized foods [3], old age and widow pensions, the 100 days employment scheme (NREGS) [4], the Mid-Day Meal in primary schools, supplementary nutrition for pregnant and lactating women and for 6- to 59-month-old children provided by the Integrated Child Development Services (ICDS) [5] and health care services provided by the National Health Mission [6]. These are meant to cover all categories of the population, but in reality, there are high levels of exclusion, as these programs were used as incentives by politicians. As a result, though there has been a tremendous increase in the coverage of villages under the ICDS in the past decade, including significant improvements in PDS, increases in fund utilization by the NREGS and improvements in health service coverage based on government reports, India continues to host the highest number of undernourished children in the world. Despite the tremendous economic progress made by India, there has been a limited reduction in poverty, as 32.7% of people in India live on less than USD 1 a day (NLiS) [7]. Malnutrition in the form of anemia, stunting, low birth weight, low BMI among women of reproductive age and wasting among children 0–3 years old continues to prevail despite India's opulence.

Evidence shows that there is little or no information regarding these entitlements and that the complicated procedures of applying for benefits hampers vulnerable communities. Village development plans and fund allocations are controlled by people with vested interests who are supported by powerful middlemen (contractors) and control the villages' economies. The commitment and motivation of the grassroots providers is also affected by the corruption among officials and elected representatives.

Runi's and Pramila's villages are no exceptions. Though all programs and services are officially being implemented in the villages, the trajectory of their lives remains gloomy. Village Health and Nutrition Days (VHNDs), mandatory events in every village that provide health services to women of reproductive age and children between 0 and 5 years old, are not observed in Pramila's village in Jharkhand. 'No one attends, and the service providers idle around the whole day without a single woman or child showing up', says Pramila. According to nongovernmental organization (NGO) worker Rajesh Jha, 'people like Pramila had no idea about the VHND because they had never witnessed such an event in their village'. A 2011 study of 3,700 households carried out by a group of NGOs working on this health crisis highlighted the fact that every 12th child in the Deoghar district (where Pramila lives) is severely malnourished. Pramila was in fact not the only one who was cooking a carbohydrate-rich meal in the region: 'The reality is that people were not aware of the need to have an adequate and balanced diet: it was only quantity that mattered', continued Rajesh. Health and nutrition education is the prerogative of ICDS centers, which were set up under the Ministry of Social Welfare to address the nutritional needs of all pregnant women and children between 0 and 5 years old. In Pramila's village, however, only 55.3% of pregnant women were registered with the local ICDS, and most of them received the daily supplementary nutrition only once during their entire pregnancy.

Similarly, in Hikini village in Odisha, where Runi and 63 other tribal families live, the ICDS was never very popular. Deepa Mundika, a mother of 2 infants, says: 'The ICDS worker had always been irregular, and the community just had no idea of what she was supposed to do or what the benefits of a functioning anganwadi [local term for an ICDS center] were.'

Money is a constraint for Pramila, because her husband, Nirmal Majhi, is a daily wage laborer and manages to find work based on the National Rural Employment Guarantee Act only occasionally, as the NREGS is malfunctioning. No one applies for jobs, as payments are irregular and compensation is not given when there are no jobs.

The PDS shops are marred with irregularities in supply, quality and compromised quantities. 'We lost hope that we could ever get cheap rice. We are illiterate and poor and cannot raise our voice against the officials', said Rajibo Pusika, a lady living in Runi's villages.

These and many other anecdotes make it clear that in India, the main problem of malnutrition is not a lack of schemes and programs but rather the exclusion of marginalized communities and poor implementation due to bad governance and corruption. The best way to overcome this is to empower communities to fight for their rights and entitlements. Indian citizens need to understand the mandate of the government to respect, protect and fulfill the rights of its citizens.

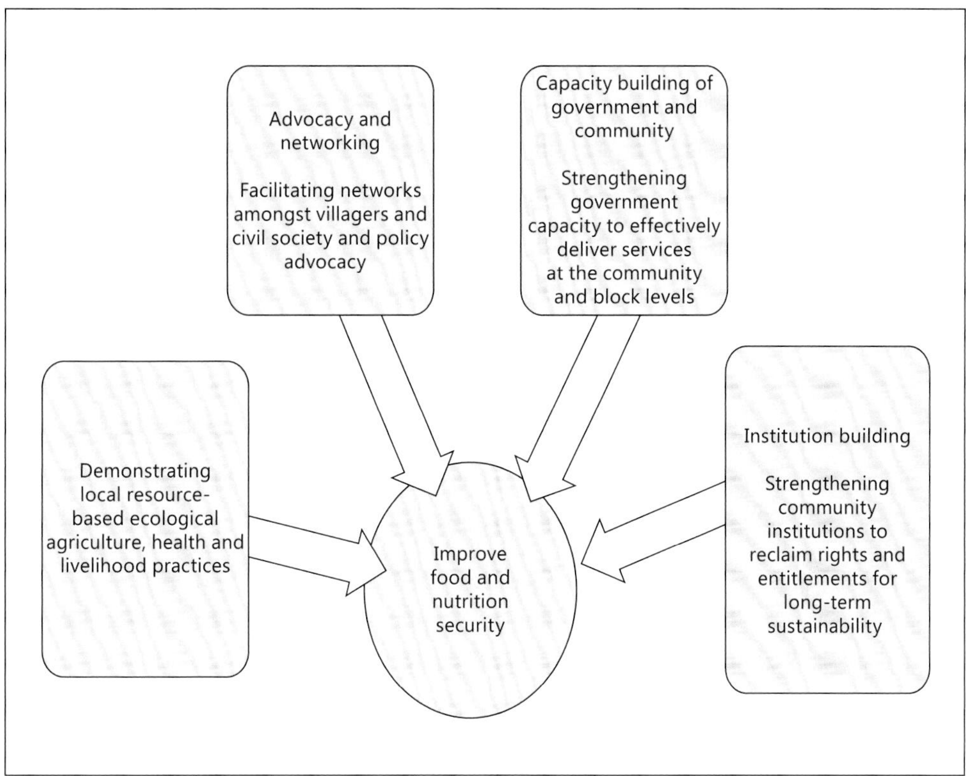

Fig. 1. The strategic approach of the FHFI to improve the quality and coverage of government services and utilization of the existing resources to improve food and nutrition security.

The Fight Hunger First Initiative

The Fight Hunger First Initiative (FHFI) in South Asia is a rights-based, long-term program implemented by Welthungerhilfe (one of Germany's largest nongovernmental aid organizations, fighting against hunger and poverty since 1962), which focuses specifically on improving income, food and nutrition security in deprived communities in India by ensuring that adequate welfare systems are in place and that basic rights are fulfilled. Only then can people break this vicious cycle and can the new generation of disadvantaged groups look forward to a new and better future in which growth benefits the entire society.

The FHFI project, started in 2011, was implemented in three states of India covering approximately 196,000 people, particularly those from low castes and tribal populations, including 38,000 households in 299 villages. The project aims to make women like Pramila and Runi aware of their existing rights and entitlements and enable them to access these entitlements by holding service providers accountable.

Table 1. Malnutrition in India (2005–2006)

- Stunting in children under 3 years of age: 44%
- Wasting in children under 3 years of age: 22.9%
- Anemia in children under 3 years of age: 78.9%
- Vitamin A deficiency among preschoolers: 62%
- Anemia among women of reproductive age: 56%
- BMI <18 among women of reproductive age: 33%
- Exclusive breastfeeding of infants under 6 months old: 71.6%

Data source – National Family Health Survey (NFHS-3) 2005, Government of India.

The initiative has been successful in making food available for 2 additional months and generating a 25% enhancement in income for farmers who tried out new techniques in 3 years. Household diet diversity moved from 'poor' to 'average'. Village institutions like women's groups, farmers' groups, youth groups and networks have been strengthened and are now able to take up issues with the local administration. People's participation in village-level planning and budgeting has increased. Access to quality mid-day meals and supplementary nutrition has improved, with more than 80% of target groups receiving these benefits.

The formation of community-based organizations and the support offered to formal committees like the Panchayati Raj Institution [8] has led to community empowerment through people's institutions. Existing committees on forest protection, school management, village health sanitation and nutrition, etc., have been strengthened. To prioritize women's issues, women have been encouraged to actively participate in such collectives. Since 2012, 20 women from Patangpahar, near Runi's village, have come together and formed 4 informal groups of 5 members each, who collect forest produce and firewood on a rotating basis. They safeguard the area from miscreants as well as the timber mafia and have come up with certain informal rules for the community to follow while gathering forest products [9].

When school teachers in Madanpur, Jharkhand, went on a 2-month strike in late 2012, a group of young girls from the village formed the 'Jyoti Yuvati Club' and convinced the school management to let them oversee the day-to-day functioning and teaching at the local Madanpur primary school to avoid disruptions in the education provided.

'Community scorecards' have proven to be a successful social accountability tool to bring community and service providers together to resolve problems and remove obstacles, and this tool has been used effectively by the community. In Devipur the Community Score Card (CSC) tool helped to strengthen government schemes and monitoring committees like the 'Village Health Sanitation and Nutrition Committee', the school Mid-Day Meal program and the performance of the health workers, etc. As a result, the ICDS center in Pramila's village is now open 6 days a week, and VHNDs are organized monthly at the center.

Extensive training and capacity building for service providers of government departments and elected representatives have considerably enhanced the quality and coverage of services. Demonstrations on recipes for low-cost weaning foods, awareness generation and capacity-building of cadres who support grassroots service providers have also been carried out to improve services.

Village-based institutions were brought together as federations and networks. There are district-, state- and national-level federations, like the Right to Food Network, the Coalition for Sustainable Nutrition in India [10], the Right to Education Network, and farmers' networks. State- and national-level consultations have been conducted to reach out to civil society and government departments to influence political manifestos and bring about policy changes. Women's groups from Odisha came together to negotiate terms with the Forest Department [11]. 'We told them that we don't want these useless trees in our forest. If you want to regenerate the forest, please plant trees that we want – those that will give us food, fodder and shelter', recalls Tamba Tuika, a woman from Patanga Pahar. The entire village stood up to the Forest Department, which finally agreed to provide saplings of mango, jackfruit, mahua, guava, etc. According to Bichitra Biswal, an NGO worker, 120 women across 60 villages in Bissam Cuttack and Muniguda are currently part of the forest protection movement.

The concept of integrated farming systems – an improved version of mixed cropping – has been introduced to the communities to demonstrate the benefits of using not only crops but also varied types of plants, animals, bird, fish and other aquatic flora and fauna for production. Improved water harvesting systems using local resources have been mainstreamed to increase crop production and reduce hunger periods.

Micro-level planning and linkages with government schemes have been proven successful in increasing knowledge about the procedure for accessing entitlements and in ensuring better utilization of government resources. School sanitation and other water, sanitation and hygiene interventions have been used to educate schoolchildren and youth. Kitchen gardening, school nutrition gardens and use of wastewater have also been promoted to improve the availability of food throughout the year. 'The kitchen garden model has proven to be a godsend. Earlier, the students used to get only khichdi (rice and lentils) and potatoes. However, with our girls maintaining the garden, where they grow green leafy vegetables as well as gourds and beans, the children get the best vegetables in their daily meals', says Basudev Singh, the father of Mamata Kumari, 14, another member of the Jyoti Yuvati Club at Mandanpur in Devipur. In Madanpur, 364 families have created kitchen gardens, and 1,024 farmers have introduced improved farming technologies to enhance their production and dietary diversity: the majority of households in Pramila's village, including hers, now consume 5–8 food groups a day.

Stories from the Ground

When Runi had declined to visit the local health center, a fellow village member, the septuagenarian Draupadi Pidikaka, stepped in. She spoke to the couple and pointed out that it did not cost much to reach the health center and that all the services would be free of charge. Women from the village group accompanied the couple and lent them some money. The service providers also accompanied Runi to the hospital. The women's group members had learnt about these health services and care practices from the Participatory Learning and Action (PLA) [12] village meetings cycles carried out under the FHFI program. Once Runi, after this experience, realized the significance of the PLA meetings, she has been a regular member. 'It was my first child, and I had no idea how to care for a baby. However, through the PLAs, I have learnt many things about motherhood and newborn care, like thermal protection, early breast feeding and proper diets for mother. Now, I am well trained, and I tell others about it, as well', says the confident young mother. The group used community scorecards [13] to urge the ICDS worker to distribute food packets. When she did not listen to them, the women marched to the office of the Child Development Project Officer to protest. 'All the village women got together and went to the CDPO [Child Development Project Officer] and informed her of the irregularities. The ICDS worker was given a strict warning, and ever since, she has been carrying out her duty diligently', concludes Deepa, a women from Runi's village, with a satisfied smile.

When activists and nutritionists of the local NGO first came to Parmila Hembram to talk to her about including all three colors of the Indian national flag 'Tiranga' (tricolor) – orange, white and green – in her family's daily diet, she was confused. Today, Pramila, who is expecting her second child, is conscious of what she eats and makes it a point to incorporate foods rich in iron and calcium in every meal. 'I know I need to eat "tiranga bhojan" (tricolor food) in order to be a healthy mother', she explains. 'We get yellow from the lentils; the green comes from leafy vegetables and white from the rice and milk. I ensure that the tricolor is present in all our meals. I have seen the difference it has made to my child! He has definitely grown taller; his skin is clearer and his hair is black and thick.' For a steady supply of greens and other veggies in her kitchen, Parmila has created a small food garden. The leafy pumpkin and gourd creepers hang temptingly from her rooftop. And whatever is surplus she sells in the weekly village market to make some quick money. What Pramila did not know at the beginning was that a sustained imbalanced intake was making her family vulnerable to ill health and putting her 4-year-old son, Pramod, at risk of malnutrition. Information is power.

Table 2. Rights-based approach: a shift in mindset

From	To
Beneficiary	Citizen
Needs	Rights and responsibilities
Consultation	Decision making
Improving living conditions	Improving living conditions and making structural changes
Micro level	Integration of the micro, meso and macro levels
Project	Policy

Conclusions

The rights-based approach is about information, empowerment and accountability. Such an approach is time-consuming, as the mobilization of the community and the strengthening of community-based organizations involves a lot of planning and strategizing. Collectivization and information sharing are often resisted by local leaders, as ignorance is the easiest way to control people. Often, different political parties get elected at the different tiers of the 3-tier local governance structure, which may cause difficulty or obstruction in the sanction of development funds for the villages. Advocacy and liaison with government departments and the local authorities can minimize the impact of conflicts and bridge gaps between the community and the service providers. The 3 major lessons from the first phase of the program are the following:

1 Promotion of LANN using the PLA methodology is useful in sensitizing and generating action on the immediate, underlying and basic causes of malnutrition
2 Changing mind-set: shift from community development to rights-based approach
3 Empowering community institutions through skill-based training on village microplanning, the role of the village assembly, government schemes and budget allocations.

Further Reading

1. Economist: Daily chart: India's malnourished infants. 2015. http://www.economist.com/blogs/graphicdetail/2015/07/daily-chart-0.
2. Bose P: India is breaking the vicious cycle of poverty, malnutrition. 2014. pratimview.blogspot.com/2014/.../india-is-breaking-vicious-cycle-of.htm.
3. Chellan R, Paul L, Kulkarni PM: Incidence of low-birth-weight in India: regional variations and socio-economic disparities. 2007. http://www.academia.edu/4276402/Incidence_of_Low-Birth-Weight_in_India_Regional_Variations_and_Socio-Economic_Disparities.
4. Women's Feature Service – WFS: Women news. www.wfsnews.org/.
5. Welthungerhilfe South Asia: Fight hunger first initiative. http://welthungerhilfesouthasia.org/our-programmes/initiatives/fhfi/#!/post-1188/.

References

1 National Food Security Act 2013. 2013. India.gov.in/national-food-security-act-2013. www.righttoinformation.gov.in (accessed February 8, 2016).
2 Extreme poverty. http://scroll.in/article/740875/670-million-people-in-rural-india-live-on-rs-33-per-day (accessed February 8, 2016).
3 Department of Food and Public Distribution. 2015. dfpd.nic.in/?q=node/101 (accessed February 8, 2016).
4 Ministry of Rural Development: Mahatma Gandhi National Rural Employment Gurantee Act 2005. 2014. www.nrega.nic.in/ (accessed February 8, 2016).
5 Ministry of Women and Child Development: Integrated child development services. 2015. http://india.gov.in/official-website-ministry-women-and-child-development-0 (accessed February 8, 2016).
6 National Rural Health Mission. 2013. http://nrhm.gov.in/nhm/nrhm.html (accessed February 8, 2016).
7 Nutrition Landscape Information System: Nutrition Landscape Information System (NLIS) country profile. 2015. www.who.int/nutrition/nlis/en (accessed February 8, 2016).
8 Wikipedia, The Free Encyclopedia: Panchayati raj. 2015. https://en.wikipedia.org/wiki/Panchayati_raj (accessed February 8, 2016).
9 Forest Rights Act, 2006 – Ministry of Tribal Affairs. tribal.nic.in/WriteReadData/.../201211290332077861328File1033.pdf (accessed February 8, 2016).
10 Coalition for Sustainable Nutrition Security in India. 2013. http://www.nutritioncoalition.in/ (accessed February 8, 2016).
11 http://www.wfsnews.org/whh-wfs_fhfi_inside-2013.html (accessed February 8, 2016).
12 Thomas S: What is participatory learning and action (PLA): an introduction. idp-key-resources.org/documents/0000/d04267/000.pdf (accessed February 8, 2016).
13 http://www.care.org/sites/default/files/documents/FP-2013-CARE_CommunityScoreCardToolkit.pdf (accessed February 8, 2016).

Sweta Banerjee, Nutritionist
Welthungerhilfe
South Extension Phase II
New Delhi 110049 (India)
E-Mail sweta.banerjee@welthungerhilfe.de

Biesalski HK, Black RE (eds): Hidden Hunger. Malnutrition and the First 1,000 Days of Life: Causes, Consequences and Solutions. World Rev Nutr Diet. Basel, Karger, 2016, vol 115, pp 203–210
DOI: 10.1159/000442106

What Political Framework Is Necessary to Reduce Malnutrition? A Civil Society Perspective

Bernhard Walter

Brot für die Welt – Evangelischer Entwicklungsdienst, Berlin, Germany

Abstract

Around 800 million people worldwide are still starving. Around 2 billion are somehow able to allay their hunger yet remain malnourished because their food does not contain sufficient nutrients. There are many reasons for this: for people living in poverty and precarious conditions, the priority is to fill their stomach, and the quality of food seems less important. Since the 1960s, global food production has been focused on increasing yield, not food quality. Mass-produced convenience food with high fat and carbohydrate contents but containing few nutrients is on the rise and – as a result of price wars – often replaces healthier locally grown products. To overcome global hunger and malnutrition, civil society organizations urge governments to turn towards sustainable and human rights-based development, including sustainable agricultural and fishing policies, to contribute to the eradication of poverty. This development is first and foremost guided by the right to food. In a policy that enables farmers to produce enough food that is healthy and rich in nutrients, the following principles should be fulfilled. Governments should assume responsibility for the international impacts of their agricultural policy decisions. The food sovereignty of other countries should be respected. Policies should enable self-supply of the population with healthy food and should promote the protection of resources, the climate, biodiversity and animal welfare. Strengthening rural structures, local economies, labor rights and small-scale food producers, establishing public programs that provide locally produced food, applying stringent standards for food labeling and the regulation of unhealthy products and paying special attention to the first 1,000 days of life as the starting point of a good and healthy well-being are core elements of such a political framework.

Eating enough, eating healthily and having a balanced diet are essential prerequisites for human development. Nevertheless, 800 million people worldwide are still starving. A further 2 billion are somehow able to allay their hunger yet remain malnourished as their food does not contain sufficient nutrients.

There are many reasons for this: for people living in poverty and precarious conditions, the priority is to fill their stomach, and the quality of food seems less important. Since the 1960s, global food production has been focused on increasing yield, not food quality. Mass-produced convenience food with high fat and carbohydrate contents but containing few nutrients are on the rise and – as a result of price wars – often replace healthier locally grown products. Knowledge about nutrition is a prerequisite for healthy eating, even more so when old eating habits and traditions have been destroyed or replaced. Understanding what is good for one's body and what is not requires at least a basic awareness of food quality and nutrient requirements.

Malnourished people are less able-bodied and mentally productive and are also more prone to illness. This particularly affects children: the lack of proper nutrition in early childhood causes long-lasting harm. Therefore, it is very important to raise the population's awareness of the importance of a balanced, healthy and affordable diet, of nutritional requirements and of the available information about crop cultivation, resource conservation and natural fertilizer use. As many people as possible should get a chance to learn how to grow their own healthy food – especially women, as within their families, women are mainly responsible for food and nutrition.

The Whole World Can Eat Healthily

Still, malnutrition is also increasing in our part of the world. Malnutrition causes illness, contributes to the waste of resources and sets a poor example by establishing unsustainable trends all over the world. Imitating a Western lifestyle hugely promotes diseases of civilization, such as diabetes, in the countries of the Global South. The corresponding treatments, however, are affordable only for the very few.

Worldwide, around 800 million women, men and children are suffering from chronic hunger. An additional 2 billion suffer from malnutrition and, although they consume enough calories so as not to go to bed hungry, they are still a long way from a healthy, active and dignified life. To achieve such a life would require important micronutrients such as vitamins, iodine, iron, protein and zinc. Even overweight people may be affected by nutrient deficiency if they consume too many empty calories in the form of white flour, saturated fats and sugar. Their number is increasing in all parts of the world. About 1.4 billion people are overweight, 500 million of whom are obese. Thus, almost half of the seven billion people worldwide suffer from hunger and malnutrition. This is a man-made problem. In the past, politics and the economy have focused too heavily on increasing food production. The Green Revolution of the 1960s relied on technological solutions, monocultures, chemical fertilizers and pest management. Staple foods such as rice, corn, wheat and potatoes were cultivated, and these foods are rich in starch but contain very few dietary elements.

Uniformity over Diversity

Contemporary plant breeding is going in the same direction. The priority is to produce first and foremost very large crops. The variety in the fields and on our plates, however, is decreasing. Our food is being turned into a uniform mash. Instead of varied and nutritious crops, people throughout the world primarily consume carbohydrates, fats and sugar. Pizza, fried food and soft drinks have conquered the world and, in particular, the cities.

Humankind is paying a high price for the industrialization of its agricultural and food systems. The economic, social and ecological costs are tremendous: the population is becoming sicker and less efficient, straining the sustainability of health systems. Biodiversity is diminishing, the soil structure is being destroyed, greenhouse gas emissions are impacting the environment, and the climate is changing. Land grabbing has assumed gigantic proportions. The booming meat industry requires more and more land for the cultivation of fodder. Our oceans are overfished. Food produced in this way does not reach the people who need it. Crop losses are too high, crop transportation distances are too long, and crop prices are too high for the poor. In rich countries like Germany, vast quantities of food end up in waste bins. To a large extent, this is caused by inappropriate subsidies, unfair trade structures, and the power of advertising and lobbying work by multinational corporations.

Strengthening Rural Structures

Rural development is the key to fighting hunger and malnutrition. Seventy to 80% of all people suffering from hunger live in rural areas. Smallholder farmers and fishermen would be able to feed their families adequately if they had the requisite knowledge, an intact infrastructure and fair trade conditions. They could even supply the urban population with healthy local products. Thus, rural structures have to be strengthened. Ecological agriculture based on soil conservation, biodiversity, home-grown seeds, traditionally cultivated plants and social cohesion can provide the world with sustainable, healthy food. One of the focal points is the advancement of women. Women usually assume the caretaker role in families: they take care of supplies for the smallholding farmer, manage the house and the farm, and take responsibility for the health, hygiene and diet of their children. Nevertheless, women are dramatically disadvantaged in most societies. If the goal of qualitatively adequate and sufficient food for everyone is to be achieved, then it is indispensable to take a stand for equal opportunities. A world without hunger and shortages is possible but requires the enormous political willpower of everyone involved. This applies to both rich and poor countries worldwide and to multinational corporations as well as consumers. Everyone can contribute.

Why the First 1,000 Days Are so Important

The problem of malnutrition begins in the womb. The first 1,000 days of life are decisive for the opportunities a person will have later in life. If a child does not receive adequate calories and nutrients from the beginning of pregnancy until its second birthday, its physical and mental development may be irretrievably damaged. Long-term (health) effects such as blindness, learning disabilities or anemia as well as chronic diseases like diabetes are potential consequences of malnutrition. To seriously combat hunger and malnutrition, it is important to start with the nutrition of pregnant women and mothers. If mothers eat healthily, their children will benefit, too: they will be born with a normal birth weight and be less prone to diseases and developmental delays. A mother who breastfeeds her infant will increase her child's chances for a healthy, active and self-determined life. Malnourished mothers, however, will pass on their deficits to the next generation, perpetuating the cycle of hunger, malnutrition and poverty.

Food Is a Human Right

Nutrition is at the center of human rights. Everyone is entitled to adequate food and nutrition, and an understanding of nutrition is the expression of culture, traditions, and social relations; therefore, the right to adequate food can only be fulfilled in the context of food sovereignty. Civil society organizations (CSOs) understand food sovereignty to be a precondition for food security and the achievement of sustainable nutrition. Food sovereignty is the right of people to define their own policies and strategies for sustainable production, distribution, and consumption of food, with respect to their own identities and systems of managing natural resources. The interdependencies of a healthy environment, food sovereignty, food security and nutrition should not be underestimated. Therefore, CSOs are deeply concerned about the impacts of the agro-industrial model, which result in the degradation, contamination and severe affectation of ecosystems, soil, water and other productive resources. All people have the right to healthy, safe and chemical-free food.

CSOs recognize the relationship between existing threats to reproductive and maternal health, environmental violence and contamination. Women and girls are disproportionately affected by malnutrition and by the realization of the right to adequate food and nutrition. Globally and across the rural-urban continuum, socio-economic inequalities between men and women have direct impacts on nutrition. Nutrition starts with women. Their sexual and reproductive rights need to be respected and guaranteed. In many communities, women are responsible for much of the work of food cultivation, harvesting and processing, as well as for providing meals for the family, but many women lack access to adequate food and nutrition education. CSOs support the inclusion of the issue of breastfeeding as a matter of not only nutrition and early childhood development but also traditional and inherent rights of infants and women. These rights have been compromised due to discrimination, harassment, and false information about the nutritional value of breastmilk and manufactured, chemically enhanced formula. Breastfeeding represents the very first guarantee of the human right to healthy food and nutrition.

CSOs demand a human-rights based approach to nutrition and food, which is understood through the lens of existing human rights standards, including but not limited to the International Covenant on Civil and Political Rights, the International Covenant on Economic and Social Rights, the Universal Declaration of Human Rights, the Convention on the Elimination of All Forms of Racial Discrimination, the Convention on the Elimination of All Forms of Discrimination against Women, the Convention on the Rights of the Child, the International Convention on the Protection of the Rights of All Migrant Workers and Members of the Their Families, the United Nations (UN) Declaration on the Rights of Indigenous Peoples and the Convention on the Rights of Persons with Disabilities.

In the near term, CSOs urge state governments and corporations to act on the UN Guiding Principles on Business and Human Rights, including the state obligation to protect human rights, the corporate responsibility to respect human rights, and the right to a remedy for victims of business-related abuses. Regarding this point, CSOs are concerned about the content of the UN Global Compact on Business and Human Rights and the concept of 'corporate social responsibility', which can be manipulated to shield corporations from true accountability with the complicity of state governments. CSOs are deeply concerned with the corporate takeover of food systems, wherein nutrition has become an industry unto itself, creating business and generating revenue not through the provision of real nutritious food but rather through the replacement of nutritious food with expensive supplements that do not meet the nutritional needs of people.

Strengthening Local Economies

The characterization of nutritional 'emergencies' in situations of urgent and protracted crises has promoted and reinforced international and regional aid programs and 'solutions' that tend to be carried out without consulting local communities and that do not meet the real nutritional needs of affected communities. This has the effect of demoralizing and devastating local economies while undermining social movements and potentially creating new conflicts. UN agencies, donors, NGOs and states must endeavor to understand the consequences of such projects and work towards more integrated solutions and approaches. This is particularly important in light of the current state of refugees and internally displaced persons, as well as the potential of future natural disasters due in part to climate change and the insufficiency of measures to address climate change.

CSOs note with alarm the ongoing diminishment of governance, particularly the capture of policy space by governments and correlated corporations at the local, regional, national, and international levels. This includes public-private partnerships, which frequently result in strengthened corporate lobbies and influence. Weakened governance and corporate capture of policy space directly contradict the rights-based advocacy of social movements all over the world. Furthermore, shrinking space for governments is resulting in a loss of accountability of governments in relation to food, nutrition and beyond. Finally, corporate capture of policy space related to nutrition and food poses substantial risks to human and environmental health, social welfare, and the future of agriculture and fisheries. Public policy must be in the public interest, and conflicts of interest need to be fully addressed.

Public Procurement from Local Producers

Governments at all levels should implement public procurement policies that source food from local small-scale producers. Regional and inter-governmental bodies should similarly adapt their policy frameworks for regulating public procurement. International regimes should also promote sustainable food systems by not adopting policies that prohibit local procurement. It is necessary to formally establish adequate mechanisms for consumers to have access to healthy fresh foods from small producers.

Standards in Food Labeling and Regulation of Unhealthy Products

The role of communications, information and media is vital to the appropriate development of public policies. As such, all information, communications and media of transnationals and other corporations require regulation and monitoring. The rights of consumers include adequate information and consumer education free of corporate influence that alerts people of risks. In this regard, we need more stringent standards in food labeling that address risk rather than disclosure of misleading benefits. Food labeling must go beyond the current minimum standard requirements and disclosures as commonly agreed.

CSOs demand regulations that prohibit all marketing of unhealthy, ultra-processed products high in sugar, fat and/or salt, including formulas, infant and small-children foods promoted to parents, children and youth. In poor communities, a lack of access to healthy food combined with a barrage of highly processed food from transnational and other food corporations is fueling the epidemics of obesity, diabetes and other diet-related diseases. Effectively tackling issues of hunger and malnutrition in all its forms and diet-related diseases would encourage communities to become active participants in shaping food systems in cooperation with small-scale food producers in surrounding areas while contributing to food sovereignty. CSOs emphasize the fundamental role that nutrition has to play as a preventive measure in the achievement of good health. Food is medicine, but medicine is not food.

Strengthening Labor Rights and Small-Scale Food Producers

An adequate standard of living is inclusive of conditions that maintain healthy living, from food to water, sanitation, housing, and health. Some of those who are most disproportionately affected are the workers who grow, harvest and process food but lack a living wage to support their own household nutrition, food security and quality of life. A core prerequisite to achieving this goal is labor rights. There is a clear link between low wages and poor nutrition. The answer is not to give supplements to workers but rather to ask employers to pay all workers living wages so that they can buy nutritious foods for themselves and their families.

Small-scale food producers, including family farmers, indigenous peoples, fishing communities and pastoralists, should be at the center of any strategy to combat malnutrition, as reinforced by the Food and Agricultural Organization International Year of Family Farming. In this regard, overcoming socio-economic environmental challenges and achieving sustainable nutrition in local communities is best served through the promotion and support of small-scale sustainable and agro-ecological food production focused on local markets. CSOs imperatively demand the protection of native and peasant seeds, as well as centers of origin, from the invasion and contamination of genetically modified seeds that affect biodiversity and ecosystems and that affect humanity of the current generations, the unborn and the lives to come. CSOs and social movements are well placed to provide positive contributions in the form of best practices in sustainable nutrition using local resources. Food systems based on indigenous and traditional knowledge can offer important contributions to collective progress towards sustainable food systems and nutrition.

CSOs urge states, local governments and authorities to ensure equitable distribution of food through the creation of effectively functioning public distribution systems, such as school meal programs and maternal and child support programs. Officials need to pay specific attention to meeting the needs of vulnerable populations, including women, children, senior citizens, indigenous peoples and the chronically ill or disabled. Furthermore, education regarding nutrition and food must be widely distributed and culturally appropriate. CSOs are concerned about the appropriation of education related to nutrition, food and food systems by transnational and other corporations with the complicity of state governments.

European Countries Are Not without Responsibility

To overcome global hunger and malnutrition, CSOs urge European policymakers to consider the following principles:

- Assume responsibility for the international effects of agricultural policy decisions
- Respect the food sovereignty of other countries and help them to become independent in their food supplies
- Enable self-supply of the population with healthy food
- Promote the protection of resources, the climate, animal welfare and biodiversity

To implement such principles, the export orientation of the Common Agricultural Policy of the European Union (EU) has to be moderated. In many countries, European food exports threaten food sovereignty. European over-production is based on the import of livestock feed and agricultural commodities from developing and newly industrialized countries, where their cultivation causes land conflicts, human rights violations and loss of biodiversity. A further step is the reliable and sustainable support of small farmers and fishermen worldwide. For example, small fisheries need protected coastal zones to save resources and implement sustainable fishing techniques. In the long term, support through public funds must be adjusted to the desired aims of society: security of supply, climate protection, preservation of biodiversity, maintenance of cultural landscapes and preservation of sustainable, regional structures. The EU and its member states should make an appropriate share of their development budgets available for this purpose. Finally, the EU and its member states should support agricultural research that places a much greater focus on the promotion of smallholder farm production so that these farmers are able to produce enough healthy food for themselves and for others.

Dr. Bernhard Walter
Brot für die Welt – Evangelischer Entwicklungsdienst
Caroline-Michaelis-Strasse 1
DE–10115 Berlin (Germany)
E-Mail bernhard.walter@brot-fuer-die-welt.de

Biesalski HK, Black RE (eds): Hidden Hunger. Malnutrition and the First 1,000 Days of Life: Causes, Consequences and Solutions. World Rev Nutr Diet. Basel, Karger, 2016, vol 115, pp 211–223
DOI: 10.1159/000442107

The Role of Food Fortification in Addressing Iron Deficiency in Infants and Young Children

Jörg Spieldenner

Nestlé Research Center, Lausanne, Switzerland

Abstract

Iron deficiency, one of the most widespread nutritional disorders, affects millions of people in emerging economies and, increasingly, in industrialized countries. Due to the high iron requirements during growth and development, infants and young children are among those most severely affected by iron deficiency. Iron deficiency that occurs during the critical phases of early life development has long-lasting health consequences that are reflected in increased risk of disease, reduced economic productivity and premature death, underscoring the importance of infants and young children as a key target group for addressing iron deficiency. This chapter focuses on the use of fortified foods as a cost-effective mechanism to address iron deficiency in this particularly vulnerable subpopulation. Nutritional policies that include food fortification need to be implemented within the context of effective public-private partnerships in order to address the fundamental mechanisms of accessibility, affordability and availability of nutritious food items for those in the lowest socio-economic strata.

Hidden Hunger: An Invisible Burden with Tangible Consequences

According to the Millennium Development Goals report of 2014, the proportion of undernourished people in developing regions has decreased from 24% in 1990–1992 to 14% in 2011–2013 [1]. Nevertheless, the fact remains that 1 in 7 children below 5 years of age is moderately or severely underweight, and 162 million young children are still suffering from chronic undernutrition. Although some regions such as Eastern and Southeastern Asia have managed to curb extreme poverty and are on track to halve the proportion of people who suffer from hunger (1990–2015), other regions (notably Sub-Saharan Africa and South Asia) are unlikely to meet the 2015 targets [1].

Malnutrition is defined as the inadequate or imbalanced intake of nutrients and energy with respect to the body's demands, resulting in suboptimal growth, maintenance, and bodily functions [2]. Of note, the term malnutrition encompasses both undernutrition and overnutrition. Individuals whose diets do not provide adequate calories and/or protein to support growth and maintenance and those who are unable to fully utilize the food they eat due to illness suffer from undernutrition. On the other hand, malnutrition also affects those who consume too many calories (overnutrition). Individuals with severe protein-energy malnutrition are nearly immediately recognizable by the presence of marasmus and kwashiorkor, as well as all the intermediate states of withering or wasting. Micronutrient deficiencies, however, are more subtle and aptly termed 'hidden hunger'. Hidden hunger refers to the chronic deficiency of micronutrients essential for health, including vitamins and minerals, and results in conditions that seriously undermine human health and productivity. Although micronutrient deficiencies mainly affect low-income countries, they also play a major role in health-related problems in developed countries, particularly among vulnerable subpopulations [3]. Women of reproductive age and children are at the greatest risk of micronutrient deficiencies. Together, recent global events such as natural disasters, war, volatile food prices, and the transition from rural to urban lifestyles have resulted in a growing prevalence of micronutrient deficiencies, which affect several billion people worldwide [1, 3, 4].

Although the physical signs of micronutrient deficiencies are less overt than those of protein-energy malnutrition, micronutrient deficiency is nevertheless a clinically significant health problem [5]. The most widespread are deficiencies in iron, zinc, vitamin A, iodine, folate, and the B group vitamins. In developing countries, the same population often exhibits deficiencies in multiple micronutrients [6]. In children, deficiencies in key vitamins and minerals impair physical and cognitive development and have consequences that last throughout life. The clinical signs of micronutrient deficiency may not always be apparent, but their effects are nonetheless damaging and frequently life-threatening.

With a focus on iron deficiency in children, this chapter will discuss the role of food fortification as part of the strategy for addressing this widespread micronutrient deficiency.

Iron Deficiency: A Global Problem

Iron deficiency is listed by the WHO as the most commonly occurring micronutrient deficiency worldwide [4, 6]. Often manifesting as iron deficiency anemia, iron deficiency is estimated to affect over 1.6 billion people [6]. Amongst children aged 6–59 months, around 43% are thought to be anemic [6–8]. The WHO currently uses a he-

Table 1. Commonly used parameters for evaluating iron status [11, 35]

Parameter	Comments
Hemoglobin	Easy to measure, practical screening tool, but not a good measure of bodily iron status
Serum ferritin	Good indicator of iron deficiency, but may be affected by inflammation
Transferrin receptor	Reflects late stages of iron deficiency, but less sensitive to inflammation
Transferrin saturation	Marker of circulating iron; may be affected by inflammation

moglobin threshold of <110 g/dl as the definition of anemia for this age group [9]. It is important to note that although anemia is easier to assess, its absence should not be taken as an indicator of sufficient iron status. Indeed, a loss of 20–30% of internal iron stores is necessary for some individuals to exhibit clinical signs of anemia [10–12]. Around 60% of all anemia cases can be attributed to iron deficiency, but the prevalence of iron deficiency is estimated to be around 2.5 times that of iron deficiency anemia [11].

Iron plays an important role in a variety of cellular and biochemical processes. A central role is that of tissue oxygenation: iron is a key component of hemoglobin, a protein necessary for the generation of red blood cells [13]. In humans, hemoglobin is the most abundant iron-containing protein and sequesters over half of the body's total iron stores. The main sites of internal iron storage are the liver and macrophages. Since dietary iron is the only external source of iron, absorption from the gut must be sufficient to meet the body's needs [13]. Iron demand arises from three main processes: tissue oxygenation requirements, red blood cell production, and blood loss from hemorrhage. As the human body does not possess the capacity to actively excrete iron, absorption from the gut is the main mechanism for regulating iron balance [14]. Dietary iron is available in the forms of heme and nonheme iron. The main sources of heme iron are meat and fish. Nonheme iron is present in legumes, pulses, fruits and vegetables, as well as in iron-fortified foods [15]. Compared to nonheme iron, heme iron is more bioavailable and therefore more easily absorbed. However, heme iron represents only a small proportion of total dietary iron intake (a maximum of 15–20% of total iron intake) [16]. Nonheme iron is less readily bioavailable, and its absorption is dependent on the presence of other food components such as calcium, phytic acid and polyphenols [14]. In the absence of heavy physical activity, disease or hemorrhage, iron homeostasis is generally stable in normal adults. A summary of the most commonly used parameters for evaluating iron status is given in table 1.

Iron deficiency occurs when iron supplies are insufficient to meet iron demands and losses [10, 17]. When the body has depleted its iron stores and dietary intake of iron is not sufficient to meet the body's needs, iron supply to tissues is compromised [17–19]. Infants and young children have particularly high iron requirements, due to their rapid growth and development. At birth, normal infants possess sufficient iron stores to meet their needs for the first 4–6 months of life. However, beyond the age of 6 months, these stores become depleted and dietary intake supplies the child's iron needs [11, 14]. The increased hemoglobin production and buildup of internal iron stores mark early childhood as a period with high demand for iron. As such, young children are especially vulnerable to the effects of iron deficiency. With or without anemia, iron deficiency can result in abnormal psychomotor and cognitive development, including impairments in attention span, intelligence, sensory perception, and behavior [20]. Children with iron deficiency anemia also show a reduction in various immune parameters, including cytokine activity and humoral, cell-mediated and nonspecific immune responses [21]. Iron-deficient individuals are also at a higher risk of heavy metal poisoning due to the increased propensity of their gut to absorb other divalent heavy metals, such as cadmium and lead [22, 23]. In children, the clinical signs of iron deficiency manifest as fatigue, poor school performance and decreased work capacity. Studies have demonstrated that children with normal iron status demonstrate better performance at several levels, including in social interaction and cognition [11, 18, 24].

Taken together, these factors underscore the importance of children as a target population for addressing micronutrient deficiencies, particularly iron deficiency. Furthermore, the period comprising gestation and the first 2 years of life is an important phase of child development [25–27]. Preclinical and clinical data have shown that early-life exposure to adverse influences during this period (particularly stress, malnutrition and infection) shapes health and cognitive function throughout life [26, 28]. In terms of economic impact, the burden of micronutrient deficiency is most highly concentrated in the youngest children among the lowest socio-economic groups [29]. A recent study of Filipino children (from 6 to 59 months of age) estimated the total lifetime cost of illness due to deficiencies in iron, vitamin A and zinc to be USD 30 million in direct medical costs, USD 618 million in decreased productivity and 122,138 disability-adjusted life years (DALYs) in terms of other intangible costs [29]. Therefore, addressing iron deficiency in infants and young children would translate into the greatest overall benefits for society in terms of individual health and overall economic benefits.

The Role of Targeted Food Fortification

Addressing iron deficiency in the most vulnerable populations requires a multi-faceted approach, including raising awareness among consumers, improving local food preparation practices, increasing dietary intake of iron-rich foods, and applying fortification strategies (table 2). For most of the world's poor, however, increasing dietary intake of micronutrient-rich foods is beyond their means [30].

Table 2. Strategies for addressing iron deficiency [64]

Strategy	Relevance to low-income populations
Increase overall food consumption	May not be feasible for the poorest
Increase consumption of micronutrient-rich foods	May not be feasible for the poorest
Improve food preparation and cooking techniques	Feasible; requires education and outreach programs, may be costly
Improve food preservation and processing techniques to preserve micronutrient content	Feasible; requires education and outreach programs
Implement food fortification	Feasible; can be cost-effective
Provide food supplementation	Feasible; adverse effects, cost and adherence may be issues

Addressing the nutrient needs of populations in developing countries will be a key driver of success towards achieving the health-related Millennium Development Goals. Recently, the Copenhagen Consensus expert panel ranked food fortification with micronutrients (specifically iron and iodine) among the top 3 international development priorities [4]. The estimated cost of iron fortification (assuming the use of wheat or maize flour as food vehicles) is estimated to be around USD 0.12 per person per year. The greatest returns of iron fortification are seen in terms of increased productivity in manual labor (among adults) and improved cognition, school performance, and future earning potential (among children) [4].

Micronutrient fortification is the addition of appropriate amounts of vitamins and/or minerals to manufactured food items in order to enhance the nutritional content of these items. The goal of food fortification is to increase the intake of particular micronutrient(s) in the target population. Food fortification is an effective tool for reaching populations with poor-quality diets, as well as those whose micronutrient status is compromised by infectious diseases or parasites [4]. There is a large body of evidence that supports food fortification as a practical and cost-effective mechanism to address iron deficiency, particularly for the world's poorest. In developed countries, nationwide food fortification programs are well established and have a long track record of safety and efficacy. Folic acid fortification has been instrumental in preventing birth defects in Canada, the USA and Chile and is the method of choice for reaching the population of women at risk [31]. Over the past decade, the Canadian health authorities have implemented mandatory food fortification requirements for the addition of vitamin D to milk, folic acid to flour, and the replacement of iron or B vitamins lost during food processing [32]. In low- and middle-income countries, there is increasing consumption of certain food products (including milk products, flour, oil, sugar and salt), and the fortification of some of these items has been shown to be effective in improving the population-wide consumption of specific micronutrients such as iodine, iron, zinc and vitamin A [31]. Developing countries, such as Nigeria, that have implemented successful food fortification programs illustrate the importance of public-private sector collaboration in order for such programs to achieve a population-wide effect [31]. Two recent international workshops addressing micronutrient deficiencies in Southeast Asia underscored the central role of the private food industry as a major contributor to successful food fortification programs [31, 33, 34].

The ideal food vehicle for fortification exhibits several key features: (1) it is widely consumed in adequate amounts by the target population, (2) the added micronutrient is safe and does not adversely affect consumer acceptance of the product, and (3) there are sufficient food manufacturing facilities to ensure the feasibility and quality of food fortification [4]. The most widely used types of foods for fortification are staples (such as rice and wheat), condiments (such as sugar, salt and sauces) and commercial manufactured food items (such as dairy products and complementary foods) [35]. However, the overall success of the food fortification strategy depends on the availability, affordability and accessibility of suitable food vehicles. Targeting infants and young children poses a specific set of challenges. First, the food vehicles used must be adapted to their specific dietary needs. Second, the fortified food items must be widely consumed by this age group. Third, along with instructions for safe use, the fortified items must be clearly identified and made available to the parents. Finally, these items must be priced at a level that is financially feasible for the target population. It is known that poor feeding practices are a significant contributing factor to iron deficiency in infants and young children, particularly amongst populations in the lowest socio-economic strata [36–38].

The private food industry has played a major role in developing specific food products suitable for infants and young children, thereby addressing the issue of availability. The development of micronutrient-fortified milk and cereal-based foods is a cornerstone of efforts to address iron deficiency in infants and young children. A systematic review and meta-analysis that included 18 trials evaluated the impact of fortified versus nonfortified milk and cereal-based foods on hematologic outcomes (including the hemoglobin and ferritin levels and the risk of anemia). The total study population consisted of 5,468 children aged from 6 months to 5 years who were located in Asia, Africa, South or Central America, or Europe [39]. The authors found that fortification of complementary foods with iron together with multiple other micronutrients was more effective than fortification with iron alone. Regardless of whether the food items were fortified with other micronutrients, the authors found that children who were fed fortified milk or cereals had a mean increase in hemoglobin and ferritin levels. Similar findings were observed for the effects on anemia: consumption of fortified milk or cereals reduced the risk of suffering from anemia by 50% [39]. The same general conclusions were reported in another meta-analysis that included infants and pre-school children; food fortification was found to result in increased hemoglobin and ferritin levels and reduced risk of anemia [35]. In both meta-analyses, however, the short-term follow-up design of the majority of the primary intervention trials hampered an evaluation of functional health outcomes such as specific disease-related morbidity, weight gain, growth or cognitive development.

One of the challenges in using fortified foods to address iron deficiency in young children is getting the food vehicle to the target population (accessibility). These food items are not often included in national food fortification programs for the general population [39]. The results from the Chilean National Complementary Feeding Program in children aged 11–18 months demonstrated that consumption of iron-fortified milk improved iron status and reduced the prevalence of anemia in the long term. One year after the introduction of the Chilean National Complementary Feeding Program, the prevalence of anemia was 9% – significantly lower than the 27% observed the year before the study ($p < 0.001$). After adjusting for confounding factors, consumption of iron-fortified milk was associated with higher hemoglobin concentrations and a lower prevalence of anemia [40]. These beneficial effects were apparent 10 years after the implementation of the program, suggesting its sustained long-term efficacy in improving iron status and reducing the prevalence of anemia in children. The Chilean example provides a roadmap for a population-wide fortification program that includes infants and young children as targets for intervention, underscoring the importance of policymakers and local governments as drivers of success.

The WHO recommendations for complementary feeding suggest that this practice should begin at 6 months of age; the European Society for Paediatric Gastroenterology Hepatology and Nutrition recommendations suggest introducing complementary foods between 4 and 6 months of age [41, 42]. However, there is little evidence-based guidance on the type of complementary foods to use or how the various types of complementary foods affect infant growth, nutritional status, and long-term health outcomes. In order to effectively promote the introduction of complementary feeding by the population, complementary foods for infants need to be affordable, locally available and relevant to the food availability and dietary practices of the region. Data from studies conducted in different countries support the feasibility of using fortified local complementary foods to improve the iron status in young children [43, 44]. A 3-month study of 81 Zambian infants (6 months old) evaluated the effects of local fortified complementary food blends on growth and hemoglobin levels and assessed whether the introduction of complementary foods affected breast milk intake [45]. Control infants did not receive complementary foods. The hemoglobin concentrations were significantly higher in the infants who received the fortified complementary foods, but breast milk intake was not affected by complementary food introduction [45]. These findings suggest that locally produced fortified complementary foods were not only effective in increasing the hemoglobin concentrations but also compatible for use alongside breastfeeding, in accordance with the WHO guidelines [42].

Pre-term infants represent another subgroup with specific iron needs. Although all normal infants experience a decrease in hemoglobin levels after birth, very-low-birthweight (VLBW) infants experience a more pronounced decline in iron stores. Without sufficient dietary iron intake, normal-term infants experience iron deficiency anemia within 6–9 months of age [46–48]. One challenge in the care of VLBW infants is the lack of diagnostic tests that can be used for the diagnosis and treatment of iron deficiency; it is plausible that the clinical effects of iron deficiency manifest sooner in VLBW infants, but there is no conclusive evidence to support this [46]. A recent systematic review focusing on the effects of iron supplementation on low-birth-weight or premature infants revealed consistent findings with respect to improvements in hematological parameters with iron supplementation and supported the tolerability and safety of these interventions [49]. However, a separate randomized controlled trial in VLBW pre-term infants did not establish any additional benefits of iron supplements when used in addition to iron-fortified formula or breast milk [46]. Larger-scale controlled trials are needed in order to determine the optimal vehicles, dosage and timing of iron supplementation. In regard to pre-term infants who are not exclusively breastfed, the current data support the use of iron-fortified formulas (rather than nonfortified formulas) and that these should be used alongside other strategies, such as delayed cord clamping, in order to meet the iron requirements of VLBW infants [47, 50, 51].

The advantages of using fortified foods over iron supplements are better tolerability and adherence. In infants and young children, the use of fortified complementary foods has been shown to be more effective than the use of supplements [40]. Three large trials (conducted in Nepal, India and Africa) in children aged 1 month to 4 years demonstrated that children who received iron/folic acid and zinc supplements had more adverse effects than those who received only placebo, raising concerns about potential zinc-iron interactions [52–55]. In contrast, no safety issues were raised when iron and zinc were delivered through food vehicles [55, 56]. Adherence is another major factor which may well have affected the safety outcomes in the iron/folic acid and zinc supplementation trials [56]. A study in northern India assessed consumer adherence to two home-based fortification strategies for iron and zinc supplementation in children 6–24 months of age. The first compared a rice-based fortified complementary food with sprinkles delivered in sachets. The data from this study indicated that after 6 months, the fortified complementary food resulted in a significant increase in mean hemoglobin levels and had greater user adherence compared to the sprinkles [56]. These findings have been supported by a number of other studies, indicating the advantages of using fortified foods over micronutrient supplements, particularly for infants and young children [57, 58]. One of the few randomized, placebo-controlled, double-blind intervention trials directly compared iron supplements with food fortification in 425 Vietnamese school-aged children [58]. The study results showed that both interventions yielded significant improvements over placebo in terms of hemoglobin, ferritin and body iron levels and anemia status but that the increases in the iron fortification group were less pronounced than those in the group receiving supplements. These differences may be largely due to the lower amounts of iron received by the fortification group (than by the supplement group) [58]. Although the use of supplements may be effective in the setting of a controlled clinical trial, user adherence over the long term remains unknown. Another issue related to the use of iron supplements is safety: under some circumstances, the use of iron supplements may be associated with increased risk of death or severe morbidities, such as in young children living in regions with malaria and/or infectious diseases [54, 59, 60]. Therefore, in a population of anemic children with mild iron deficiency, iron fortification is the preferred strategy for addressing anemia [58].

Despite the beneficial effects of iron fortification on hematological parameters in infants and young children, there are several open questions that remain to be answered. First, it is unknown how hematological parameters may be extrapolated into functional health outcomes (such as growth and cognitive skills) over the long term. Second, delivery is a major limitation of the application of fortified foods, as these foods may not reach the very poor. In order for these interventions to be effective in the target populations, a combination of approaches involving raising awareness among caregivers, using different delivery channels, reducing prices, and improving product nutritional profiles may be needed. The food industry, including Nestlé, is applying nutrient profiling in order to evaluate and improve the nutrient quality of its products, taking into account nutrients to limit (such as sugars and added fats) as well as micronutrients beneficial to health (including iron). This ongoing process is part of a global effort to align the nutrient content of its food products in order to meet the nutritional needs of populations, including infants and young children, in accordance with international and local health guidelines. Nutritional profiling of foods is currently being used to drive the reformulation of food products that can be targeted to meet the needs of iron-deficient infants and young children and to raise the micronutrient density of widely consumed staple items.

The Cost Effectiveness of Food Fortification

Other key issues related to the success of these interventions are affordability and cost-effectiveness [61, 62]. However, few studies have been done in infants and pre-school-aged children. A recent study estimated the cost-effectiveness of price-based interventions using fortified powdered milk to address micronutrient deficiencies in children aged 6–23 months in the Philippines [63]. Specifically, the authors evaluated the effectiveness and cost effectiveness of different prices of the same product in reducing iron and vitamin A deficiencies. Survey-based data were collected from 1,800 low- or middle-income households with at least one child in this age range. The results from this study highlighted several key points. First, the poorer households exhibited the greatest price elasticity, in which a small change in price had a large effect on the demand for the product. Another key finding from this study was that amongst the poorer households, the nutritional awareness of the mother (who was the primary decision maker regarding foods purchased for the child) had no impact on the demand for fortified powdered milk; instead, product price was the main driver of demand [63]. These findings are especially relevant in light of how the cost burden of micronutrient deficiencies is distributed across different socio-economic strata. A health economics study that simulated the lifetime costs of micronutrient deficiencies in Filipino children (aged 6–59 months) revealed that the poorest third of households incurred the greatest estimated lifetime costs from micronutrient deficiencies (including medical costs, production losses and other projected lifetime costs from impaired mental and physical development and premature deaths) [29]. Therefore, lowering the price of a commercially available and accepted complementary food product is a feasible mechanism for making fortified food items available to the poorest subpopulations, and targeting the poorest would yield the greatest cost savings in terms of DALY gains [29, 63]. To this end, the public sector and local governments could play a role by implementing social programs that provide food subsidies or other financial support to the poorest, facilitating the distribution or purchase of fortified products to the most needy populations [33]. Such public channels, along with the support of private partners, will be important not only for increasing the availability of fortified items to those in the lowest socio-economic strata but also for disseminating awareness of the importance of a nutritious diet [33] while lowering transaction costs for the public sector.

Conclusions

At all levels, nutrition is a central element that defines well-being and success: it enables humans to achieve their physical and cognitive potential, and it is the landmark by which we chart our course towards the sustainable development goals of the future. Infants and children are among those most vulnerable to micronutrient deficiencies. Addressing micronutrient deficiencies (particularly iron deficiency) in children would have beneficial effects that cascade into later life, resulting in the greatest gains in DALYs. As a tool, food fortification provides a means to address micronutrient deficiencies for a large proportion of the world's population, especially infants and young children in developing countries. Fortified infant formulas, powdered milk and complementary foods are feasible vehicles for this target population, especially when combined with the appropriate pricing and delivery strategies. Yet, the full potential of food fortification remains untapped. Currently, there remains a lack of nationalized public-private partnerships and political commitment to drive this strategy to the forefront of the actions against micronutrient deficiencies. Effective food fortification programs must be applied in conjunction with the appropriate production, distribution, and communication to the target populations. A central element in driving these programs forward is the creation of shared values among all stakeholders. Value-driven business models will provide a sustainable platform upon which the needs of consumers and society at large can be met. This will render fortification efforts sustainable, since they will be fully integrated into business models. However, the private food industry alone cannot deliver viable fortification programs without the cooperation of the scientific community, international agencies, and governmental and non-governmental organizations. The sustainability and success of iron fortification programs are dependent upon their integration into a holistic framework that bridges the gap between public health needs and nutrition goals, particularly for the world's most vulnerable populations.

References

1 United Nations: The Millennium Development Goals Report. 2014. http://www.un.org/millenniumgoals/2014%20MDG%20report/MDG%202014%20English%20web.pdf (accessed July 26, 2015).

2 Bloessner M, de Onis M: WHO Environmental Burden of Disease Series 12. Malnutrition: quantifying the health impact at national and local levels. 2005. http://www.who.int/quantifying_ehimpacts/publications/MalnutritionEBD12.pdf (accessed September 7, 2015).

3 Tulchinsky TH: Micronutrient deficiency conditions: global health issues. Public Health Rev 2010; 32:255.

4 Horton S, Manner V, Wesley A: Micronutrient fortification (iron and salt iodization). 2008. http://www.copenhagenconsensus.com/sites/default/files/bpp_fortification.pdf (accessed July 5, 2015).

5 Muthayya S, Rah JH, Sugimoto JD, Roos FF, Kraemer K, Black RE: the global hidden hunger indices and maps: an advocacy tool for action. PLoS One 2013;8:e67860.

6 Food and Agriculture Organization (FAO): Global Hunger Index: the challenge of hidden hunger. 2014. http://ebrary.ifpri.org/utils/getfile/collection/p15738coll2/id/128360/filename/128571.pdf (accessed July 3, 2015).

7 Scott SP, Chen-Edinboro LP, Caulfield LE, Murray-Kolb LE: The impact of anemia on child mortality: an updated review. Nutrients 2014;6:5915–5932.

8 Stevens GA, Finucane MM, De-Regil LM, Paciorek CJ, Flaxman SR, Branca F, et al: Global, regional, and national trends in haemoglobin concentration and prevalence of total and severe anaemia in children and pregnant and non-pregnant women for 1995–2011: a systematic analysis of population-representative data. Lancet Glob Health 2013;1:e16–e25.

9 WHO/UNICEF: Iron Deficiency Anemia Assessment, Prevention and Control. Geneva, World Health Organization, 2001.

10 Beutler E, Waalen J: The definition of anemia: what is the lower limit of normal of the blood hemoglobin concentration? Blood 2006;107:1747–1750.

11 Burke RM, Leon JS, Suchdev PS: Identification, prevention and treatment of iron deficiency during the first 1,000 days. Nutrients 2014;6:4093–4114.

12 Zimmermann MB: Methods to assess iron and iodine status. Br J Nutr 2008;99(suppl 3):S2–S9.

13 Miller JL: Iron deficiency anemia: a common and curable disease. Cold Spring Harb Perspect Med 2013;3:a011866.

14 Abbaspour N, Hurrell R, Kelishadi R: Review on iron and its importance for human health. J Res Med Sci 2014;19:164–174.

15 McDermid JM, Lönnerdal B: Iron. Adv Nutr 2012;3: 532–533.

16 Lönnerdal B: Alternative pathways for absorption of iron from foods. Pure Appl Chem 2010;82:429–436.

17 Alton I: Iron deficiency anemia; in Stang S, Story M (eds): Guidelines for Adolescent Nutrition Services. Minneapolis, University of Minnesota Press, 2005, pp 101–108.

18 Cairo D, Castro R: Iron deficiency anemia in adolescents; a literature review. Nutr Hosp 2014;29:1240–1249.

19 Paoletti G, Bogen DL, Ritchey AK: Severe iron-deficiency anemia still an issue in toddlers. Clin Pediatr (Phila) 2014;53:1352–1358.

20 Jauregui-Lobera I: Iron deficiency and cognitive functions. Neuropsychiatr Dis Treat 2014;10:2087–2095.

21 Ekiz C, Agaoglu L, Karakas Z, Gurel N, Yalcin I: The effect of iron deficiency anemia on the function of the immune system. Hematol J 2005;5:579–583.

22 Khan DA, Ansari WM, Khan FA: Synergistic effects of iron deficiency and lead exposure on blood lead levels in children. World J Pediatr 2011;7:150–154.

23 Kordas K: Iron, lead, and children's behavior and cognition. Annu Rev Nutr 2010;30:123–148.

24 Benton D: Micronutrient status, cognition and behavioral problems in childhood. Eur J Nutr 2008; 47(suppl 3):38–50.
25 Chango A, Pogribny IP: Considering maternal dietary modulators for epigenetic regulation and programming of the fetal epigenome. Nutrients 2015;7: 2748–2770.
26 Hoeijmakers L, Lucassen PJ, Korosi A: The interplay of early-life stress, nutrition, and immune activation programs adult hippocampal structure and function. Front Mol Neurosci 2015;7:103.
27 Black RE, Allen LH, Bhutta ZA, Caulfield LE, de Onis M, Ezzati M, et al: Maternal and child undernutrition: global and regional exposures and health consequences. Lancet 2008;371:243–260.
28 Brenseke B, Prater MR, Bahamonde J, Gutierrez JC: Current thoughts on maternal nutrition and fetal programming of the metabolic syndrome. J Pregnancy 2013;2013:368461.
29 Wieser S, Plessow R, Eichler K, Malek O, Capanzana MV, Agdeppa I, et al: Burden of micronutrient deficiencies by socio-economic strata in children aged 6 months to 5 years in the Philippines. BMC Public Health 2013;13:1167.
30 Darmon N, Drewnowski A: Does social class predict diet quality? Am J Clin Nutr 2008;87:1107–1117.
31 Tulchinsky TH: The key role of government in addressing the pandemic of micronutrient deficiency conditions in Southeast Asia. Nutrients 2015;7: 2518–2523.
32 Canadian Public Health Association: Food fortification with vitamins and minerals. 2015. http://www.cpha.ca/en/programs/history/achievements/09-shf/fortification.aspx (accessed July 10, 2015).
33 Bloem MW, de Pee S, Hop lT, Khan NC, Laillou A, Minarto, et al: Key strategies to further reduce stunting in Southeast Asia: lessons from the ASEAN countries workshop. Food Nutr Bull 2013;34(2 suppl):S8–S16.
34 Gayer J, Smith G: Micronutrient fortification of food in Southeast Asia: recommendations from an expert workshop. Nutrients 2015;7:646–658.
35 Das JK, Salam RA, Kumar R, Bhutta ZA: Micronutrient fortification of food and its impact on woman and child health: a systematic review. Syst Rev 2013; 2:67.
36 Hipgrave DB, Fu X, Zhou H, Jin Y, Wang X, Chang S, et al: Poor complementary feeding practices and high anaemia prevalence among infants and young children in rural central and western China. Eur J Clin Nutr 2014;68:916–924.
37 Senarath U, Godakandage SS, Jayawickrama H, Siriwardena I, Dibley MJ: Determinants of inappropriate complementary feeding practices in young children in Sri Lanka: secondary data analysis of Demographic and Health Survey 2006–2007. Matern Child Nutr 2012;8(suppl 1):60–77.
38 Senarath U, Agho KE, Akram DE, Godakandage SS, Hazir T, Jayawickrama H, et al: Comparisons of complementary feeding indicators and associated factors in children aged 6–23 months across five South Asian countries. Matern Child Nutr 2012; 8(suppl 1):89–106.
39 Eichler K, Wieser S, Rüthemann I, Brügger U: Effects of micronutrient fortified milk and cereal food for infants and children: a systematic review. BMC Public Health 2012;12:506–512.
40 Brito A, Olivares M, Pizarro T, Rodríguez L, Hertrampf E: Chilean complementary feeding program reduces anemia and improves iron status in children aged 11 to 18 months. Food Nutr Bull 2013;34:378–385.
41 Agostoni C, Decsi T, Fewtrell M, Goulet O, Kolacek S, Koletzko B, et al: Complementary feeding: a commentary by the ESPGHAN Committee on Nutrition. J Pediatr Gastroenterol Nutr 2008;46:99–110.
42 World Health Organization: Global strategy for infant and young child feeding. 2003. http://apps.who.int/iris/bitstream/10665/42590/1/9241562218.pdf?ua=1&ua=1 (accessed August 7, 2015).
43 Fahmida U, Santika O, Kolopaking R, Ferguson E: Complementary feeding recommendations based on locally available foods in Indonesia. Food Nutr Bull 2014;35(4 suppl):S174–S179.
44 Skau JK, Touch B, Chhoun C, Chea M, Unni US, Makurat J, et al: Effects of animal source food and micronutrient fortification in complementary food products on body composition, iron status, and linear growth: a randomized trial in Cambodia. Am J Clin Nutr 2015;101:742–751.
45 Owino VO, Kasonka LM, Sinkala MM, Wells JK, Eaton S, Darch T, et al: Fortified complementary foods with or without alpha-amylase treatment increase hemoglobin but do not reduce breast milk intake of 9-mo-old Zambian infants. Am J Clin Nutr 2007;86:1094–1103.
46 Taylor TA, Kennedy KA: Randomized trial of iron supplementation versus routine iron intake in VLBW infants. Pediatrics 2013;131:e433–e438.
47 Domellöf M: Iron and other micronutrient deficiencies in low-birthweight infants. Nestle Nutr Inst Workshop Ser 2013;74:197–206.
48 Marques RF, Taddei JA, Lopez FA, Braga JA: Breastfeeding exclusively and iron deficiency anemia during the first 6 months of age. Rev Assoc Med Bras 2014;60:18–22.
49 Long H, Yi JM, Hu PL, Li ZB, Qiu WY, Wang F, et al: Benefits of iron supplementation for low birth weight infants: a systematic review. BMC Pediatr 2012;12:99.
50 Baker SS, Cochran WJ, Flores CA, Georgieff MK, Jacobson MS, Jaksic T, Krebs NF: Iron fortification of infant formulas. Pediatrics 1999;104:119–123.

51 van de Lagemaat M, Amesz EM, Schaafsma A, Lafeber HN: Iron deficiency and anemia in iron-fortified formula and human milk-fed preterm infants until 6 months post-term. Eur J Nutr 2014;53:1263–1271.

52 Bhandari N, Taneja S, Mazumder S, Bahl R, Fontaine O, Bhan MK: Adding zinc to supplemental iron and folic acid does not affect mortality and severe morbidity in young children. J Nutr 2007;137:112–117.

53 Sazawal S, Black RE, Ramsan M, Chwaya HM, Stoltzfus RJ, Dutta A, et al: Effects of routine prophylactic supplementation with iron and folic acid on admission to hospital and mortality in preschool children in a high malaria transmission setting: community-based, randomised, placebo-controlled trial. Lancet 2006;367:133–143.

54 Tielsch JM, Khatry SK, Stoltzfus RJ, Katz J, LeClerq SC, Adhikari R, et al: Effect of routine prophylactic supplementation with iron and folic acid on preschool child mortality in southern Nepal: community-based, cluster-randomised, placebo-controlled trial. Lancet 2006;367:144–152.

55 Whittaker P: Iron and zinc interactions in humans. Am J Clin Nutr 1998;68(2 suppl):442S–446S.

56 Sazawal S, Dhingra P, Dhingra U, Gupta S, Iyengar V, Menon VP, et al: Compliance with home-based fortification strategies for delivery of iron and zinc: its effect on haematological and growth markers among 6–24 months old children in north India. J Health Popul Nutr 2014;32:217–226.

57 Hieu NT, Sandalinas F, de Sesmaisons A, Laillou A, Tam NP, Khan NC, et al: Multi-micronutrient-fortified biscuits decreased the prevalence of anaemia and improved iron status, whereas weekly iron supplementation only improved iron status in Vietnamese school children. Br J Nutr 2012;108:1419–1427.

58 Thi LH, Brouwer ID, Burema J, Nguyen KC, Kok FJ: Efficacy of iron fortification compared to iron supplementation among Vietnamese schoolchildren. Nutr J 2006;5:32.

59 de Benoist B, Darnton-Hill I, Lynch S, Allen L, Savioli L: Zinc and iron supplementation trials in Nepal and Tanzania. Lancet 2006;367:816.

60 Sazawal S, Black RE, Ramsan M, Chwaya HM, Stoltzfus RJ, Dutta A, et al: Effects of routine prophylactic supplementation with iron and folic acid on admission to hospital and mortality in preschool children in a high malaria transmission setting: community-based, randomised, placebo-controlled trial. Lancet 2006;367:133–143.

61 Baltussen R, Knai C, Sharan M: Iron fortification and iron supplementation are cost-effective interventions to reduce iron deficiency in four subregions of the world. J Nutr 2004;134:2678–2684.

62 Horton S, Ross J: The economics of iron deficiency. Food Policy 2003;32:141–143.

63 Wieser S, Brunner B, Plessow R, Eichler K, Solomons N, Malek O, et al: Cost-effectiveness of price reductions in fortified powdered milk for the reduction of micronutrient deficiencies in 6–23 month old children in the Philippines. 13th Micronutrient Forum Global Conference. Addis Ababa, Ethiopia, Poster, 2014.

64 Biesalski B: Food-based approaches for combating iron deficiency. 2013. ftp://ftp.fao.org/ag/agn/nutrition/Kapitel_21_210207.pdf (accessed July 8, 2015).

Dr. Jörg Spieldenner
Nestlé Research Center
Vers-chez-les-Blancs
CH–1000 Lausanne 26 (Switzerland)
E-Mail Jorg.spieldenner@rdls.nestle.com

Biesalski HK, Black RE (eds): Hidden Hunger. Malnutrition and the First 1,000 Days of Life:
Causes, Consequences and Solutions. World Rev Nutr Diet. Basel, Karger, 2016, vol 115, pp 224–232
DOI: 10.1159/000442109

How to Achieve Transparency in Public-Private Partnerships Engaged in Hunger and Malnutrition Reduction

Manfred Eggersdorfer[a] · Julia K. Bird[b]

[a]Nutrition Science and Advocacy, DSM Nutritional Products, Basel, Switzerland;
[b]DSM Nutritional Products, Delft, The Netherlands

Abstract

Multi-stakeholder partnerships are important facilitators of improving nutrition in developing countries to achieve the United Nations' Sustainable Development Goals. Often, the role of industry is challenged and questions are raised as to the ethics of involving for-profit companies in humanitarian projects. The Second International Conference on Nutrition placed great emphasis on the role of the private sector, including industry, in multi-stakeholder partnerships to reduce hunger and malnutrition. Governments have to establish regulatory frameworks and institutions to guarantee fair competition and invest in infrastructure that makes investments for private companies attractive, eventually leading to economic growth. Civil society organizations can contribute by delivering nutrition interventions and behavioral change-related communication to consumers, providing capacity, and holding governments and private sector organizations accountable. Industry provides technical support, innovation, and access to markets and the supply chain. The greatest progress and impact can be achieved if all stakeholders cooperate in multi-stakeholder partnerships aimed at improving nutrition, thereby strengthening local economies and reducing poverty and inequality. Successful examples of public-private partnerships exist, as well as examples in which these partnerships did not achieve mutually agreed objectives. The key requirements for productive alliances between industry and civil society organizations are the establishment of rules of engagement, transparency and mutual accountability. The Global Social Observatory performed a consultation on conflicts of interest related to the Scaling Up Nutrition movement and provided recommendations to prevent, identify, manage and monitor potential conflicts of interest. Multi-stakeholder partnerships can be successful models in improving nutrition if they meet societal demand with transparent decision-making and execution. Solutions to the issue of malnutrition are available. We have the resources and knowledge, and we must act as a global community in the immediate future. Transparency about the roles and contributions of each partner may be a key factor for successful cooperation in multi-stakeholder partnerships.

Key Points

- Multi-stakeholder partnerships are important facilitators of improving nutrition in developing countries to achieve the Sustainable Development Goals.
- Individually, companies are likely to have a limited impact, but in partnership, they can address hunger and malnutrition much more successfully.
- Trust and transparency are key attributes of success.
- Successful examples of multi-stakeholder partnerships exist and can be used as models for further development.

The Issue

Hunger, food insecurity and malnutrition are major public health challenges that affect the well-being and economic capacity of current and future generations in developing countries. Deficits in macro- or micronutrients are particularly devastating in young children, as they result in adverse functional outcomes such as stunting and reduced cognitive abilities that can permanently affect the future health and productivity of individuals and populations. Stunting paradoxically places children at greater risk of obesity and associated chronic disease in later life. In adults, chronic hunger reduces work capacity and has a profound effect on quality of life. The prevalence of global stunting has declined from 40% in 1990 to 27% in 2010 and has been projected to decrease to 22% in 2020 [1]. Although progress in reducing chronic hunger has been made over recent years, 785 million people were undernourished in 2014 according to the most recent estimates [2]. The levels of stunting and hunger remain high and are important reasons why countries fail to escape the cycle of poverty.

Global agricultural production has exceeded population growth in past decades, such that per capita food availability in 2006–2008 was estimated to exceed 2,700 kcal/person/day [3]. In addition to improved access to food, the number of chronically undernourished people has fallen from 34% in the mid-1970s to 15% in recent years. Regional differences belie these global gains: 28% of Sub-Saharan Africans experience food insecurity. The unequal distribution of resources both between and within countries is the reason why food insecurity exists despite the adequate production of food to meet the world population's needs. As income and productivity are the most important drivers of food security, uneven and noninclusive economic growth has limited further reductions in malnutrition [2]. Natural and man-made disasters can cause food access emergencies in vulnerable populations.

Historically, mistrust between industry, nutrition experts and nongovernmental organizations has hampered the development of constructive solutions to malnutrition. Even though effective solutions are available, they have not been implemented well due to a lack of collaboration between diverse actors. There is a need for a frame-

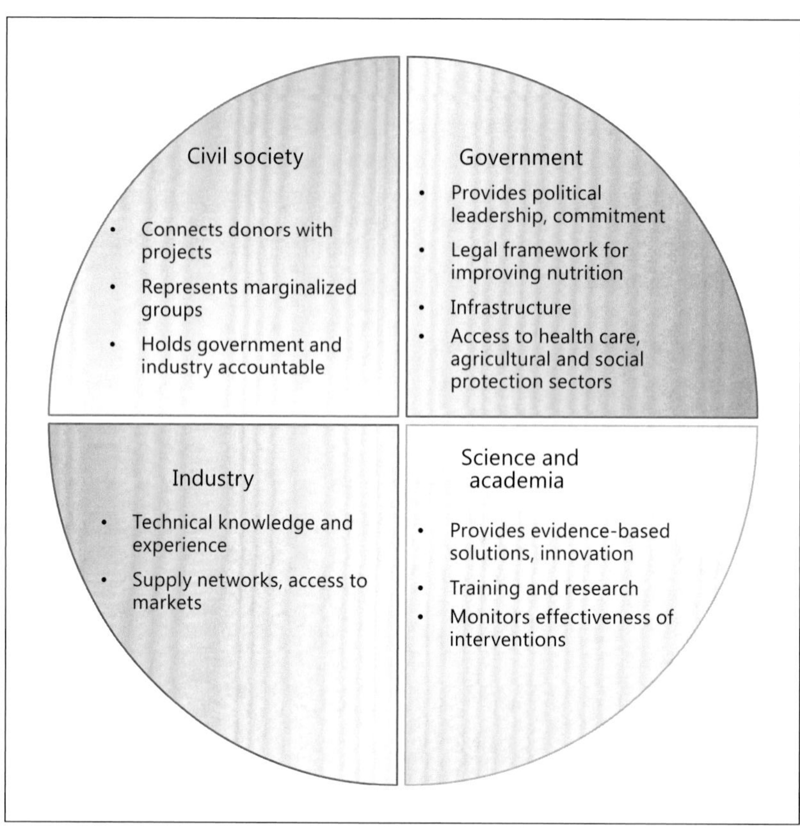

Fig. 1. Roles of stakeholders in addressing malnutrition.

work and an enabling environment in which governments provide a regulatory context that structures demand for the most vulnerable and guarantees fair competition between institutions.

Solutions

Effective solutions exist to improve access to the food supply, deliver deficient micronutrients to needy populations, and reduce food waste. The Food and Agriculture Organization (FAO) states that 'hunger, food insecurity and malnutrition are complex problems that cannot be solved by a single stakeholder or sector' [4]. Interventions that improve nutrition require the collaboration of various stakeholders for their successful implementation. The combination of the skills and resources of various sectors provides a benefit that is greater than the sum of individual contributions. Sustainable reductions in malnutrition result from productive alliances between government, industry, science and civil society (fig. 1).

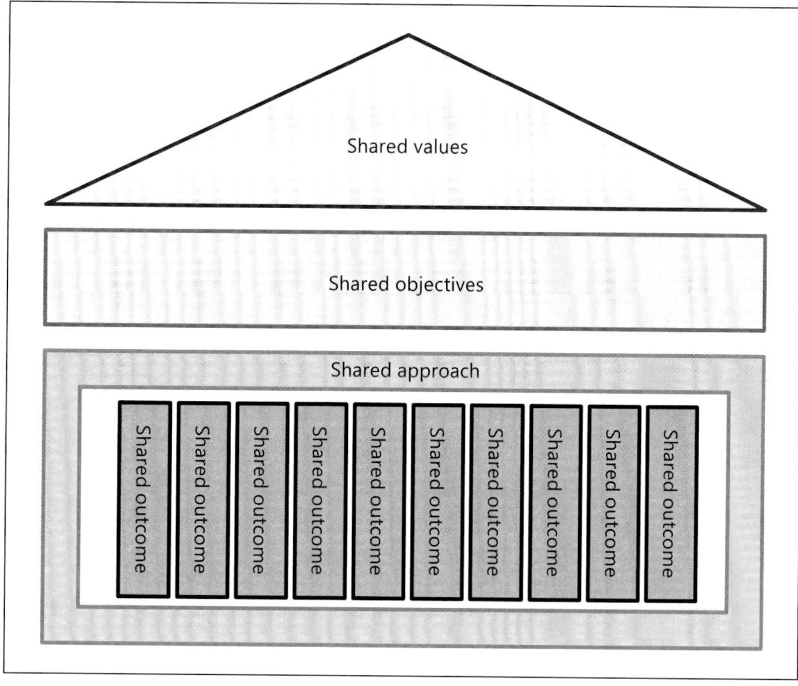

Fig. 2. Framework for successful public-private partnerships.

The Approach

We describe a framework for facilitating public-private partnerships to achieve improvements in the nutritional status of populations (fig. 2). Public-private partnerships bring together a set of actors for the common goal of improving the health of populations based on mutually agreed roles and principles. Nutrition problems are complex and diverse in nature; therefore, there is no prescribed method for setting up multi-stakeholder alliances [5]. Sharing key values and objectives provides the organizing principle around which the partnership will function: steering and strategic management.

Shared Value – Filling a Societal Need

A certain level of trust is required if organizations with differing aims are to work together to achieve reductions in hunger. Trust is achieved by committing to shared values that fulfill a societal need. An open and honest discussion about what each partner values is necessary for building trust. Agreement on a shared value is needed at an early stage of partnerships. A neutral third party may assist in developing the partnership. Written policy statements, especially regarding conflicts of interest, may be beneficial [6].

These agreed-on values will be a driving force for engagement. For the public sector, social values and partnering are drawn from its directive, politics, and a desire to improve the well-being of its represented population. Private partners' social values and partnering are driven by corporate social responsibility, brand value, or business strategy when the business is to develop social goods or services. While private partners may agree on a social value, some form of measurable economic value must be present for the private sector to become involved. That value can be measured in expected profits, cost savings, market growth, or brand value enhancements such as name recognition, goodwill or public relations benefits. It is important for the private sector to be up front about its motivations.

Shared Objective – The Factor to Be Achieved
Shared objectives are explicit goals for the partnership, expressed in concrete and realistic terms as to the target group and what will be achieved. These shared objectives represent tangible and measureable extensions of the shared values and provide a means to assess progress. Aspirational goals are generally not useful here: the objectives are intended to drive the practical aspects of the partnership, and they should be as well-defined as possible. For example, while partnerships may aim to reduce stunting in a broad sense, objectives such as these are – because of the multi-factorial causes – too diffuse to be useful. A better objective would be to improve the nutrient content of the food basket, which fulfils a societal need but is more clearly defined and able to be implemented within the partnership. Greater clarity in objective-setting facilitates the implementation of the partnership and continues to build trust and mutual accountability.

Shared Approach – How Will the Objective Be Achieved?
A roadmap for implementing the objective is defined in the shared approach. By outlining the approach in a project plan, the level of involvement, roles and responsibilities are clear from the outset. The implementation strategy lists the partners' monetary and in-kind investments into the partnership, provides a cost-benefit analysis of the investments, and defines the scale of the project and the expected bottlenecks. With approaches to address malnutrition, the public sector may provide co-funding, support in policy changes to implement the project, logistical support and capacity, and interaction with the general public. The private sector is responsible for product development, knowledge transfer and provision of services to the partnership.

Shared Outcomes – Short- and Long-Term Indicators of Success
Both long- and short-term outcomes are indicators used to measure progress and the ultimate success of the partnership. Measures of factors leading to the objective and of the success of the partnership should be considered as outcomes; outcomes that describe the benefits to both sides of the partnership are important for its continued success. These shared outcomes can be evaluated to determine the actual return on investment.

Successful Examples

DSM-World Food Programme Partnership

DSM has been in a successful partnership with the World Food Programme since 2007 [7]. By committing to a shared value of improving the vitamin and mineral contents of foods provided by the World Food Programme, this partnership has been helping to reduce malnutrition in people receiving food aid. At the start of the partnership, both parties brought together their capacities, reach, knowledge and technologies to meet shared objectives aimed at reducing micronutrient deficiencies in crisis populations. For the World Food Programme, the aims of the partnership were not exclusive to accessing additional funding and materials from DSM. Specific technical information on formulating micronutrients to improve the nutrient content of the distributed foods and the possibility to create novel micronutrient delivery applications were important to the World Food Programme. The partnership also aimed to raise awareness of the World Food Programme amongst DSM employees and within DSM's sphere of influence. DSM wanted to align a corporate social responsibility program with its business activities and to gain better market understanding in order to innovate products and fortification strategies to develop new business opportunities in underserved markets. Increasing employee engagement and improving public relations were also goals for DSM. Together, the World Food Programme and DSM defined several joint objectives:

- To increase the micronutrient content of the World Food Programme's food basket
- To reach 80% of World Food Programme beneficiaries with improved nutrition
- To raise awareness among policymakers of the importance of micronutrients to improve learning and earning capabilities and to reduce future health costs

DSM provides the partnership with scientific knowledge, innovation and development capacities, micronutrients and nutrient premixes, human resources, funding, media and private sector contacts. The World Food Programme offers logistical support, understanding of local needs, and support as a trustworthy and respected aid organization. Meeting the shared objectives is important for both parties in achieving each organization's objectives. There was a deliberate policy of building common ground between the two organizations, derived from the principle of 'common and noncompeting agendas' [8].

The partnership's approach was divided into several work streams aimed at meeting the broad objectives of the partnership. Early in the partnership, DSM was able to use its expertise to help develop MixMe™ micronutrient powder sachets – containing all vitamins and key minerals – intended for home fortification. NutriRice™ was then innovated by combining broken rice kernels, which are by-products of normal rice production, with essential vitamins and minerals to improve the nutrient content of rice. Current projects are focused on incorporating micronutrients into fortified blended foods and ready-to-use therapeutic foods to treat acute malnutrition. In 2013, the partnership was able to reach 20.6 million people in Latin America, South Asia, Southeast Asia and Sub-Saharan Africa with products containing increased nutrient contents, and the aim is to increase this to 30 million by the end of 2015. The goal of fortified food products reaching 80% of World Food Programme beneficiaries (defined as pregnant or lactating women and children under the age of 5 years) was met in 2013 [8]. Key success factors in the partnership are complementary competences and the establishment of objectives in a manner that was transparent from the beginning.

Sustainable Evidence-Based Actions for Change
Public-private partnerships are only possible when organizations have a clear understanding of the issues and shared values in the approach. An important factor in partnerships' success is the synergy arising from the competencies of each stakeholder's organization. The Sustainable Evidence-Based Actions for Change initiative aims to bring key stakeholders from government, academia, the food and ingredient industry, donors and nongovernmental organizations from the South-East Asia region together to catalyze multi-sectoral partnerships to improve nutrition in pregnant women and children under 2 years old. These workshops bring together relevant experts to assess country-specific issues and co-develop concrete local programs involving all stakeholders. With this approach, a couple of impactful national nutrition improvement programs are currently in development.

The National Complementary Feeding Program in Chile
The National Complementary Feeding Program in Chile dates back many years. The starting point was when the Chilean Ministry of Health recognized an increasing rate of overweight and obesity in its population, especially in children. The Chilean Ministry of Health started a call to action and invited stakeholders to develop solutions. The agreed-on goals include preventing and correcting nutritional deficiencies, promoting exclusive breastfeeding until infants reach 6 months of age, and preventing overweight and obesity. In particular, intake of long-chain omega-3 fatty acids in Chile was low, and this was considered to be a restricting factor in the cognitive development of children in the population (supplementation with docosahexaenoic acid was found to increase IQ by 4 points in a clinical study [9]). A public-private partnership was created between the Chilean Ministry of Health, the University of Chile, a major food producer and a food ingredient producer. Each partner provided various competences to meet the overarching goal of increasing micronutrient intake in pregnant women:

A. Knowledge of the importance of adequate consumption of long-chain omega-3 fatty acids for normal neurological development of infants
B. Political will and ownership of the project
C. Scientific research resources
D. An industry partner that is technically competent and interested
E. An ingredient manufacturer with product application expertise and the right product
F. Scientific and analytical support

The final product was a beverage containing cereals, dairy, a mixture of vitamins and minerals suitable for pregnant and lactating women, and 80 mg of long-chain omega-3 fatty acids per serving. The product was shown to increase the long-chain omega-3 fatty acid and micronutrient concentrations in the target group when consumed as directed [10], to increase birth weight, and to reduce the rate of very preterm birth [11].

This product is distributed free of charge to expectant mothers, although there is an emphasis on low-income mothers. Over 100,000 pregnant and lactating women receive the product annually. For the industry partners, there is an opportunity to gain a new market if the final product is acceptable and meets the needs defined by the partnership. As the product is intended to not only improve the health of infants but also increase the IQ of the population, there is a clear return on investment in terms of increased work ability in later life resulting from the increase in the IQ of the population. In particular, it was calculated that the return to society based on IQ improvement was almost 200 times higher than the initial cost.

Conclusions

Public-private partnerships are an effective means of solving complex nutritional problems. Nutrition targets cannot be achieved by government or civil society alone; the private sector also plays an important role in creating sustainable access to good nutrition for all. Partnerships exemplify what can be achieved when the public and private sectors work together. When governments establish an environment enabling food fortification, the private sector can implement food fortification programs, and entire countries benefit from access to healthier and more nutritious diets. The food industry and internationally operating companies are important stakeholders in improving nutrition in developing countries and in achieving significant and sustainable improvements. By combining the strengths of each partner, organizations can achieve more than if they had worked individually. An important consideration for partnerships is the definition of shared values, goals and objectives during the initial phase. A certain level of trust and transparency is needed, and all parties should be direct about their expectations at the outset of the partnership. The establishment of written documents that define the framework of the partnership, individual and combined goals, and the approach to be taken is valuable. It may be advisable to initiate discussions on shared values from a neutral position, potentially with the help of a mediator. Consideration of potential conflicts of interest may avoid complications as the partnership starts to implement the plan of action. Facilitating the cooperation of multiple stakeholders is vitally important in effectively implementing established effective solutions for preventing malnutrition.

References

1 de Onis M, Blossner M, Borghi E: Prevalence and trends of stunting among pre-school children, 1990–2020. Public Health Nutr 2012;15:142–148.

2 FAO, IFAD, WFP: The state of food insecurity in the world 2015. Meeting the 2015 international hunger targets: taking stock of uneven progress. Rome, Food and Agriculture Organization of the United Nations, 2015.

3 FAO: FAO Statistical Yearbook 2012. Rome, Food and Agriculture Organization of the United Nations, 2012.

4 FAO, IFAD, WFP: The state of food insecurity in the world 2014. Strengthening the enabling environment for food security and nutrition. Rome, Food and Agriculture Organization of the United Nations, 2014.

5 Scaling Up Nutrition: Scaling up nutrition in practice: effectively engaging multiple stakeholders, 2014. Issue 1. http://scalingupnutrition.org/wp-content/uploads/2014/03/Sun-in-Practice-issue-1.pdf (accessed July 8, 2015).

6 Global Social Observatory: Consultation process on conflict of interest in the SUN Movement. The main conclusions and next steps for sustainability, April 2015. http://gsogeneva.ch/wp-content/uploads/GSO-COI-Project-Main-Conclusions-and-Next-Steps.pdf (accessed July 17, 2015).

7 DSM: DSM/WFP Partnership factsheet 2015. http://www.dsm.com/content/dam/dsm/cworld/en_US/documents/dsm-wfp-partnership-factsheet.pdf (accessed July 17, 2015).

8 Bahl K, Jayaram S, Brown B: DSM-WFP: a partnership to advance the global nutrition agenda. Washington, Results for Development Institute, 2014.

9 Helland IB, Smith L, Saarem K, et al: Maternal supplementation with very-long-chain n-3 fatty acids during pregnancy and lactation augments children's IQ at 4 years of age. Pediatrics 2003;111:e39–e44.

10 Atalah SE, Araya BM, Rosselot PG, et al: Consumption of a DHA-enriched milk drink by pregnant and lactating women, on the fatty acid composition of red blood cells, breast milk, and in the newborn (in Spanish). Arch Latinoam Nutr 2009;59:271–277.

11 Mardones F, Urrutia MT, Villarroel L, et al: Effects of a dairy product fortified with multiple micronutrients and omega-3 fatty acids on birth weight and gestation duration in pregnant Chilean women. Public Health Nutr 2008;11:30–40.

Prof. Dr. Manfred Eggersdorfer
Wurmisweg 576
CH–4303 Kaiseraugst (Switzerland)
E-Mail Manfred.eggersdorfer@dsm.com

Biesalski HK, Black RE (eds): Hidden Hunger. Malnutrition and the First 1,000 Days of Life: Causes, Consequences and Solutions. World Rev Nutr Diet. Basel, Karger, 2016, vol 115, pp 233–238
DOI: 10.1159/000442110

Public-Private Partnerships and Undernutrition: Examples and Future Prospects

John Hoddinott[a, b] · Stuart Gillespie[b] · Sivan Yosef[b]

[a]Cornell University, Ithaca, NY, and [b]International Food Policy Research Institute, Washington, DC, USA

Abstract

In this chapter, we clarify what is meant by public-private partnerships (PPPs), provide examples of both successful and less successful PPPs and describe some broad lessons. We see scope for PPPs that would reduce aspects of undernutrition. However, this optimism comes with significant caveats. First, while there would appear to be a large body of evidence on this topic, closer examination shows that there are few independent, rigorous assessments of the impact of commercial sector engagement in nutrition. Considerable caution is therefore warranted when assessing either commendations or criticisms of PPPs in nutrition. Second, progress in this area requires that the private sector recognize that past and current actions by some firms have created an environment of mistrust and that the public sector accept that sustainable PPPs permit private firms to generate profits. Progress also requires recognition that PPPs involving multiple firms can be problematic either because such partnerships force competitors to collaborate or because they create the potential for the involved firms to lock out firms that are not members of the partnership. Lest this all sound too negative, from a nutrition perspective, we note that there may be significant scope for the involvement of the private sector in driving innovations that could reduce undernutrition. More speculatively, there may also be scope for the private sector to act as a financier of investments to improve children's nutritional status. For PPPs to succeed, there must be open discussions of the objectives, roles and expectations of all parties along with potential conflicts of interest.

Introduction

In recent years, political commitment to reducing undernutrition has risen globally. Nutrition features prominently in developmental agendas, in prime ministerial speeches, in international development discourse and in the media. The multi-sectoral nature of nutrition is best recognized with the corresponding need for engagement by multiple actors in different sectors and at different levels. Markets are increasingly important as sources of nutrition-relevant goods and services for all income groups, while malnutrition also remains a problem for all income groups. This has thrown a spotlight on the issue of private sector engagement in nutrition-relevant actions and the relationships between public and private sector actors.

Yet, looming over new initiatives that engage the private sector is a deeply suspicious nutrition sector. This deep suspicion is rooted in continued violations of the International Code of Marketing of Breast-Milk Substitutes [1]. In 2013 alone, the International Baby Food Action Network reported violations of the code – ranging from labelling to product promotion, advertising and bribing of health workers – by 26 companies in a 237-page report [2]. This suspicion is accentuated by the aggressive marketing of ultra-processed foods by food and beverage manufacturers [3, 4] and well-documented examples in which selected firms distorted or attempted to influence research on nutrition [5, 6].

This chapter, an abridged version of a report by Hoddinott et al. [7], speaks to both optimists who see public-private partnerships (PPPs) as an important means of reducing aspects of undernutrition (such as stunting, wasting and micronutrient deficiencies) in developing countries and pessimists who see PPPs as fraught with dangers. We clarify what is meant by PPPs, provide examples of both successful and less successful PPPs and describe some broad lessons.

PPPs for Undernutrition: Definitions and Examples

Confusion surrounding PPPs begins at the definitional level. For example, the World Health Organization [8] gives the following definition: 'A collaboration between public- and private-sector actors within diverse arrangements that vary according to participants, legal status, governance, management, policy setting, contributions and operational roles to achieve specific outcomes'. Yet, as Hawkes and Buse [9] suggest, there is an important distinction between interactions characterized by 'shared decision-making power among partners' and those characterized simply by the 'participation' of both sectors. Mindful of this distinction, we propose that discussions regarding PPPs and undernutrition distinguish between two types of partnership arrangements: noncontractual and contractual. In noncontractual PPPs, representatives from the public and private sectors coalesce around a set of shared goals [10]. Partners contribute time, money, expertise, or other resources to the partnership and share decision-making and management responsibilities. However, there is no legally binding contract between partners, and the partnership can be dissolved at any time. Contractual PPPs, as the name suggests, are characterized by a formal contract between public and private sector entities. They are further characterized by an objective of advancing a public goal; long-term partnership arrangements; often, but not always, a bundling of activities, and a blurring of lines between financier and implementer and a concomitant shift of risk from the public sector to the private sector.

As described in the report by Hoddinott et al. [7], we undertook a systematic review of the impact of PPPs on undernutrition. We found 24 studies, suggesting a relatively rich body of case studies and evidence. However, we also found that this evidence base was weak. In reviewing potential case studies, we needed to be careful to weed out cases that appeared to be little more than company public relations statements to focus only on examples with documented impact. This narrowed the field considerably, as – while there are many non-peer-reviewed 'capsule stories' in glossy company brochures (especially on food fortification) – there is not much at all in the way of independently generated evidence of the impact of PPPs in reducing child undernutrition. Further, many of the studies listed above are descriptive rather than analytical; few considered counterfactuals. However, there were some instructive examples, two of which are summarized below.

The Fortify West Africa (FWA) initiative is an example of a noncontractual PPP that appears to have been successful. FWA had two specific goals: ensure 70% coverage of vitamin A-fortified cooking oil and 70% coverage of wheat flour fortified with iron, zinc, folic acid and B vitamins. This description is taken from Sablah et al. [11].

Inception work on FWA began in 2000 with diagnostic work identifying foods that were both suitable for fortification and widely consumed and determining the extent to which these would need to be fortified. Gradually, national alliances were established. Members of these alliances typically included government ministries of health, commerce, industry and finance, United Nations agencies, nongovernmental organizations, domestic food industries, food importers, local research organizations and the media. These partnerships had four functions: to develop national standards and directives on mandatory fortification of cooking oil and wheat flour; building the capacity of large-scale cooking oil and wheat flour milling industries to implement fortification in the region as well as the ability of regulatory agencies to monitor compliance; to develop and implement social marketing campaigns built around branding fortified foods, and to monitor program implementation, support public sector enforcement of standards, and ensure that quality assurance systems are in place. As of late 2011, approximately 55 million people in West Africa were consuming fortified wheat, and the same number were consuming fortified vegetable oil.

In looking at this case study, it is striking how much time it took before meaningful scale-up occurred. Exploratory work started in 2000. While some initiatives began in 2003 or so, it took another 4 years before substantial implementation took place.

Much of this was time was taken up with a laborious process of getting agreement from national governments both in principle and in substance, for example, establishing regulatory regimes for food fortification and enforcement of standards. National and regional private sector firms were enthusiastic. Food fortification represented new, profitable opportunities to sell a higher value commodity. Regulations regarding fortification created both a trade barrier – effectively excluding importing firms that did not meet regional and national standards – and an additional barrier to the entry of new firms into the processed food market, thus giving incumbent firms more market power. Foreign firms that assisted in this process, for example providing pre-mix and technical assistance, were also supportive, as this created a new market for their products. However, despite these benefits, private sector firms would not make investments in new equipment or staff training until regulations were promulgated, technical standards were agreed upon and enforcement systems were put in place.

Poor-quality complementary foods, monotonous and lacking in caloric density, contribute to growth failure [12]. An attempt to address this issue in Bangladesh involved Grameen Danone Foods Ltd., a joint venture between a large multinational food and beverage firm, Danone, and the Grameen Bank. Beginning in 2006, this partnership revolved around the development and marketing of a fortified yoghurt called 'Shokti Doi', which was rich in protein and calcium [13]. The yoghurt, developed by nutrition experts at the Global Alliance for Improving Nutrition and Danone, was initially distributed solely in rural areas by Grameen saleswomen [14]. Grameen Danone owns some assets, such as the plant, brand, and product formula, while the acquisition of raw materials relied on partners such as local dairy farmers, BASF SE for nutrients, International Cap for packaging materials, the Global Alliance for Improving Nutrition for social marketing, and CARE for salespeople. Initially, the venture intended to cover its costs but not make profits or generate revenues that would sustain payouts or dividends to either Danone or Grameen. Accordingly, the yoghurt was priced at a level below the cost of production [13]. The long-term goal was to create 50 dairy factories by 2020. While not a PPP in the strictest sense of the term (Grameen is a nongovernmental organization, not a public sector entity), this joint venture had all the characteristics of a contractual PPP: there was a formal contractual arrangement between entities that shared a common objective, a long-term partnership arrangement and a bundling of activities.

The joint venture lost a considerable amount of money – more than USD 0.6 million – in its first 2 years of operation [13] largely because of low demand for the product by poor rural households to whom the product was initially marketed. Subsequently, the saleswoman program was cut, the yoghurt was distributed solely through retail outlets, distribution was expanded to more urban areas, and product prices were increased by 60% in order to subsidize the sales in rural areas.

Broad Lessons for PPPs and Undernutrition

We see scope for PPPs that would reduce aspects of undernutrition, including chronic undernutrition and micronutrient deficiencies, in developing countries. However, this optimism comes with significant caveats.

First, while there would appear to be a large body of evidence on this topic, closer examination shows that there are few independent, rigorous assessments of the impact of commercial sector engagement in nutrition. Considerable caution is therefore warranted when assessing either commendations or criticisms of PPPs in nutrition. While there are some instructive case studies, there is simply not an evidence base to support statements. More and better evidence needs to be generated.

Second, progress in this area requires that the private sector recognize that past and current actions by some firms have created an environment of mistrust and that the public sector accept that sustainable PPPs permit private firms to generate profits; the Danone yoghurt example is illustrative of this. Progress also requires recognition that PPPs that involve multiple firms can be problematic either because this arrangement forces competitors to (at least notionally) collaborate or because it creates the potential for these firms to lock out firms that are not members of the partnership. The challenges associated with Fortify West Africa illustrate these challenges. All of these issues take time to resolve.

Lest this all sound too negative, from a nutrition perspective, we see that PPPs are best placed to operate where the benefits (to nutrition) are the greatest, where public sector solutions are not readily available, effective or sustainable and where there is the least risk (to nutrition). In particular, we see significant scope for the use of the private sector in driving innovations that could reduce undernutrition, and there are both push and pull mechanisms that could be adapted to achieve these innovations (see Hoddinott et al. [7] for a discussion of these topics). More speculatively, there may be scope for the private sector to act as a financier of investments to improve children's nutritional status. Underpinning all of these partnerships must be open discussions of objectives, roles and expectations of all parties, along with potential conflicts of interest, an open space or platform where issues and challenges can be discussed and addressed, promotion of the pro-nutrition roles of the private sector, establishment of strong, transparent, well-enforced monitoring processes and serious, independent evaluations of these activities.

Acknowledgements

Work on this paper has been supported by the Department for International Development (UK) through its funding of the Transform Nutrition consortium.

Conflict of Interest Statement

We declare that we have no conflicts of interest.

References

1 Save the Children UK: Superfood for Babies: How Overcoming Barriers to Breastfeeding Will Save Children's Lives. London, Save the Children, 2013.

2 IBFAN: Breaking the Rules, Stretching the Rules. Penang Malaysia, International Baby Feeding Action Network, 2014. http://www.ibfan-icdc.org/files/Jan_2014.pdf (accessed February 16, 2014).

3 Hawkes C: Uneven dietary development: linking the policies and processes of globalization with the nutrition transition, obesity and diet-related chronic diseases. Global Health 2006;2:4.

4 Moodie R, Stuckler D, Monteiro C, Sheron N, Neal B, Thamarangsi T, Lincoln P, Casswell S: Profits and pandemics: prevention of harmful effects of tobacco, alcohol, and ultra-processed food and drink industries. Lancet 2013;381:670–679.

5 Bes-Rastrollo M, Schulze M, Martinez-Gonzalez M: Financial conflicts of interest and reporting bias regarding the association between sugar-sweetened beverages and weight gain: a systematic review of systematic reviews. PLoS Med 2013;10:e1001578.

6 O'Connor A: Coca-Cola funds scientists who shift blame for obesity away from bad diets. New York Times, August 9, 2015. http://well.blogs.nytimes.com/2015/08/09/coca-cola-funds-scientists-who-shift-blame-for-obesity-away-from-bad-diets/?_r=0 (accessed September 27, 2015).

7 Hoddinott J, Gillespie S, Yosef S: Public-Private Partnerships and the Reduction of Undernutrition in Developing Countries. Mimeo. Washington, International Food Policy Research Institute, 2015.

8 World Health Organization: Public-private partnerships for health. 2011. http://www.who.int/trade/glossary/story077/en/index.html (accessed April 23, 2013).

9 Hawkes C, Buse K: Public health sector and food industry interaction: it's time to clarify the term 'partnership' and be honest about underlying interests. Eur J Public Health 2011;21:400–401.

10 Relave N, Deich S: A guide to successful public-private partnerships for youth programs. New York, The Finance Project, 2007.

11 Sablah M, Klopp J, Steinberg D, Baker S: Private-public partnerships drive one solution to vitamin and mineral deficiencies: fortify West Africa. SCN News 2011;39:40–44.

12 Black RE, Victora CG, Walker SP, Zulfiqar ZA, Christian P, de Onis M, Ezzati M, Grantham-McGregor S, Katz J, Martorell R, Uauy R: Maternal and child undernutrition and overweight in low-income and middle-income countries. Lancet 2013; 382:427–451.

13 Garrette B, Karnani A: Challenges in marketing social useful goods to the poor. California Management Review 2010;52:1–19.

14 Bapat P: Failure or success waiting to happen? The case of Grameen Danone. The Hunger and Undernutrition Blog, June 6, 2011. http://www.hunger-undernutrition.org/blog/2011/06/failure-or-success-waiting-to-happen-the-case-of-grameen-danone.html (accessed January 22, 2014).

John Hoddinott
Savage Hall, Room 305, Division of Nutritional Sciences
Cornell University
Ithaca, NY 14853 (USA)
E-Mail Hoddinott@cornell.edu

Author Index

Subject Index

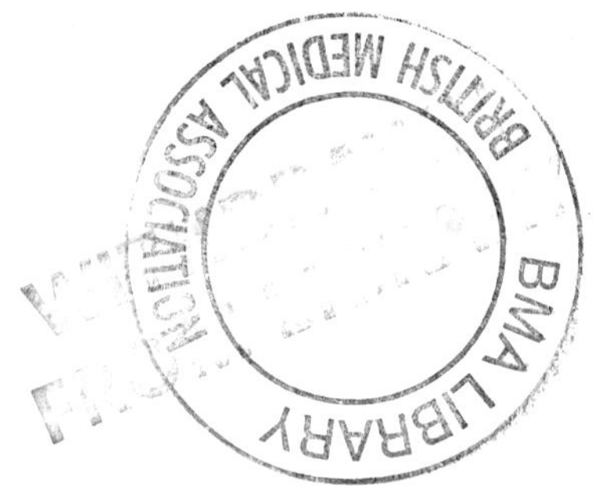